HIPPOCRATES IN A WORLD OF PAGANS AND CHRISTIANS

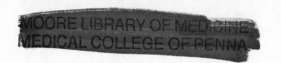

OWSEI TEMKIN

Hippocrates in a World of Pagans and Christians

THE JOHNS HOPKINS UNIVERSITY PRESS
BALTIMORE AND LONDON

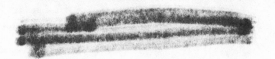

© 1991 The Johns Hopkins University Press
All rights reserved
Printed in the United States of America

The Johns Hopkins University Press
701 West 40th Street, Baltimore, Maryland 21211
The Johns Hopkins Press Ltd., London

The paper used in this book meets the minimum requirements
of American National Standard for Information Sciences—Permanence
of Paper for Printed Library Materials, ANSI Z39.48-1984.

LIBRARY OF CONGRESS CATALOGING-IN-PUBLICATION DATA

Temkin, Owsei, 1902–
    Hippocrates in a world of pagans and Christians / Owsei Temkin.
        p.   cm.
    Includes bibliographical references and index.
    ISBN 0-8018-4090-2 (alk. paper)
    1. Medicine—Religious aspects—History. 2. Hippocrates.
3. Paganism—History. 4. Spiritual healing—History. I. Title.
BL65.M4T35 1991
610′.9′015—dc20   90-45564

CONTENTS

VII HIPPOCRATIC MEDICINE AND TRIUMPHANT CHRISTIANITY

PREFACE AND
ACKNOWLEDGMENTS

How did the fame of the Greek physician Hippocrates fare during the first six centuries of our era, during which a pagan culture was transformed into a Christian one? How, during this period, was Hippocratic medicine—that is, medicine that looked to Hippocrates and the works attributed to him for inspiration and guidance—reflected in the thoughts of pagans and Christians? And how, grounded in a pagan Greek world, did it find a *modus vivendi* in a world dominated by the Christian church?

To answer these questions is the task of the present work, in which the name Hippocrates stands for the historical person; for any of the authors of the collection of some sixty medical works, the so-called Hippocratic Corpus or Hippocratic Collection; and for medicine in the Hippocratic tradition.[1] A similar broad meaning will be attached to the adjective "Hippocratic." Thus, physicians who accepted the medical ideas of Hippocrates will be called Hippocratic physicians. A quotation from the works of Hippocrates, literal or paraphrased, a theory or practice ascribed to him by one or another author, will be taken as representing Hippocratic medicine. For example, according to an author of the early fifth century, when dealing with delirious patients,

1. On the concept and the history of the Hippocratic tradition, see Smith (629).

"physicians . . . use fetters and forcibly foment [their] heads."[2] What appears here as common medical practice was ascribed to Hippocrates somewhat earlier by Jerome, who spoke of "the fetters of Hippocrates" for raving madmen, and of "the fomentation of Hippocrates by which a melancholic monk would be served better than by admonitions."[3] Both statements will be taken as Hippocratic, though in this exact form the practice cannot even be traced in the Collection.

Hippocrates in a World of Pagans and Christians is a work of medical history dealing with one particular theme, not a history of medicine in late Antiquity. The role of Hippocrates in the medical works of this period has been discussed elsewhere.[4] The aim of the present book, however, is to contribute to the understanding of the relationship between a form of secular medicine and religion. Where all secular medicine was condemned, there was no place for its Hippocratic subspecies. Nevertheless, a considerable part of this study will have to discuss the Jewish and Christian attitudes toward secular medicine as such.

The intrusion of a medical historian into the history of religion may evoke the warning *Ne sutor supra crepidam* ("Let not the cobbler overstep his last").[5] As far as possible, the intrusion has been limited to the interpretation of texts, with no discussion of theological questions such as the personality and the mission of Jesus, and the nature of the cures attributed to him and to the apostles and saints. Throughout the work, the sources will be given great latitude to speak for themselves, so that their voices can be heard (even if only in translation), a feeling for the temper of their time communicated, and misleading paraphrases of important passages avoided. Greater attention has been paid to the *how* than to the *why* of events. Beliefs have been treated as historical facts, without any judgment regarding their ultimate truth. In this manner, pagan, Jewish, and Christian beliefs could be dealt with on a basis of equality.

The focus on Hippocratic medicine will be further narrowed by a concentration on the variety of Hippocratism that found its basis in natural philosophy and "science." Those Hippocratic physicians who rejected the study of "science" and placed their trust in experience, their own or that of others, also demanded a study of the literature that embodied the clinical knowledge of past ages, beginning with certain

---

2. Theodoretus (676), *Graecarum affectionum curatio* 1.4; p. 105, ll. 4–5.
3. Jerome (339), *Epistulae* 109.2; 55:353; and idem, 125.16; 56:135. On medicine in the writings of Jerome, see Pease (535). On John Philoponus as another who failed to mention Hippocrates by name, see Todd (688), p. 105 and n. 16.
4. Temkin (668).
5. This translation is offered by Brewer's *Dictionary of Phrase and Fable.*

of the Hippocratic works.[6] Learning was a hallmark of all Hippocratic medicine, and it relied heavily on books. All through the centuries, the Hippocratic works remained authoritative,[7] to be supplemented by additional knowledge but not to be discarded. Just as the Homeric epics could still be cited in serious "scientific"[8] discourse, so could the Hippocratic works. This involved interpretation; and commentaries on the Hippocratic writings—and later, on the works of Galen—were an essential part of medical activity and medical teaching.

Most of the Hippocratic works were probably written between the late fifth century and the middle of the fourth. The fact that a few books, written around the first century A.D. were incorporated into the Hippocratic Collection is proof enough that there was no hiatus between the old and the new in the form in which "historical" and "currently valid" are distinguished today. "The ancients," and Hippocrates as "the ancient," could carry greater weight than more recent authors.

Hippocratic medicine was well suited to its primary clientele, the educated and well-to-do strata of Greek and Roman society. The educated doctor and his educated patients spoke the same philosophical language. The dietetic therapy he favored presupposed patients who could afford to have their food and drink, their exercise, and their whole manner of life regulated by him. This does not mean that doctors were necessarily motivated by the desire for a lucrative practice. The authors of the Hippocratic Collection did not refuse to treat slaves and poor people, and dietetic medicine could be—and was—accommodated to the demands of people who had neither the means nor the freedom to control their regimen or their time.[9] There were physicians who practiced merely for the sake of money, but this was not a Hippocratic ideal. The congruence of Hippocratic medicine and its clientele permits a greater reliance on the extant Graeco-Roman literature (which, the Bible and hagiography excepted, reflects the life and outlook of an educated readership) than would a work of secular medicine as such.

Just as the scope of the present work is limited to Hippocratic med-

6. See Smith (629), pp. 204–15.

7. Except among the Methodists; see below, chap. 1.

8. The Greeks spoke of medicine as a techne (a term corresponding to the Latin ars), a combination of theory, practice, and craftsmanship, for which English has no equivalent. It would be better to speak of techne and shun words such as "science" and "scientific," with their modern connotations. However, this would lead to cumbersome consequences, and the consistent use of quotation marks would be pedantic. Quotation marks will therefore have to be added mentally wherever appropriate.

9. See Edelstein (198), p. 305.

icine, so is its consideration of Christianity limited to the orthodox faith of the churches of Constantinople and Rome. Interesting as the interrelationships between medicine and Gnosticism, Manichaeism, and other heresies may be, they will not be considered. Some attempt will be made at some specificity in the use of the words "Christian" and "Christianity," which, like "pagan" and "paganism," are liable to obscure the diversity behind them. The words "pagan" and "paganism," as used here, include all religious forms whose followers do not submit to a single, all-powerful God. Philosophers who, in theory, assumed the existence of one god without, in practice, giving up the cult of other deities, remained pagans in spite of their philosophical monotheism.

More than twenty years ago, the *Reallexikon für Antike und Christentum* asked me to contribute an article on Hippocrates.[10] This article left me with some material which went beyond Hippocratic biography, and which I intended to use for an essay, "Hippocrates in a World of Pagans and Christians."[11] Slowly, very slowly, the intended essay grew into the present book.

The long gestation time has been due to prolonged study and repeated reinterpretation of my sources. The dissertation by Frings,[12] a treasure trove of information regarding the medical opinions of early patristic authors, had left no doubt about their favorable and receptive attitude toward Hippocratic medicine. Nevertheless, I assumed that the conversion from paganism to Christianity, with its revolutionary consequences for the cultural and social life of the Roman empire, had forced far-reaching accommodations upon Hippocratic medicine in spite of the continuation of the ancient tradition in substantive scientific matters. Gradually my sources convinced me that this was not the case. I had underrated the strength of popular support for secular medicine. I had overrated the influence of philosophical and religious creeds, and I had not sufficiently realized the latitude that medicine left to the physician regarding his private life.

Some sixty years ago, essential differences between the thinking of ancient and modern doctors had often received scant attention. Because all were doctors, pursuing the same goal of healing, they were believed to share the same outlook. Increased awareness of the "otherness" of

10. Now vol. 15, cols. 466–81. I take this opportunity to thank the editors of the *Reallexikon* for valuable references that have also been helpful in writing the present book.

11. Under the same title I have on several occasions read papers on various topics covered in the present book.

12. Frings (239).

former periods in dealing with the history of medicine—for which Ludwig Edelstein deserves major credit—led to an intensified study of the philosophical, religious, and social conditions under which ancient medical ideas and medical practice evolved. However, the quest for new insight tended to overrate the tutelage over medicine of the general ideas and creeds that dominated the times, and tended to underrate the autonomy of medicine.[13] Also, it did not always allow sufficient leeway for the physician as an individual whose life was not totally defined by his profession. As the member of a family, as a citizen, as a religious person, and as an emotional being, he might follow a course that his art did not prescribe to him.

The ancients realized that the professional sphere had its limitations. As a physician, a man would not harm an enemy, though as a good citizen and soldier he would fight him, said a Roman medical author of the first century.[14] A Roman philosopher of the same period thought that a doctor, like a cook, need not be a good man.[15] This meant that moral good and evil were outside the scope of medicine. A Greek commentator of the very end of Antiquity listed the character traits that a doctor ought to possess "not only as a human being but also as a physician." He should cultivate them "as a human being more than as a physician," whereas otherwise he must be accomplished primarily as a doctor.[16]

Objective reasons were not alone in delaying the completion of this book. Advancing age and its concomitants also played their part. They formed an obstacle to my reaching the libraries. I am, therefore, all the more grateful to all those who sent me copies of their publications or otherwise facilitated my work. In particular I wish to thank Darrel Amundsen and Gary Ferngren, Gerhard Baader, Gert Brieger, Gerhard Fichtner (who sent me the proof of his article "Christus als Arzt" as well as excerpts from various ancient authors), Georg Harig, Huldrych Koelbing, Linda C. Cork, Fridolf Kudlien, Vivian Nutton, Joanne H.

13. Kudlien (390), p. 91, criticized Edelstein for concentrating on the philosophical guidance of medical ethics and for overlooking "the common stock of non-philosophical values and rules which may rightly be called 'popular' or 'vulgar' ethics and of which *all* members of any society are indeed participants, be it consciously or not."

14. Scribonius Largus (614), *Compositiones,* Epistula dedicatoria, art. 4; p. 2, ll. 13–16.

15. Seneca (615), *Epistulae* 87; 2:332.

16. Stephanus (646), *Commentary on Hippocrates' Aphorisms* 1.2; pp. 42 (l. 28)–44 (l. 1). see also Westerink's translation, idem, pp. 43–45.

Phillips, John Scarborough, Hans Schadewald, Heinrich Schipperges, Wesley Smith (to whom I owe a photocopy of Putzger's edition of the Hippocratic Letters), Gotthard Strohmaier (for a copy of his tentative translation from the Arabic of chapter 23 of Galen's commentary on the Hippocratic *On Airs, Waters, Localities*), and Leendert G. Westerink (for a copy of his unpublished essay "Academic Practice about 500: Alexandria").

It gives me pleasure to express my appreciation to the Johns Hopkins University Press: to its director, Jack Goellner, without whose gentle, very gentle, reminders the book might not yet have been completed; to the anonymous reader to whom I am indebted for many corrections and for valuable suggestions; and to my copy editor, Miriam Kleiger, who has labored very hard on the improvement of my manuscript. Thanks are also due to the secretaries of the Johns Hopkins Institute of the History of Medicine, especially Mrs. Mary Moore and Mrs. Dolores Sawicki, for word processing my longhand manuscript. Last but not least I thank my wife, C. Lilian Temkin, for scrutinizing the text of my manuscript for idiomatic and stylistic blunders.

OWSEI TEMKIN
The Johns Hopkins University
Institute of the History of Medicine

NOTE TO THE READER

The numbers in parentheses or brackets in the footnotes, usually following authors' or editors' names, refer to items in the Bibliography. Citations of ancient works often specify the relevant subdivisions of the original work, followed by the location within the modern edition. The following example cites book 1, article 11, and volume 1, p. 164: Hippocrates (302), *Epidemics* 1.11; 1:164. Cross-references such as "see text to n. 14" refer to the text to which n. 14 applies.

To facilitate chronological orientation while avoiding repetitiousness, biographical dates of historical personages are included in the Index.

Where no translator's name is added in the notes, the translation is to be considered mine even if the edition cited carries an English translation, with the exception that, unless otherwise indicated, all English Biblical references are to the Authorized (King James) Version (hereafter, AV).

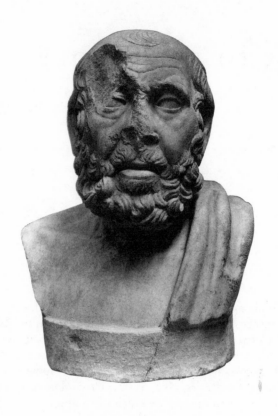

Roman bust (after a Hellenistic Greek original) found at Ostia,
alleged to represent the historical Hippocrates. Ostia Museum.
From John Scarborough, *Roman Medicine*, plate 49 (opposite
page 137).

I

Background

Background

1

INTRODUCTION

The Roman Republic came to an end with the battle of Actium in 31 B.C. The victor, Augustus as he was to be called, gave Rome a constitution that, with modifications, prevailed for about two hundred years. The Early Empire upheld many republican forms; nominally, the emperor shared his rule with the senate, and the Greek cities retained a considerable degree of administrative autonomy. The city of Rome was the undisputed capital of the realm within whose frontiers the civilized western world during the second century enjoyed an unprecedented period of peace. At the end of the second century, peace and stability collapsed, and for about a hundred years political conditions close to anarchy disrupted cultural and economic life.

With the reorganization effected by Diocletian (A.D. 284–305), a

For the entire period covered by this book, Gibbon's (259) classic *Decline and Fall of the Roman Empire,* though it has been superseded in many details, still holds the first place. Chadwick (138), *The Early Church,* provides an orientation to the history of the Christian church till about the sixth century; Daniélou and Marrou (160) and Frend (236) provide detailed accounts. For the history of medicine, Iwan Bloch's (102) article on Byzantine medicine, and the pertinent chapters in Neuburger's (480) *Geschichte der Medizin* can still be read with profit, while Scarborough (605), *Symposium on Byzantine Medicine,* represents the present state of our knowledge. On Roman medicine, see Scarborough's (604) work of that title, supplemented by Gourevitch (267) and Kudlien (397).

third period, that of the Later Empire, began.[1] The emperor was a monarch; rule was increasingly centralized and did away with municipal autonomy. Earlier tendencies came strongly to the fore: burdensome taxation, the reduction of small and weak landowners to a state near serfdom, and the increasing replacement of Romans by barbarians in the army and elsewhere. Devastating incursions of barbaric tribes were often followed by the settlement of these tribes on Roman soil. The city of Rome lost its central role, and in A.D. 330, the emperor Constantine made Byzantium (which he renamed Constantinople) his capital, so that the empire now had two political centers. After the death of the emperor Theodosius in 395, the empire was permanently divided into East and West. In the Latin West, province after province had to be evacuated; Rome itself was sacked in 410, and the last Western emperor was dethroned in 476.

While the West was on its way to the Latin Middle Ages, the Greek East preserved its ancient heritage. Justinian even succeeded in reconquering Italy, Africa, and part of Spain, and reuniting the Roman Empire. But the reunification did not long outlast him. Culturally, Antiquity faded away slowly, but politically the East, even before the onset of the Arab conquests in 634, had become the Byzantine Empire.

The three periods in the history of the Roman empire during the approximately six hundred years of its existence coincided with distinct stages in the history of Christianity as well as that of medicine. The world of the Early Empire, Jewish Palestine excepted, was undisputedly pagan, with Greek, Roman, and oriental deities being syncretically fused. The cult of the deified Roman emperors, from which only the Jews were exempted, put a political stamp on paganism as a religious form of life. As yet, Christianity was of little account; persecutions, though they could be savage, were sporadic and locally limited. It was during the third century that the growth of the Christian church made itself felt, and the beginning of the Later Empire marked a decisive turn of events. Only a few years separated the thoroughgoing persecution under Diocletian and Galerius from Constantine's edict of Milan (A.D. 313), which proclaimed toleration and restored Christian property.

Tolerated and favored by the state, Christianity was still far from having won the hearts of all the people, so that Julian's attempt (A.D. 361–63) to restore pagan dominance was not as hopeless as it may seem in retrospect.[2] Pagans interpreted the disaster of the sack of Rome

1. For the Early Empire and the third century, see Millar et al. (461); for the Later Empire, see Jones (349), Brown (117), and idem (120).
2. See Herbert Bloch (101).

as a punishment for having forsaken the old gods who had helped to make Rome great. Augustine countered with *The City of God*. The old gods were evil demons; all power and hope lay with the true God, whose city he, Augustine, was defending against the earthly city of His enemies. The history of paganism in the fifth and sixth centuries is the history of its retreat toward gradual extinction. When Boethius, in prison, awaited his execution (A.D. 524), he invoked philosophy, that is, reason, rather than faith to console himself.[3] But when, a few years later (A.D. 527), Justinian closed the Neoplatonic school of Athens, where a mystical pagan theology was taught, paganism lost its intellectual center, though not all its followers. Even afterwards, some outstanding personalities were still pagan, and in enclaves outside the mainstream, paganism survived into the seventh century.

From its beginnings into the fifth century, Christianity had to accept a pagan ambience, diminishing and unevenly distributed though it was. During the centuries of persecution, Christians had to defend themselves against accusations, of which that set forth by Celsus, around 180, probably is the best remembered because it was answered by Origen.[4] After persecution had ceased, the fourth and fifth centuries saw the appearance of the great Christian theologians Basil, Gregory of Nazianzus, Gregory of Nyssa, John Chrysostom, Theodoret in the East, and Ambrose, Augustine, and Jerome in the West.[5] But this was also the time of great pagans: of Libanius the teacher of rhetoric, of Symmachus the prefect of Rome, and of the Neoplatonists Iamblichus and Proclus. Hagiography gives a very vivid picture of the struggle of the saints against heathens who, when seen as demons, were believed to harm Christian folk.

In the first century, when Christianity had its origin, Hippocrates was already famous and his medicine well established. The historical Hippocrates was born on the island of Cos in or around 460 B.C., a member of the Asclepiads, who thought of themselves as descendants of Asclepius.[6] Hippocrates was of small stature, willing to teach medicine for a fee, and well known at the time of his younger contemporaries Plato and Aristotle, to whom the above scanty data are due. How prominent he was is a moot question, as is the question of whether any book of the Hippocratic Collection was actually written by him. His fame, embellished by legend, grew during the Hellenistic period; by the

---

3. Boethius (105), *Consolation of Philosophy* 1.3; p. 140.
4. Origen (509) and idem (510).
5. For these and other Fathers of the Church, see Quasten (576).
6. For Asclepius and the Asclepiads, see below, chaps. 7 and 14.A.

beginning of the first century, admiration for him seems to have been widespread among physicians. Not all of them admired him for the same reasons. There was considerable variety, often even contradiction, among the teachings of the works of the Collection. Two main sects had formed among his followers. For the so-called Dogmatists, or Logicians, Hippocrates was the founder of a scientific medicine based on natural philosophy, anatomy, and physiology—in short, on hidden causes, as their opponents, the Empiricists, contended.[7] In the opinion of the latter, nature could not be fathomed; hence speculation about these hidden causes, which included elements, humors, and pneuma, was useless. They held that medicine had to make do with a knowledge of obvious causes, such as hunger, cold, and sleep, and with clinical experience supported by analogy from similar cases. The Empiricists thought of Hippocrates as himself an Empiricist, their great clinical teacher of the past.[8]

The first century brought an innovation with the rise in Rome of still another sect, the Methodists. They believed that medicine needed no science and should rest not on experience but on direct diagnosis on the basis of the symptoms, which indicated whether the body or its parts were in a condition of constriction, of relaxation, or of a mixture of the two. They did not think of Hippocrates as the head of their sect, which they considered a new departure in medicine.

These three sects only represented the main divisions within medical belief, for none of them was homogeneous in itself. Their significance can best be assessed by realizing that they presented themselves as three kinds of medicine, among which a doctor had to choose.[9] The rejection of sects in favor of a single medical science, guided exclusively by the search for what reason and experience proved to be true, was one of Galen's main historical contributions.[10]

Little is known of medicine in the anarchic third century,[11] so that

7. Cf. Celsus (137), *De medicina*, prooemium, arts. 27–44; 1: 15–25.

8. On Hippocrates in general, see Edelstein (200), and for the later interpretation of Hippocratic opinions and writings, see Smith (629). Edelstein's views are not generally accepted; see, for instance, Joly (345); also Lichtenthaeler (421) on Edelstein's interpretation of the Hippocratic oath.

9. See Edelstein (198), pp. 436–40.

10. See ibid. Galen had a model in Posidonius, of whom he wrote, "Whereas [the Stoics] made up their mind to betray their fatherland rather than the tenets [of their sect], Posidonius [would prefer to betray] the Stoics [rather] than the truth" (Galen [242], *Quod animi mores corporis temperamenta sequntur* 11; 2:77(l. 20)–78(l. 2).

11. Cf. Kudlien (398). As shown by Fox (230), our general knowledge of the third century has increased greatly in recent years.

Galen's death toward the end of the Early Empire[12] closes a chapter in the history of medicine. Galen had thought of himself as the follower of the great master whose work, correctly interpreted, he had brought to completion.[13] In the East, the Later Empire accepted Galen, Hippocrates, and Hippocratic medicine as seen through Galen's eyes as authorities representing true medicine.

This short outline of political, religious, and medical developments, offering no more than a rough framework, indicates that what follows will be heavily slanted toward developments in the Greek East. Much will be said about the differences between pagan and Christian attitudes. In spite of the differences, however, it must not be forgotten that pagans and Christians, living together,[14] also shared some traditional ways of thought and were confronted by the same realities of life. Up to a point, pagans and Christians had a common notion of the principles of Hippocratic medicine, its relation to body and mind, and its goal regarding human health and disease. Also, both had to make use of the physician, unless they rejected secular medicine altogether.

12. Nutton (490), pp. 322–24, has drawn attention to a remark by the Arabic historian Sulaymān as Sijistānī, which places Galen's death sometime after A.D. 210.

13. See Temkin (667), pp. 32–33 and 58. On Galen as philosopher of nature, see Moraux (470).

14. Fox's (230) monumental *Pagans and Christians* has added a wealth of information to our understanding of the religious and civic life of late Antiquity. I regret that I have not been able to do full justice to this book.

2

THE MEDICINE OF THE
BODY AND THE MEDICINE
OF THE SOUL

Aristotle noted that it was the task of the natural philosopher to look into the principles of health and disease. "Therefore, most natural philosophers end by going into matters that concern medicine, while of physicians those who exercise this art philosophically take their departure from what concerns nature." [1] By late Antiquity, this view had crystallized into the belief that "medicine and philosophy are sisters." [2]

About fifty years before Aristotle, however, Democritus, a contemporary of Hippocrates, had said, "The medical art heals diseases of the body, whereas wisdom relieves the soul of passions." As if to illustrate the apophthegm, he also said, "Banish [the] uncontrolled grief of a benumbed soul with reasoning!" [3] By late Antiquity, it had become a commonplace to say that "medicine is the philosophy of the body and philosophy the medicine of the soul." [4] The idea of two forms of medicine, one of which heals the diseases of the body and employs diet, drugs,

1. Aristotle (48), *Parva naturalia* 1; 436a19–436b1.
2. For sources and discussion, see Temkin (665), pp. 187–88.
3. Diels (174), Democritus, frags. B31 and B290; 2:71 and 120.
4. See Temkin (665) p. 187. For the relationship of body and soul in Antiquity, see Pigeaud (546) and Brown (115). On the origin of the treatment of diseases by reasoning, see Laín Entralgo (410). On the relationship of medicine and philosophy, see Edelstein (198), pp. 349–66, and on the relationship of doctors to the two medicines, see Kudlien (382); see also below, chaps. 11.C and 13.

and surgery, while the other heals the troubles of the mind by reasoning and sundry psychological techniques, was popular among pagans and Christians and is still with us.[5]

Aristotle's comment envisaged a close relationship between the pre-Socratic philosophers of nature and physicians such as many of the authors of the Hippocratic Collection. Even works such as the Hippocratic *Epidemics,* famous for its empirical character, combined theoretical aspects with clinical observations.[6] In judging an individual illness, its author took into consideration

> the common nature of all diseases and the particular nature of each, the illness, the patient, what had been prescribed, and who prescribed it—these cause improvement or deterioration—the whole and the partial cosmic constitution and the constitution of each region, the habits, regimens, pursuits, and age of every [patient].[7]

Human beings were here seen in cosmic and geographic context; disease in general had a nature, and so had every single disease; food, drink, and medicines could change illness for the better or the worse, and the individual's age and pursuits were factors not to be overlooked. However much this may have been the result of empirical knowledge, all together it delineated the author's general approach to the sick. The absence of any mention of the traditional gods is as significant as is the stress on cosmic phenomena and "the nature" of disease and of diseases.

Next, the author listed what he observed at the bedside:

> Speech, behavior, silence, thoughts, sleep, absence of sleep, dreams—of what kind and when, plucking, itching, tears upon exacerbation, bowel movements, urine, sputum, vomiting, how many transitions of disease from one kind to another, as well as abscessions toward a fatal or a critical issue, sweat, chill, frigidity, coughing, sneezing, hiccupping,

5. It was given a metaphysical basis by the Cartesian view of the soul as a purely spiritual entity, as compared to the body as a *res extensa.* When Heinroth, in 1818, used the term "psychiatry," he was met with the objection that the soul was not liable to diseases in any but a metaphorical sense. Today, too, many (and not laymen only) think of the doctor's domain as extending over diseases with a somatic basis, whereas purely mental troubles should be left to psychiatrists (as distinguished from "real" doctors), psychologists, psychoanalysts, and priests. In this view, psychiatry will become a truly medical discipline when merged into neurology.

6. Lloyd (426), p. 154, speaks of the "theory-laden" terms used in the descriptions of the cases in *Epidemics.*

7. Hippocrates (302), *Epidemics* 1.23; 1:180. The distinction between general nature and individual nature has been discussed by Pigeaud (546), pp. 65–67.

breathing, belching, flatulence silent or noisy, hemorrhages, and hemor-
rhoids. These things and what they bring must be considered.[8]

Here too, theoretical notions entered the field of observation: during
the course of an illness, disease could change its character; diseases had
crises; and the sequestration of morbid matter (abscession) pointed toward a fatal issue or a salutary crisis. The whole range of observations,
covering both somatic and mental phenomena, was viewed dispassion-
ately.

Then, as now, a doctor had to note any deviations from the healthy
form and function of the body, as well as from usual behavior and
perception—for instance, hallucinations, illusions, and delusions. The
Hippocratic doctor took it upon himself to treat mental diseases that
he thought to be concomitant with somatic abnormality. The allocation
of the soul or of psychic functions to certain parts or constituents of the
body, such as the diaphragm (φρήν), the heart, or bile, was ingrained
in archaic Greek thought,[9] and the concept of diseases springing from
these components of the body may have been bequeathed to Greek
medicine and taken up by Hippocratic doctors. Phrenitis (a name that
has survived in the word "frenzy") became feverish hallucinations;
mania and melancholia were associated with bile or black bile; and
"the sacred disease," manifested by seizures (epilēpsiai), became "epilepsy" (epilēpsia) and was attributed to a surplus of phlegm in the brain
by at least one author of the Collection.[10]

What then was the Hippocratic philosophy of the body? Toward the
beginning of the fifth century B.C., the introduction of correct regimen
as a treatment of disease added a new dimension to medicine, supple-
menting the older forms of treatment: drugs and surgery.[11] How to find
the diet that would maintain the body in health and free it from disease
was a problem that invited speculation about the constituents of body
and of food, as well as about the structure, the functions and the activities of the body and its parts. It invited scientific hypotheses of all
kinds, and it allowed more or less extensive borrowing from natural
philosophy.

The writings of the Hippocratic Collection, which extend over al-

8. Hippocrates (302), *Epidemics* 1.23; 1:180.
9. See Onions (503), p. 84, for χόλος as bile as well as wrath. According to
Smith (630), p. 555, χόλος in Homer "is not precisely bile . . . it is the emotion
anger, or the cause of anger, *kotos* and *mēnis*."
10. The author of *On the Sacred Disease.* The ancient pathology of mental
diseases has been discussed in detail by Pigeaud (546), pp. 70–138.
11. On pre-Hippocratic Greek medicine, see Kudlien (383).

most all branches of medicine, display a great variety of hypotheses and show the doctor's wish to be able to predict the outcome of an illness. This wish stemmed neither from exclusively therapeutic nor from purely scientific interests. It was largely motivated by the doctor's need to protect himself from suspicion and accusations in case of an unfavorable outcome. Moreover, in a time when therapeutic results tended to be uncertain, a doctor's reputation was enhanced by his ability to foretell the course an illness would take, or to describe a patient's past and present illnesses without asking about them. These social motivations stimulated the study of favorable and unfavorable prognostic signs.[12]

The founding of Alexandria was an important event in the history of ancient scholarship, science, and medicine. From the third century B.C. until its conquest by the Arabs in A.D. 642, Alexandria was the foremost center of medical study and especially of anatomy. For a time, it seems, anatomy could be studied on human bodies, until Roman law put an end to such study and confined anatomy to animal dissection. Surgery profited greatly by the anatomical advances. As late as about 500, the narrow streets of Alexandria were said to count "more surgical butcher stalls than dwelling places."[13]

By the end of the first century A.D., Empiricism and the rise of the Methodists brought the rivalry of the medical sects to its height. Methodism, which had grown out of a corpuscular theory, a legacy of Epicurus, inclined toward mechanistic thinking. Stoic philosophy, which stressed the role of the pneuma in natural processes, was popular at the time and left its mark on medicine, as had Aristotelian philosophy earlier. In this situation, Galen's personality and his work appear as a turning point in the history of medicine in late Antiquity. By nature Galen was a fierce fighter and not without vanity; by his long and careful education, he was a physician and a philosopher; by his indefatigable industry, a master of nearly all branches of medicine; and by fate the last of the creative medical scientists of Antiquity. In the ongoing discussion of genuine, doubtful, and spurious Hippocratic works, Galen's opinions became all but decisive. His presentation of Hippocratic principles in a light that favored Hippocrates even in comparison with Plato, and his boundless admiration for Hippocrates as a great master and a paragon in medicine and philosophy, all helped to create out of the diversity of the Collection a picture of the Hippocratic philosophy

12. See Edelstein (204), chaps. 2 and 3, and the corresponding English translation in idem (198), pp. 65–110. I believe Edelstein's thesis of the Hippocratic doctor as a craftsman to be basically sound, though presented in sharper contours than our knowledge of ancient life allows.

13. Fulgentius (240), *Mitologicae* 1; p. 9, ll. 10–17.

of the body. Galen's interpretation defined Hippocratic medicine as the great patristic authors were to see it. Its main points were the basic roles of the four "classical" humors, and an allopathic principle of therapy.[14]

According to the theory of the humors as interpreted by Galen, matter and four qualities combine so as to form four elements: fire, which is warm; water, which is cold; earth, which is dry; and air, which is moist.[15] In different proportions, these elements and qualities constitute all material things, including food and drink, as well as medicines derived from vegetable, animal, and mineral substances. In the human body, four types of humors correspond to the elements: gall or bile (warm and dry); phlegm (cold and moist); black bile (cold and dry); and blood (warm and moist). Food and drink, when digested, maintain the humors, from which (especially from the blood) the parts of the body take their appropriate nourishment. The mixture of the qualities determines the temperament of the body and of its parts. In health, the qualities and the humors are properly proportioned; in disease the proportion is upset so that there is a surplus or a deficiency of a quality or of a humor.

Not only must human beings eat and drink, they also depend on the surrounding air, which they inhale. The inhaled air, or an airlike substance, the pneuma, is distributed through the body; apart from cooling, it is the vehicle of vital and psychic functions. The air can also carry diseases and cause epidemics, especially when polluted by a miasma. The climate of a place and the yearly seasons are determining factors in the incidence of disease, and the seasons too have their temperaments, summer (like yellow bile) being warm and dry; winter (like phlegm) moist and cold; autumn (like black bile) cold and dry; and spring (like blood) moist and warm.[16]

Rational Hippocratic therapy consisted in correcting, by diet and drugs, any imbalance of the humors. This was achieved by opposing any deviation in one direction by its opposite. For instance, a cold and moist condition had to be met by a regimen (or drug therapy) that was warming and drying. According to Galen, this was the truly Hippo-

14. See Neuburger (480), 2:48, and Temkin (667) pp. 62–64.

15. These are the four elements in their pure, ideal form, in contrast to the existing, impure elements; cf. Moraux (470), pp. 89–90.

16. For the outline of Hippocratic humoral medicine as conceived by Galen, see Hippocrates (302), *On the Nature of Man* 5 and 7, which Galen held to be genuinely Hippocratic; Stephanus (646), *Commentary on Hippocrates' Aphorisms* 1.1; pp. 34–39; and idem 1.22; pp. 96–99. For a detailed discussion of Galen's doctrine of elements and qualities, see Moraux (470).

cratic therapeutic principle, best known in its Latin version: *Contraria contrariis curantur.*[17]

Dietetics, built as it was on natural philosophy, was the speculative core of Hippocratic medicine. To a minor degree, dietetics applied to surgery, too. Moreover, in his attempt to bring back to the structural norm any deviation from it, the Hippocratic surgeon, like other doctors, used the theoretical notions of that which is "according to nature" (normal), and "that which is contrary to nature" (abnormal); as well as anatomical knowledge; the surgeon also used empirically developed practices, many of which had probably originated before Hippocrates. Books on surgery formed a large and very important part of the Collection, and it is that part which comes most easily to modern understanding, because much of it leaned on anatomical and mechanical thinking.

The foregoing is a rough approximation of the basic medical doctrine of Hippocrates as constructed by the late second century. Many features of this picture had been anticipated by earlier authors. An edition of the works then current under the name of Hippocrates was published in the days of Emperor Hadrian (A.D. 117–38). If a coherent synthesis of Hippocratic medicine existed before Galen, it has not yet been recaptured.

To use a modern expression, Hippocratic medicine was psychosomatic insofar as conditions of the body were recognized to affect mental states and the latter, in turn, to affect the body. Galen wrote a short treatise with the title *That the Faculties of the Soul Follow the Temperament of the Body,* and Hippocrates, together with Plato and other philosophers, served him as witnesses for his thesis. One author of the Collection thought that human intelligence could be changed by diet,[18] and Galen also believed that he could similarly improve sundry mental functions. If the soul was a material substance or, as Galen intimated, the temperament of the brain, this was a logical consequence of dietetic medicine and not so very far from Feuerbach's notorious dictum *Der Mensch ist was er isst.*[19]

17. Hippocrates (306), *On Breaths* 1; p. 92, l. 8.
18. Hippocrates (302), *On Regimen* 1.35; 4:280–94.
19. "Man is what he eats." See Buchmann (124), pp. 187 and 231. Regarding the psychosomatic character of ancient medicine, cf. Pigeaud (547), especially pp. 430–32. Pigeaud rightly stresses the difficulties arising from the distinction between diseases of the body and diseases of the soul. Nevertheless, I still believe that the notion of a radical (i.e., Cartesian) gulf between body and soul was foreign to ancient doctors. Such a notion would have cast a doubt on the possibility of an interaction as outlined by Posidonius (see idem, p. 431); cf. above, n. 5.

Unwholesome habits concerning food, drink, exercise, and visual and acoustic impressions, including music, corrupted the disposition of the soul by producing undesirable changes in its material substratum. Therefore, Galen argued, "he who pursues the art of hygiene must be experienced in all these things, and he must not think that it is for the philosophers alone to shape the disposition of the soul; it is for [the philosophers] to shape the health of the soul itself because of something that is greater, whereas it is for the physician to do so on behalf of the body, lest it easily slip into disease." [20]

This expressed the essential difference between the doctor as the physician of the body and the philosopher as the physician of the soul. The doctor's concern remained with the body even when he acted upon the soul, as he might do in musical therapy. The philosopher's concern was with the soul and its aspiration to knowledge, virtue, and beauty. Vices, including uncontrolled passion, crime against man, and sin against the gods, were diseases of the soul, which the philosopher had to cure. The doctor's primary concern with the soul was with the diseases from which it suffered concomitantly with the body as well as with the reactions its perturbances provoked in the body. Galen mentioned "passion, weeping, anger, grief, immoderate worry, and much sleeplessness" as bringing on "fevers and the beginnings of severe diseases . . . just as, on the other hand, a sluggish mind and mindlessness, and an altogether spiritless soul often produce lack of color and atrophies." [21] Whatever their individual explanations were, most authors of the Collection would probably have accepted this interrelationship of body and soul. The two were not felt to be separated by as deep a gulf as Descartes later envisioned.

Ordinarily, his patients' morals were not the doctor's business; he did not comment on them in his case histories. He might, however, turn moralist and meet with the philosopher if he reflected on the responsibility of his patients for their diseases. A modern doctor will warn against smoking, overweight, lack of exercise, and other threats to health. The Hippocratic physician, to an even higher degree, found

20. Galen (243), *De sanitate tuenda* 1.8; p. 19, ll. 24–30; cf. Temkin (667), p. 19, and Pigeaud (546), p. 64. Diels (174), Democritus, frag. B187; 2:99, already had advised caring more for the soul than for the body, and Galen, with his Platonic and Stoic leanings, considered the physician's concern for the soul to be on a lower level than the philosopher's. Cf. Pigeaud (546), pp. 69–70.

21. Galen attributed the latter symptoms to the lack of "innate heat," a concept that, although not absent from the Hippocratic Collection, came to prominence later. Unfortunately I am unable to remember the exact reference for the Galenic passage. It resembles Posidonius's list (see Pigeaud [547], p. 431).

many diseases to be caused by disregard for a reasonable way of life or by the lack of control of one's desires. Such diseases could be tagged with a moral blemish, as Galen did with gout, severe arthritis, stone and ulcer of the bladder, and abdominal pain.[22] To insist on a rational, wholesome way of life was the task both of the philosopher and of the physician. But it was not, nor is it now, the doctor's duty to moralize about his patients' dietary trespasses.

The doctor was supposed to dispel the sick person's fears and inspire courage. He may also have tried to assuage overweening desires and other passions. But as the following story—current in different versions, involving different great doctors—shows, he confronted passion as a skillful psychologist rather than as a moral philosopher. He was not expected to treat those diseases of the soul that had no somatic origin.[23]

In the version of the story told by both Plutarch and the historian Appian,[24] Erasistratus was the medical hero. A Seleucid prince was hopelessly in love with his old father's young wife. Accusing himself for his terrible yet unconquerable desire and thinking of himself as incurably ill, the prince decided to seek release from life. By neglecting himself and abstaining from food, he would slowly enfeeble his body, pretending to suffer from some disease. Erasistratus found the prince very ill; yet in the absence of any signs of a somatic illness, he concluded that it was a disease of the soul, and that love was at its core. The prince had not responded to his questions, and whereas grief, anger, and desires other than love were usually admitted, chaste persons would not admit love.[25] Erasistratus now closely watched the prince's "face and paid attention to those parts and movements of the body which are mostly affected together with the soul's turmoil."[26] Whenever his father's wife entered the room, "shame and his conscience made him particularly troubled in mind and silent, while his body, against his will, became more vigorous and lively, yet weaker again when she left."[27] Very dip-

---

22. Galen (243), *De sanitate tuenda* 5.1; pp. 137–38. Cf. Temkin (667), pp. 39–40.

23. The "verbal and psychological part of the treatment [as in Celsus and Caelius Aurelianus] is only ancillary to the physical treatment" (Gill [262], p. 320).

24. Plutarch (561), *Demetrius* 38.906–7; 9:92–97; Appian (35), 10.59–61; 2:216–23. For the Greek text with German translation, see Müri (474), pp. 40–45. Ciavolella (141), p. 23, cites the story after Valerius Maximus (early first century), where the changing pulse rate is diagnostically decisive. For the pulse in love, see Pigeaud (546), p. 251; and Galen (250), *On Prognosis* 7.10; p. 104, ll. 20–23.

25. According to Appian's version.

26. Plutarch (561), *Demetrius* 38.3; 9:92, ll. 21–23.

27. Ibid.

lomatically, Erasistratus informed the king of the state of affairs and succeeded in making him yield his wife to his son, who then recovered. In all versions, the doctor cured the patient. He did so not by treating the illness, as he would in the case of a somatic disease, but by helping to gratify an illicit desire, a procedure of which a philosopher would hardly approve.

Thinking of the soul in medical terms as potentially healthy or sick enabled the philosopher (and the prophet and the priest) to draw analogies from the concrete and the observable to the abstract and the invisible. It allowed the transfer of the physician's authority to the philosopher, and it supported the demand that those sick in soul bear their treatment as willingly and patiently as did the sick in body. This way of thinking was not exclusively Greek; it also had its independent existence among the ancient Jews (and possibly other nations).

To a degree of intensity and with a power of poetical expression hardly matched by the Greeks, the Jews used wounds and diseases as symbols of sin and disobedience to the Lord.[28] Isaiah (1:5–6) was not speaking of the body when he said: "The whole head is sick, and the whole heart faint. From the sole of the foot even unto the head there is no soundness in it; but wounds, and bruises, and putrifying sores." And speaking of the people of Judah, Isaiah (6:10) declared that they could be healed were they to "understand with their hearts and convert." Jews and Christians could thus draw on the philosophical tradition of Greece as well as on their own religious tradition. Jesus himself justified his eating with publicans and sinners by saying, "They that be whole need not a physician, but they that are sick" (Matt. 9:12), thereby comparing himself to a physician, and publicans and sinners to sick people whom he had come to heal by being merciful and calling them to repentance (Matt. 9:13).

Some examples may suffice here to illustrate the use that pagans and Christians could make of the analogy between the therapy of the body and that of the soul. The popular philosopher Epictetus of the late first century insisted that the philosopher's lecture room was a surgery: "You ought not to walk out of it in pleasure, but in pain."[29] In quite a different form, the analogy that suffering could benefit the soul as painful surgical treatment benefits the body is to be found in the work of Prudentius, a Christian poet who wrote in Latin during the late fourth century. According to Prudentius, Saint Romanus, describing his mar-

28. See Hempel (296); and Kee (358), pp. 12–16.
29. Epictetus (206), *Discourses* 3.23.30; 2:180–81 (Oldfather's translation). See also Edelstein (198), p. 365.

tyrdom, compared his suffering with that due to gout and arthritis, and his torturers with surgeons: "You will shudder at the handiwork of the executioners, but are doctors' hands gentler, when Hippocrates' cruel butchery is going on? The living flesh is cut and fresh-drawn blood stains the lancets when festering matter is being scraped away." [30] The saint exhorted those around him to think of the executioners as surgeons using their knives for his health. "That by which health is restored is not vexatious. These men appear to be rending my wasting limbs, but they give healing to the living substance within." [31]

Later examples will confirm that the analogy between medicine of the body and medicine of the soul served Christians as a means of clarifying their beliefs as it had served pagans long before them. But these examples will also show the parting of the ways.

30. Prudentius (574), *Peristephanon* 10.496–505; 2:263 (Thomson's translation). For a general reappraisal of Prudentius, see Smith (628). For other examples, see Frings (239). The comparison of surgery with the torturer's work strikes me as a revulsion against operative surgery (without anesthesia!) rather than as an invective against medicine as it has been interpreted by Kudlien (382), p. 17, n. 19. As attested by Fulgentius (see above, n. 13), the comparison of surgery with butchering was not uncommon then—nor is it uncommon now.

31. I.e., the soul.

3

THE HIPPOCRATIC
PRACTITIONER

Physicians of the soul, be they philosophers, prophets, priests, or theologians, would hardly compare their task with that of the doctor if they believed that medicine was a worthless art and successful cures were due to chance. Radical criticism of medicine was not lacking in Antiquity; it found strong expression at the time of Hippocrates, only to be skillfully countered by an author of the Hippocratic Collection.[1] But on the whole, radical criticism remained relatively subdued; the Greeks seem to have had considerable confidence in their medicine. The same cannot be said without qualification of their attitude toward its practitioners, whose expertise and moral character people were not willing to accept on trust. In the absence of academic degrees and of licenses, the laymen's suspicion is very understandable, and in view of the corresponding importance of a good reputation, good doctors desired to see themselves distinguished from the black sheep. There was not much of a medical *esprit de corps* in Antiquity. Both pagans and Christians showed far-reaching agreement as to who were the "outstanding," "excellent," or "best" doctors, as a frequently used Greek term (οἱ ἄριστοι) may be rendered.

When Galen spoke of "the best doctors" (often coupled with "the

---

1. According to Hippocrates (302), *Regimen in Acute Diseases* 8; 2:68, the art had a bad reputation, and its very existence was denied. Hippocrates (306), *On the Art*, provided a rebuttal of such accusations; see also below, n. 19.

best philosophers"), he was usually thinking of men of outstanding accomplishments. Similarly, when Emperor Julian asked his friend and physician Oribasius to "go through the works of all the best doctors and gather what is most opportune and all that is serviceable for the aim of medicine,"[2] Oribasius surveyed the works of the authors who had dealt best with medical subjects. Galen was assigned the first place "because he uses the most accurate methods and definitions by following the Hippocratic principles and opinions."[3]

Outstanding practitioners might belong to any sect; from the laymen's point of view, efficient performance and good character were more important than adherence to a particular sect or doctrine. In one of his works, the Christian Methodius had someone ask: "Do you not call him an excellent doctor who has already proved himself in severe diseases and has healed many [people]? . . . Moreover, do you not call him entirely unfit who has not yet accomplished anything and has never had sick people in hand?"[4]

Long before the division of medicine into sects, and before the Hippocratic oath and the other deontological writings of the Collection, the good craftsman obeyed the basic rules of his calling. Thucydides reports that when the plague invaded Athens (in 430 B.C.), "the physicians were of no avail. At first they treated without any knowledge; but they themselves were most likely to die inasmuch as they were the ones who chiefly visited [the sick]."[5] These doctors who perished in the practice of their profession did so at a time when the books of the Collection were only beginning to appear. Yet one of these books contains a passage that reflects on the hard life of a doctor. Medicine, it complains, is one of the arts that are profitable to those who make use of them, yet toilsome for their practitioners: "The physician sees terrible things, touches what is loathsome, and from others' misfortunes harvests troubles of his own."[6]

Thucydides took it for granted that doctors would visit the sick, regardless of the possible danger for themselves; he did not praise their behavior as heroic. The doctors may not yet have known how deadly the disease was. However, the craft of medicine had its risks and unpleasantnesses, and a true doctor had to take these upon himself. This tenet was and remained the backbone of medical ethics, before and

2. Oribasius (505), *Collectiones* 1, preface; 1:4, ll. 7–9.
3. Ibid.; 1:4, ll. 17–18.
4. Methodius (456), *Convivium* 11.3; col. 217D.
5. Thucydides (685), 2.47.4; 1:119, ll. 28–30.
6. Hippocrates (306), *On Breaths* 1; p. 91, ll. 5–7. I do not suggest that this passage was written with a view to the Athenian plague.

after philosophical notions of philanthropy made an impact.[7] It can be read into the first of the duties that the Hippocratic oath imposed upon medical practitioners.

Inscriptions from Hellenistic times show what a community valued in its doctors. In Cos, at the time of an epidemic, public honors were to be bestowed upon one Xenotimus on account of his "good will and care." The citation pointed out that even previously he had given medical care to the citizens, showing himself zealous in saving the sick. "Now, when many life-threatening illnesses were rampant and the public physicians in the city ill because of overexertion in the care of the sick, Xenotimus, of his own free will, constantly rendered assistance to those who needed it; intent upon bringing recovery to all the sick indiscriminately, and toiling for all citizens equally, he saved many."[8]

"Good will and care" for their people prompted the Athenians to honor a man who had offered "to serve gratis as public physician."[9] To these examples of doctors honored for their unselfish dedication to the general welfare may be added that of a public physician of whom it was said that he served "fairly all alike, whether poor or rich, slaves or free or foreigner," and that "he maintained a blameless reputation in all respects, providing proper attendance, which was open to all, as befits a man of culture and moral sense."[10]

Such inscriptions give some reality to the demands of the deontological writings of the Collection, demonstrating that there were doctors who came very near to embodying the ideal as the Greeks saw it. These were the kind of men the cities sought for the post of public physician.[11] The candidates for this post were examined by a body of laymen. The name of the teacher or of the place of study (Alexandria ranked highest)[12] were testimonials for the man's knowledge, and his reputation and the impression he made established his moral character. It may sound strange that knowledge and morality could be compared, and yet Erasistratus not only did so but supposedly gave the palm to morality. "It is fortunate indeed," he said, "wherever it happens that the

7. This general rule is not invalidated by the reluctance of Hippocratic physicians to get involved in awkward situations.

8. From the Greek text in Müri (474), p. 40.

9. Ibid., p. 39.

10. Quoted from Hands (283), p. 205. Here, as well as in *Precepts* (see below, text to nn. 84 and 87), foreigners receive special mention.

11. On public physicians in Greece, see Cohn-Haft (154). In Roman times the appointment was left to the prominent citizens of the provincial cities, who had to assure themselves of the moral probity and medical skill of the candidates; see Below (88), p. 41; and Nutton (487), p. 168.

12. Ammianus Marcellinus (12), 22.16.18; 2:306. For the translation of this passage, see Nutton (487), pp. 165–66 and 173.

physician is both, perfect in his art and most excellent in his moral conduct. But if one of the two should have to be missing, then it is better to be a good man devoid of learning than to be a perfect practitioner of bad moral conduct, and an untrustworthy man—if indeed it is true that good morals compensate for what is missing in art, while bad morals can corrupt and confound even perfect art." [13]

The pagan Scribonius Largus and a Christian commentator on Job (13:4) illustrate how this could be meant. Scribonius Largus could think of only two reasons why physicians would refrain from the use of medicaments: either ignorance of pharmacology or deliberate withholding of drugs, in which case their guilt was even greater. [14] The Christian observed that either ignorance or wickedness could make a physician so worthless that he would administer bad medicines. [15]

Wickedness of all sorts was certainly not absent among physicians in the centuries before the Romans became the masters of the Hellenized world. The Hippocratic oath (which was written before the first century A.D., when it is first mentioned in the extant literature) [16] made the future physician swear to act "for the benefit of the sick" and made him forswear certain practices. He will not give "a deadly drug to anybody even if asked for it," nor will he suggest it, nor will he give an abortifacient to a woman. He "will not use the knife, not even on sufferers from stone [of the bladder]." [17] There would be little sense in solemnly forswearing murder, cooperation in suicide, abortion, and euthanasia if doctors had never been known to participate in such deeds. Also, the physician will enter any household solely for the sake of helping the sick person. He will keep himself aloof from all intentional wrongdoing and harm, and especially from sexual relations with men and women, whether free or slave, and he will not speak about anything he hears or sees that ought not to be spread abroad.

Modern medical ethics has retained the demand for confidentiality

13. Edelstein's ([198], p. 334) translation, modified, from pseudo-Soranus, *Quaestiones medicinales*, in Rose (590), fasc. 2, p. 244, ll. 17–23. The authenticity of this quotation, accepted by Edelstein, has been questioned by Deichgräber (167), p. 103, n. 1, but has been reasserted (for the initial sentence) by Gourevitch (267), p. 268.

14. Scribonius Largus (614), *Compositiones*, epistula dedicatoria, art. 3; p. 2, ll. 5–10.

15. Didymus Alexandrinus (173), *Fragmenta in Job* 13.4; col. 1147 C–D.

16. The date and the origin of the oath are a matter of dispute. By the first century, it was accepted as the authoritative work of the great Hippocrates. Edelstein (201), Harig and Kollesch (287), and Lichtenthaeler (421) mark three distinct positions in the discussion of the Hippocratic oath. Together with Triebel-Schubert (693), they provide ample bibliographical information.

17. Edelstein's ([198] pp. 5–6) translation.

and the prohibition of sexual relations as far as the patient is concerned. But not only did the oath go farther by including all persons of the household in the sexual prohibition, it also demanded abstinence from any wrongdoing. A hint as to what may have been implied is given elsewhere in the Collection: "[Sick people] put themselves into the hands of the doctors, and at all hours these meet with women, maidens, and possessions very precious indeed. So toward all these self-control must be used." [18]

Again, elsewhere in the Collection, the absence of any penalty for malpractice in the Greek states was held responsible for the ignorance of the practitioners. Medicine, the most illustrious art, had sunk far below the others. Dishonor was the only penalty, "and it does not hurt those who are the embodiment of dishonor." [19]

Fear of the doctor as a poisoner certainly existed. The extent to which it was justified is uncertain, however, because of the Roman distrust of Greek doctors.[20] Galen, a proud Greek, practiced in Rome, and what he tells of his fellow practitioners in that city makes the Romans' distrust of them not unreasonable. He was harassed by his colleagues and his very life was threatened, so that he wished to return to his native Pergamum. The smaller cities, he thought, where everybody knew everybody else, were not infested with so much rascality.[21] If a Roman layman who wrote about a hundred and fifty years later is to be trusted, conditions in the provinces were bad enough:

> On my travels it frequently was my lot to experience various fraudulent acts of physicians, be it in connection with my own illness or that of members of my household. Some sold quite worthless [vilissima] remedies at horrendous prices; others, because of [their] greed, undertook to heal what they did not know how to cure. Indeed, I have certain knowledge of some physicians who act so as to prolong diseases which might be driven out in a very few days or even hours, in order to derive an income from their patients for a long time, and they [thus] show [themselves] more savage than the very diseases.[22]

18. Hippocrates (302), *On the Physician* 1; 2:313 (Jones's translation, modified).

19. Hippocrates (306), *Law* 1; p. 7, ll. 6–7. On liability and malpractice in Antiquity, see Amundsen (15) and idem (19).

20. See Kudlien (390), pp. 97–107, and Gourevitch (267), chap. 4 ("L'Anti-Hippocrate, ou le roman noir de la médecine"), pp. 347–414. Gourevitch's work rightly emphasizes the disparity between Greek medicine and Greek medicine in Rome.

21. Galen (250), *On Prognosis* 4.9; p. 90, ll. 23–26.

22. Pseudo-Pliny (558), p. 4, ll. 2–8. This work (the so-called *Medicina Plinii*),

It is not necessary to take all such stories at face value. Nor, on the other hand, will it do to underestimate the number of bad physicians and the frequency of doubtful practices. "What medical man," asked the theologian Irenaeus, "anxious to heal a sick person, would prescribe in accordance with the patient's whim, and not according to the requisite medicine?"[23] The answer to Irenaeus's rhetorical question would be that no good physician would act so. But Galen, Irenaeus's contemporary, commented on physicians in Rome who did just that, prescribing according to the whims of their powerful patients.[24]

There were outstanding doctors and there were worthless and wicked ones, and there were those who fell somewhere between the extremes. "In name there are many doctors, but in fact there are very few."[25] This sentence expressed the layman's predicament, regardless of whether its Hippocratic author saw it in this light. It did not suffice that a doctor be good, his integrity and competence also had to be recognizable. Only thus could the interests of both doctor and layman be met.

The Hippocratic oath was an ethical document demanding that life and art be guarded "in purity and holiness."[26] Other deontological writings of the Collection presented a combination of ethics and etiquette that seems to mix the ideal with the trivial, unless it is realized that by his proper demeanor the good practitioner helped the layman to make the right choice. Ethics and appearance were both of social importance.[27]

In a similar vein, the Collection contains a short introduction to surgical practice whose author deemed it desirable that the surgeon look healthy and well nourished, because otherwise the populace would think that he could not take proper care of others.[28] He should be clean

---

written around A.D. 300, belongs to the Western part of the empire at the time barbarization was beginning. For the East, cf. the similar complaint of Oribasius, below, chap. 16, n. 85. The accusation of dragging out the patient's illness was also known to the later Middle Ages; see Amundsen (14), p. 34.

23. Irenaeus (330) *Against Heresies* 3.5.2; 1:267 (Roberts and Rambaut's translation).

24. Galen (241), *Methodus medendi* 1.1; 10:4.

25. Hippocrates (306), *Law* 1; p. 7, l. 10.

26. Edelstein (198), p. 6, translates ὁσίως by the literal "[in] holiness." For a discussion of various translations, see Kudlien (404), who denies the religious character of ἀγνός and ὅσιος and interprets "integer und rechtschaffen." Cf. Lichtenthaeler (421), pp. 153–63.

27. This is also suggested by Edelstein (198), pp. 87–88.

28. Hippocrates (306), *On the Physician*, pp. 20–24. Jones's edition of Hippocrates contains the first chapter only (Jones [302], 2:303–13). Whereas Edelstein (198), p. 329, and Diller (310), p. 87, assign the book to the fourth century B.C., Kudlien (393) suggests the third century B.C. or a later date.

and well dressed, and the ointments he used should be pleasant, for this was agreeable to the sick.

Regarding his mental qualities, he should be prudent not only in re-straining his tongue but also in being altogether disciplined in his man-ner of life, for these things are of great value for [his] reputation. [His] behavior should be gentle and noble,[29] being dignified and humane [φιλάνθρωπον] toward all. For an over-forward obtrusiveness is de-spised, even though it may be very useful.[30]

He must look thoughtful but not stern,

for [then] he seems to be unfeeling and misanthropic [μισάνθρωπος]. But if he freely indulges in laughter and is too gay, he is taken to be vulgar, something to be very much guarded against. He must be fair in all his dealings, for on many occasions fairness has to be of help to him.[31]

The relationship between physician and patients is close; they put them-selves into his hands, and he must exercise self-control.[32]

All this advice seems to be aimed at producing superficial results. Yet the subsequent chapters disprove the suspicion that the sole aim was to make a favorable impression in the surgeon's interest. The author's purpose was to educate craftsmen,[33] and his instructions demanded that, as the product of good craftsmanship, medical treatments must be beneficial for the recipient.[34] For instance, the light in the surgery must not harm or cause discomfort to the patient's eyes.[35] Incisions must be made so as to cause the least pain.[36]

Except for the instruments, nothing should be used that is made of bronze, for it seems to me vulgar display to make use of such equipment

29. Hippocrates (306), *On the Physician* 1; p. 20, ll. 11–12: καλὸν καὶ ἀγαθόν. This is a formula used largely for persons of noble rank.

30. Ibid.; p. 20, ll. 9–14. The translation of the last sentence follows Jones (302), 2:311–13.

31. Hippocrates (306), *On the Physician,* 1; p. 20, ll. 16–19. In the last clause I read δικαιοσύνην and follow Diller's ([310], p. 88) German translation.

32. Hippocrates (306), *On the Physician,* 1; p. 20, ll. 20–23. For translation, see the text to n. 18, above.

33. Ibid. 2; p. 20, l. 25: τεχνικόν.

34. See Edelstein (198), p. 95, and his chapter "The Hippocratic Physician," especially pp. 87–96. Because of its relatively late date (see above, n. 28) and the demand that the doctor be humane (φιλάνθρωπον) to all, Edelstein (198), pp. 320–22, separated *On the Physician* from those writings that express the ethics of pure craftsmanship. See also Kudlien (393).

35. Hippocrates (306), *On the Physician* 2; p. 21, ll. 3–9.

36. Ibid. 5.

. . . [37] Dressings that are elegant and showy but of no benefit should be rejected, for the like is vulgar and outright pretentious and often brings harm to the patient. The sick person looks not for embellishment but for what is salutary.[38]

Patient and surgeon alike are affected by incorrect methods. Discussing the best way to avoid undue hemorrhage in operations, the author adds, "and it is rather shameful when the operation does not succeed as expected."[39] Venesection that results in a hematoma or in suppuration causes twofold harm: "pain for the person operated upon and much disrepute for the operator."[40]

This introduction to surgery, which teaches the ethics of medical craftsmanship, probably hailed from the fourth century B.C. or even later. It has been remarked that its ideal of the good doctor was not very far from the ideal of the good Athenian citizen of about that time.[41]

The Collection also contains two late writings bearing the significant titles *Decorum* and *Precepts,* which were expressive of medical ideals at the time of Jesus and the Apostles. Here, as in other deontological works, what should be done is often stated or made explicit by a description of what should not be done. Both works open with philosophical deliberations about the foundation of medicine, and in both, the influences of Stoicism and perhaps Epicureanism are noticeable.[42]

Decorum begins by praising the kind of wisdom that has manifold uses in human life. Wisdom that has its origin in useless learning may, unless downright idle and misdirected, be stimulating, sharpen the intellect, and contribute to the beauty of life. But wisdom that has been fashioned into an art (techne) is more refined, especially if the art aims at decorum and good repute.[43] "Indeed, all wisdom that is free of sordid love of gain and of indecency is good[44] if it possesses method and operates in a craftsmanlike manner."[45] The author is contemptuous of those who have succumbed to temptation, who go from city to city and

37. Ibid. 2; p. 21, ll. 11–13.
38. Ibid. 4; p. 21, ll. 32–35.
39. Ibid. 6; p. 22, ll. 19–20. Hippocrates (309), *De morbis* 1.6; 6:150–52, gives a list of techniques that a doctor must have mastered. See also below, n. 64.
40. Hippocrates (306), *On the Physician* 8; p. 23, ll. 14–15.
41. Diller (177), p. 87. However, see above, n. 28, for the date of this book.
42. The text of *Decorum* and of *Precepts* is badly corrupted, and the interpretation of many passages relies on conjecture.
43. Hippocrates (306), *Decorum* 1; p. 25.
44. I accept the reading of καλαί, ᾗσι given by Littré (309), 9:226, and adapted by Jones (302), 2:278.
45. Hippocrates (306), *Decorum* 2; p. 25, ll. 11–12.

deceive people with their cheap trickeries.[46] These practitioners of the wrong kind of wisdom are recognizable by their dress—but dress is important for practitioners of the right kind, too. Whereas the former may be overadorned, the latter adopt dress that is simple, respectable rather than overelaborate, and "suitable for men of thoughtful disposition as well as for walking."[47] Their personal qualities mark them as men of the world rather than as lonely thinkers. Among other things, they are

> sharp in encounter, skillful in repartee, severe when meeting with opposition, well-intentioned and affable when meeting with like-mindedness, good tempered toward all . . . considerate of their food and moderate . . . putting into well-chosen words all the arguments, using eloquent language, being endowed with grace. Relying on the reputation that results from these [qualities], they accept the truth once it has been proved.[48]

Natural disposition is of the utmost importance, but it is the task of wisdom to make known the work of nature. Education must be thorough, and reasoning, the source of all true craftsmanship, must not be mere opinion, artfully presented yet unrelated to practice. Especially in medicine, opinions that are not founded on practice bring blame to those who propound them and are fatal for those who use them.[49]

A basis has now been laid for the demand that wisdom (philosophy) be applied to medicine and medicine to wisdom,[50] "for a physician who is a philosopher is godlike."[51] This famous phrase is not an endorsement of any and all philosophizing in medicine. Only a pragmatic philosophy represented by the right kind of people will do.[52]

After philosophy has received due recognition, unstinted praise is given to medicine. Actually, medicine includes all the features of wis-

46. This seems to be the approximate meaning of ibid.; p. 25, ll. 11–17; cf. Jones (302), 2:279–81.

47. Hippocrates (306), *Decorum* 3; p. 25, ll. 23–24.

48. Ibid., ll. 25–26. Translated with some borrowings from Jones (302), 2:281–83.

49. This is the gist of chap. 4; cf. Jones (302), 2:284, n. 1, and idem, 2:286, n. 1. Hippocrates (306), *On the Art* 13; p. 19, ll. 6–7, also distinguished between that which is demonstrated by acts and that which is demonstrated by oratory. Similarly Hippocrates (306), *Law* 4; p. 8, ll. 9–10. Polybius (565), *Histories* 12.25d; 4:372–75, described the representatives of "logical," i.e., theoretical, medicine, who had no practical knowledge. They went from town to town to the detriment of the sick.

50. Hippocrates (306), *Decorum* 5; p. 27, ll. 1–2.

51. Ibid., l. 3: ἰητρὸς γὰρ φιλόσοφος [literally "a lover of wisdom"] ἰσόθεος.

52. Cf. Edelstein (198), p. 331.

dom: "lack of avarice, modesty, a sense of shame,[53] reserve, opinion, judgment, calm, neatness, principle, knowledge of the things useful and necessary for life, rejection of what is not clean, lack of superstition, [and] divine excellence."[54] And this "in opposition to licentiousness, vulgarity, greediness, lust, thievery, shamelessness."[55] Although not stated in so many words, medicine emerges as the ideal form of philosophy, and the virtues that medicine represents are those of practical philosophy. Even "awareness of the gods" is seen as immanent in medical thought.[56]

From philosophy, morality, and prudent behavior,[57] the author proceeds to detailing the particulars that make for good practice, such as bedside manner, and those things that must be prepared and ready at hand. The author is a practitioner who thinks of pragmatic philosophy as the elevation of an honest craft to an art with insight into what it does and what ought to be done. He has little interest in contemplative philosophy or in the lonely thinker. His philosopher-physician is a public figure with his feet on the ground.

The great rhetorical skill demanded of the physician was a desideratum of medical practice because opinions had to be justified to the patient and his relatives and friends, and defended against objecting bystanders and colleagues. The Hippocratic Collection contained examples of such controversy in very practical matters.[58] Galen described the scene in which he gave an opinion to the ailing emperor Marcus Aurelius, dissenting from the opinion of the physicians already attending him.[59] Apollonius of Tyana compared doctors at the bedside of the patient with a herd of elephants surrounding a wounded member.[60] Theodorus Priscianus, a physician of the fifth century with an empirical bent, accused his arguing colleagues of vainglory and a lack of compassion. He made Nature say, "The patient does not die, he is killed, and I am accused of weakness."[61] In Alexandria, the physician Magnus, who

53. Hippocrates (306), *Decorum* 5; p. 27, l. 5: ἐρυθρίησις, literally "blushing."
54. Ibid. 5; p. 27, ll. 4–7.
55. Ibid. 5; p. 27, ll. 8–9.
56. Ibid. 6; p. 27, l. 13.
57. See especially ibid. 7.
58. For instance, controversy about the proper extension in fractures and dislocation (Hippocrates [302], *On Fractures* 1; 3:94). See also Edelstein (198), pp. 99–100.
59. See Brock's ([113], pp. 217–18) English translation from Galen's *On Prognosis* 11.
60. Philostratus (543), *Life of Apollonius of Tyana* 2.16; 1:160.
61. Theodorus Priscianus (678), *Euporiston* 1.2; p. 3, ll. 6–7; see also the preceding lines.

enjoyed great fame about the middle of the fourth century, was so powerful a disputant that he could prove that those cured by other doctors
were still sick. Yet his own reputation as a healer did not equal his
prowess as a lecturer and a dialectician.[62]

"To help or not to harm" was an avowed maxim of Hippocratic
medicine and expressive of the good craftsman's pride and caution.[63]
Orthopedic appliances must serve their purpose well or not be used at
all, for to use them and to fail is "shameful and unworthy of the art." [64]
Harm to the patient must be avoided, as the Hippocratic oath implied—not only bodily harm but also mental harm that would affect
health. As an example of a harmful approach, Galen related the anec-
dote of the doctor who quoted to a suffering and complaining patient
the Homeric words "Patroclus also had to die, and he was much better
than you" (*Iliad* 21.107).[65] More than that, the doctor should try to
make matters as pleasant as possible. *Epidemics* contains a somewhat
disjointed list of

> amenities for the sick: for instance, keeping clean: drink, food and what
> he sees; soft: what he touches. Others: [allowing] what does not do
> great harm and can easily be set right again, like something cold when
> indicated. [The doctor's] visits: words, posture, dress—all [to be] agree-
> able to the patient—[as are] hair, nails, smells.[66]

This note was expanded by Galen and later commentators.[67] *Epidemics*
was highly respected and carried authority among doctors. Its advice
was probably taken as part of the philanthropy the doctor owed his
patients.

While philanthropic considerations are not absent from *On the
Physician* and *Decorum*, it is in *Precepts* that philanthropy plays a key
role, adding an accent of its own. Not unlike *Decorum*, the introductory chapters of *Precepts* warn against exclusive reliance on reasoning
in medical practice. "Experience together with reason" is needed.[68]

---

62. Eunapius (209), *Lives of the Philosophers and Sophists;* pp. 530–33. Cf.
above, n. 49. On dialectic in medicine, see Kudlien (384).
63. Hippocrates (302), *Epidemics* 1.11; 1:164.
64. Hippocrates (302), *Fractures* 30; 3:168; see also above, n. 39.
65. Galen (246), *In Hippocratis Epidemiarum librum sextum* 4.10; p. 203; also
Deichgräber (165), frag. 357. For comment see Deichgräber (167), p. 33.
66. Hippocrates (309), *Epidemics* 6.4.7; 5:308. Müri (474), p. 31, gives a
slightly paraphrased German translation.
67. Stephanus (646), *Commentary on Hippocrates' Aphorisms* 1.2; p. 42, ll.
16–31; see idem, apparatus, the references to Galen and Palladius. To these, add
John of Alexandria (327), pp. 198–205.
68. Hippocrates (306), *Precepts* 1; p. 30, ll. 4–5. For a translation of *Precepts*,
see Jones (302), 1:303–33.

Facts[69] must constantly be kept in one's memory, for only thus can the mind arrive at the truth. This approach will be to the advantage of both practitioner and patient, whereas reliance on unfounded opinions makes innocent patients already in the grip of the disease suffer from their doctor's inexperience as well.[70] Indeed, the doctor should not hesitate to learn from laymen when this would be helpful at the time of treatment.[71]

For physicians to question laymen was nothing unheard of; Rufus of Ephesus, around the same time, had written a book on the subject.[72] But it was not generally accepted by doctors, many of whom wished to impress the public by their omniscience. *Precepts'* insistence that colleagues be consulted in a perplexing case was a still stronger thrust against letting the doctor's selfish interest prevail over that of the patient. *Precepts* was quite outspoken on this matter. Faced with a condition with which they were unable to deal, it was ignoramuses— quacks[73] who were not dedicated to healing—who did nothing and, in their wicked disregard for providing help, shunned calling in other doctors.[74] There was nothing shameful in learning from others and joining with them in providing help;[75] consultation did not redound to the discredit of the art. But doctors meeting in consultation must not engage in rivalry and the exchange of insults, and they must be free of jealousy. Such behavior showed weakness and smacked of the business of the marketplace.[76] The author of *Precepts* had a high opinion of medicine and wanted its dignity preserved. The principles of the art were irreproachable, and by following them a good doctor, a so-called "fellow of the art," [77] might excel.

Precepts urged that everything possible be done for the healing of the sick. But then as now, the demand for complete dedication to the art conflicted with the doctor's need to make a living by its practice. How to resolve this conflict is a problem of medical ethics for which *Precepts* found its answer in adjusting self-interest to philanthropy. It advised the physician not to start out by discussing his fee with the

69. Hippocrates (306), *Precepts* 1; p. 30, l. 11: τῶν . . . ἐπιτελεομένων; and idem 2; p. 31, l. 3: τῶν γινομένων.

70. Ibid. 1; p. 30, ll. 19–21.

71. Ibid. 2; p. 31, ll. 6–7.

72. Rufus of Ephesus (596), *Quaestiones medicinales.*

73. Hippocrates (306), *Precepts* 7; p. 32, l. 15: ἀνίητροι, literally "not-physicians."

74. This seems to be the meaning of ibid. 7; p. 32, ll. 22–24.

75. Ibid. 8; p. 33, ll. 5–9.

76. Ibid. 8; p. 33, ll. 11–15.

77. Ibid. 7; p. 32, l. 19: ὁμότεχνος καλεόμενος. Jones (302), 1:321, translates this as "a brother of the art"; cf. below, n. 81.

suffering patient. In case of disagreement, the latter will think that the doctor will leave without heeding him and prescribing something for his immediate need.[78] Worrying about the fee does the patient no good, particularly in cases of acute illness. "Not the striving for profit but rather the thought for [his] reputation spurs on the man who treats properly. Thus it is better to reproach [patients] who have been saved than to snuff out [the life of] those in danger of death."[79]

There are sick people who demand the impossible. They should not be heeded, yet should not be punished.[80] Unfortunately, the condition of the text of the following few sentences is such that the only thing that can be said with some assurance is that the author there doubts the existence of a "brother doctor"[81] so hardened as to refuse to examine any case and to prescribe treatment. The reward also must not be overlooked, "to say nothing of the desire that makes a man ready to learn."[82] The author obviously does not believe that accepting a fee demeans a doctor. But he advises

> not to give way to excessive inhumanity [ἀπανθϱωπίην] but to have a good look at [the patient's] affluence and means, sometimes also treating gratis, remembering a previous favor or in view of present satisfaction.[83] And when the occasion arises to support somebody who is an alien and without resources, such people in particular must be helped.[84]

This culminates in the famous sentence "For if love of men [φιλαν-θϱωπίη] is present, love of the art [φιλοτεχνίη] is also present."[85]

78. Hippocrates (306), *Precepts* 4; p. 31, ll. 16–20. According to idem 3, all illnesses go through many stages before reaching a state in which a definite treatment can be prescribed. See above, chap. 2, text to n. 8, regarding changes during the course of an illness.

79. Ibid. 4; p. 31, ll. 23–25. For the translation of πϱομύσσειν, see Temkin (672), p. 8 and p. 21, n. 10.

80. Hippocrates (306), *Precepts* 5; p. 31, ll. 26–27.

81. Ibid. 5; p. 32, l. 1: ἠδελφισμένος (or ἠδελφισμένως ἰητϱεύοι); the word seems to have the same meaning as "fellow of the art" (see above, text to n. 77) and to correspond roughly to our "colleague."

82. I follow Jones's ([302], 1:318, ll. 9–10) arrangement of the text and his translation in preference to Heiberg's ([306], p. 32, ll. 4–5). The wish to gather experience is attributed to Hippocrates by Galen (see below, chap. 5, text to n. 4) as well as by the legend (see below, chap. 6, text to n. 15 and text following n. 86). *Precepts* takes it for granted that a good doctor desires to add to his experience.

83. Edelstein (198), p. 99, interprets this as meaning "the patient's gratitude and . . . the reputation [the doctor] gains for also treating the poor." One manuscript actually reads εὐδοκιμίην, i.e., good repute (Hippocrates [306], *Precepts* 6; p. 32, apparatus to l. 7), instead of εὐδοκίην, i.e., satisfaction.

84. Hippocrates (306), *Precepts* 6; p. 32, ll. 5–9.

85. Ibid., l. 9.

To paraphrase: Regarding the fee, humanity demands a consideration of the patient's economic condition. At his discretion the doctor
may demand much, less, or little. As a *quid pro quo,* free treatment
may be given if the doctor has some previous obligation to the patient
(hospitality easily comes to mind), or if he is presently receiving some
satisfaction from the patient.[86] A third occasion for liberality is the case
of destitute aliens, that is, persons outside the bond of citizenry. To go
out of one's way to help such people is a particularly striking piece of
philanthropy, yet in line with the Hellenistic inscriptions.[87]

A doctor who has such love for humanity will also love his art and
will, therefore, be a dedicated and successful practitioner. His very decency may have therapeutic results. "For some patients," the above
quotation continues, "though aware that their condition is not without
danger, yet recover their health simply through their satisfaction with
the decency of the physician." [88] The doctor's obligations are then summarized: "It is indeed well to take charge of the sick for the sake of
their health and to give thought to the healthy for the sake of their
freedom from disease, also [it is well] to give thought to the healthy for
the sake of decorum." [89]

Precepts contains additional, more detailed, advice on how to behave.[90] To a degree, a doctor can do things, for instance regarding dress
and perfumes, that will please, as long as he remains in good taste.[91]
But nothing must be done that will counteract the doctor's authority
and dignity, which are important for lifting the patient's morale.[92] The
author frowns on lecturing in order to attract a crowd. At the least,
poetic citations should not be used as evidence, since this shows a lack
of application to medicine.[93] Doctors who hold forth at length vehe-

86. Perhaps from the patient's singing the doctor's praises; cf. above, n. 83.

87. See above, n. 10. The attention paid to foreigners can be connected with the
later rise of inns for those "who were separated from their families, solitary persons
and foreigners" (Uta Lindgren, quoted by Volk [707], p. 26).

88. Hippocrates (306), *Precepts* 6; p. 32, ll. 9–11. I am no longer able to accept
Edelstein's ([198], p. 321) interpretation of φιλοτεχνίη as referring to the patients'
love of the art. Ἐπιείκείη, however translated (cf. Gourevitch [267], p. 282, n. 80),
is a personal quality of the doctor. A doctor who loves people will also be devoted
to his art. Besides, the verb φιλοτεχνέω in Hippocrates (306), *Precepts* 14; p. 35, l.
3, can hardly refer to anybody but the physician.

89. I see no need for replacing "the healthy [ὑγιαινόντων]" in the last clause of
Hippocrates (306), *Precepts* 6; p. 32, ll. 11–13, by "one's own self [ἑωυτῶν]," as
done by Jones (302), 1:318, 319. *Precepts* gives two reasons why the doctor should
care for the healthy: it is intrinsically right, and it is also seemly.

90. See Hippocrates (306), *Precepts* 9–14.

91. Ibid. 10.

92. Ibid. 9.

93. Ibid. 12.

mently and mindless of propriety might arouse the admiration of laymen; the author, however, would not welcome them as consultants.[94]

This, then, is the description of a humane Hippocratic practitioner of about the first century, seen from a Greek doctor's point of view: Dedicated to his art and to healing his patients, he is willing to learn from laymen and to consult other doctors. He values his reputation, and he claims a right to his fee. But whenever the need arises, his concern for the fee must yield to consideration for the patient's welfare. He does not worry his sick patients by arguing about his fee; he considers their circumstances and their means, and even assists aliens who lack resources. Nor is he so hardened as to refuse help to recalcitrant patients.

It is unwarranted to consider a doctor's regard for his reputation as no more than subservience to the judgment of the outside world. To be sure, the doctor can be a mere conformist. But as a member of the society that molds his reputation, he will not entirely escape sharing its values. For the Hippocratic doctor, the opinion of the educated stratum of society, influenced by Stoic and Epicurean philosophy, counted for much, and philanthropy was one of the demands of the Stoic ethics. It can therefore be assumed that the emphasis on philanthropy in *Precepts* was not quite free from Stoic influence.

Seneca (to quote a contemporary Stoic philosopher, though a Roman) maintained that no other philosophical school was "kinder and milder, none more full of love [*amantior*] of man and more concerned for the common good, so that it is its intent to be useful and helpful not only for oneself but to be mindful of all as well as of the individual." [95] Seneca said this in defense against the accusation that Stoicism denied to a sage "the feeling of pity [and] forgivingness." [96] But there has to be reason in what is being done; mere pity (*misericordia*) must be avoided: "It is the blemish of a weak mind that succumbs at the sight of others' misfortunes." [97]

There is no indication that the author of *Precepts* was a "bleeding heart," ruled by sentiment unbridled by reason. On the other hand, there is no reason to deny offhand that he felt pity and compassion for the sick. His emphasis on philanthropy shows that he was in harmony with the concepts of his time, but this does not add much to what the text itself reveals. It will not do to declare him a Stoic and hence to

94. Ibid. 13. See also above, n. 49, and below, text to n. 110.
95. Seneca (616), *On Mercy* 2.5.3; 1:438–39 (Basore's translation, modified). Cf. Pohlenz (564), 1:30, but also Hands (283), p. 82.
96. Seneca (616), *On Mercy* 2.5.2; p. 438.
97. Ibid. 2.5.1; p. 438.

deduce what he felt and thought.[98] But feelings apart, his behavior does not compare unfavorably with that of a decent modern doctor.

Closer dependence on Stoic ethics is found in the writings of Scribonius Largus, a medical practitioner of about the middle of the first century. Envy, he believed, "is especially sinful among physicians, for unless theirs is a heart full of mercy and humanity [*misericordiae et humanitatis*], in accordance with the will of the medical profession itself, they are rightly hated by all the gods and men." [99]

It has plausibly been argued that Scribonius Largus accepted Cicero's notion of humanity, derived from the Greek Stoic Panaetius.[100] There is more to it, however. Scribonius Largus declared compassion, which in *Precepts* can only be surmised,[101] to be a desideratum of the medical profession. Whatever may have led him to this statement, the presence of compassion among doctors was taken for granted by authors of the first century. The Roman encyclopedist Celsus thought that a surgeon should be "filled with pity, so that he wishes to cure his patient" without, however, being moved by the patient's cries to too great a hurry or to cutting less than required. He will do "everything just as if the cries of pain caused him no emotion." [102] Even too great an emotional involvement was to be feared.

Toward the turn of the second century, the Methodist Soranus took it as a matter of course that a good midwife ought to have compassion with the mother's pain in childbirth. But contrary to a prevailing opinion, he did not think it necessary that she herself have borne children in order to feel compassion.[103] Possibly also in the first cen-

98. Modern authors usually interpret *Precepts* within the conceptual confines of deportment and Stoic philosophy; see Amundsen and Ferngren (26), pp. 1–4; idem (23), p. 28; Baader (65), p. 309; Hands (283), pp. 131–32; and Gourevitch (267), pp. 283–84. In his ground-breaking essay "The Ethics of the Greek Physician" (Edelstein [198], p. 319–48), in which he elaborated his view on the close relationship of medical ethics and philosophy, Edelstein spoke of philanthropy in *Precepts* and *On the Physician* as "a proper behavior towards those with whom a physician comes in contact during treatment; it is viewed as a minor social virtue, so to say" (idem, pp. 321–22).

99. Scribonius Largus (614), *Compositiones*, epistula dedicatoria, art. 3; p. 2, ll. 10–13. Quoted from Hamilton's ([282], p. 213) translation.

100. Edelstein (198), pp. 337–43.

101. Edelstein finds charitableness especially in the help for "a stranger in . . . financial straits" (ibid., p. 329). Still, to Edelstein this is no more than a philosophically postulated "kindly and tolerant *attitude*" (idem, p. 330; emphasis mine); cf. above, n. 98.

102. Celsus (137), *De medicina* 7, prooemium, art. 4; 3:297 (Spencer's translation).

103. Soranus (636), *Gynaeciorum* 1.2.4; p. 5, ll. 21–23. For translation, see

tury,[104] Aretaeus, an author of the Pneumatist sect, bewailed the fate of the victims of tetanus and the helplessness of the doctor: "With them, then, who are overpowered by the disease, he can merely commiserate." [105]

Because the remarks of Celsus, Soranus, and Aretaeus were made in passing, they are credible testimonies to historical reality. They make it doubtful that compassion among doctors sprang into existence in response to a new trend of Stoic philosophy. Seneca, who rejected pity (*misericordia*) as justifying any action, still admitted that "most people praise it as a virtue and call a compassionate [*misericordem*] man a good man." [106] Physicians long before the first century probably thought so too, so that Scribonius Largus could think of compassion as rooted in medical ethics.

The medical code imposed restrictions, such as forbidding complicity in suicide. (In Antiquity there was no general objection to suicide.) A Latin novel of the second century tells of a doctor who was asked to provide poison, allegedly on behalf of a man desperate to end his life because of his unbearable suffering. The doctor did not know that he was to be used for murderous purposes, and his compliance would not have been punishable. Yet he did not comply, both because he was suspicious of the purchaser, and because the art to which he was sworn demanded respect for life, not its destruction.[107]

The practice of Hippocratic medical ethics can be understood as a physician's living up to the rightful demands and expectations of the world, as well as to the principles that his profession and his conscience imposed upon him. Praise of wisdom—fashioned into the kind of art

---

Soranus (637), p. 6. For *Precepts,* Scribonius Largus, Celsus, Soranus, and pseudo-Soranus, cf. Gourevitch (267), pp. 266–76.

104. Kudlien (401), p. 22, has proposed the hypothesis that Aretaeus was an author of the Pneumatist sect living in the middle of the first century.

105. Aretaeus (39), *Acute Diseases* 1.6; p. 7, ll. 22–23. Quoted in modified form from Adams's ([40] p. 249) translation. Schubring (612), p. 455, comments on the doctor's personal chagrin in hopeless cases. Kudlien (395), col. 1108, believes that Aretaeus may well stand closer to the Christians than to the Stoics.

106. Seneca (616), *On Mercy* 2.4.4; p. 436. The compassion of pagan doctors for their patients has been well recognized but has been seen as something new, belonging to Roman times; see Amundsen and Ferngren (23), p. 28. Gourevitch (267), pp. 285–86, is very explicit: "φιλανθρωπία va prendre un sens nouveau ainsi que sa traduction latine *humanitas* . . . Et cette philanthropie nouvelle va devenir un véritable constituant de la vocation médicale, parallèlement à l'amour de la gloire ou l'amour de l'argent." I wonder whether the impression of something quite new may be due to the paucity of medical sources from the three pre-Christian centuries. I do not believe that Seneca's "most people [*plerique*]" was limited to the followers of the new trend in Stoic ethics, represented by Panaetius and Cicero's *humanitas*.

107. See Amundsen (20), p. 325.

that aimed at decorum and repute—thus loses its seeming priggishness and comes to mean praise of the art which, instructed by wisdom, leads to an ethical life and deserved renown.

None of the Hippocratic deontological writings quite expressed this idea, which is a synthesis of their individual tendencies. There obviously were many doctors whose behavior was unethical, and there were others whose practice was not remarkable in either direction. It is impossible to tell how many were outstanding as judged by the standards of Hippocratic craftsmanship and deontology. To speak of Hippocratic practitioners is to speak of practitioners who took or were expected to take the deontology of the Collection as their guide. These included more than the followers of Hippocratic medicine as a doctrine, and in this sense Scribonius Largus, for instance, also was a Hippocratic practitioner, whatever his orientation otherwise may have been.

Actually, *Decorum* and *Precepts* show little concern with medical theories, and this in spite of the praise of wisdom and method in *Decorum* and the emphasis on experience in both works. *Decorum* holds that in the case of doctors whose behavior is without reproach, exposure to actual experience can make up for deficient knowledge.[108] *Precepts* describes the medical art as a "ready and infallible habit" acquired by attention to facts,[109] and maintains that those who present subtle theories with fluent oratory but lack the calm assurance of skill should be listened to, but not followed.[110] Yet the author's brief remarks on pneuma, heat, humors, and nature[111] suggest that he was not an Empiricist. If anything, the deontological writings discourage thinking of the sects as pigeonholes into which all practitioners must fit neatly.

The Hippocratic practitioner as described here was a pagan. Yet Christians used the same criteria for distinguishing between good, bad, and outstanding practitioners. Moreover, the deontological writings of the Collection became an important source for a literature of late Antiquity and the early Middle Ages that has come down in Greek, Latin, and Arabic versions.[112] What was to distinguish the sincere Christian doctor from the pagan was a new relationship to his faith and its church rather than a fundamental change in his professional ethics.[113]

108. Hippocrates (306), *Decorum* 18; p. 29, ll. 34–35.
109. Hippocrates (306), *Precepts* 2; p. 31, ll. 3–5. Quoted from Jones's ([302], 1:315) translation.
110. Hippocrates (306), *Precepts* 13; p. 34, ll. 22–23. Cf. above, nn. 49 and 94; also Dio Chrysostom (180), *Discourses* 33.6; 3:278; and Kee (358), pp. 63–64.
111. Hippocrates (306), *Precepts* 9.
112. See below, chap. 11, n. 84.
113. For further comments on this point, see below, chap. 17.B and the Epilogue.

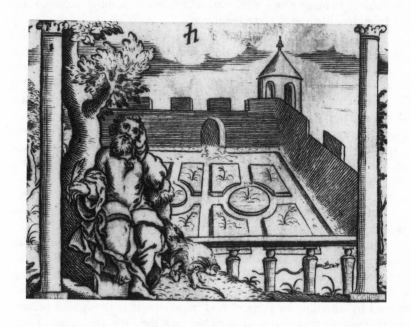

Democritus of Abdera. From the title page of *The Anatomy of Melancholy*, by Robert Burton. London: Peter Parker, 1676.

II

Hippocrates in the
Pagan World

4

THE GREAT, HUMANE,
AND WISE AUTHOR

That a fetus born in the seventh month is perfect has now been accepted owing to the authority of that very learned man, Hippocrates. Hence, a son born in the seventh month following a legitimate marriage must be held to be legitimate."[1] This opinion, rendered by the jurist Paul in about A.D. 200, testifies to the great authority Hippocrates enjoyed, even outside the ranks of the physicians and the natural philosophers.

It is fair to date Hippocrates' fame among educated Greeks to a much earlier time. Readers of Plato would remember Hippocrates of Cos, the Asclepiad, a physician who taught medicine for a fee.[2] They would also remember Socrates and Phaedrus discussing the nature of the soul and whether it could be understood "without the nature of the whole."[3] Socrates agreed with Phaedrus that Hippocrates was right in contending that even regarding the body, it was impossible to obtain knowledge without knowing the nature of the whole. "However," he added, "besides Hippocrates one must also question reason and see whether it agrees." Phaedrus consenting, Socrates continues, "Well

1. *Corpus iuris civilis* (156), *Digesta* 1.5.12; p. 7. The editor, Theodor Mommsen, refers to Hippocrates' *On Diet* 1.26 (see Hippocrates [309] 4:265), as the source.

2. Plato (554), *Protagoras* 311B; p. 98.

3. It is a matter of debate whether "the nature of the whole [τῆς τοῦ ὅλου φύσεως]" refers to the body or to the universe.

then, see what Hippocrates as well as true reason say concerning nature," and he outlines a method for investigating the nature of whatever it may be.[4] To the present day, commentators, Galen prominently among them, have tried to trace this method in the Hippocratic works.[5]

In the time of Nero, the Greek lexicographer Erotianus listed as Hippocratic a large number of the writings that now constitute the Hippocratic Collection. Erotianus counted Hippocrates among the classical authors, on a literary par with Homer, Democritus, Herodotus, Thucydides, and "the Ancients" in general.[6] He recommended the study of the Collection as useful for all persons with a claim to intellectual culture, and above all for those physicians who did not repudiate the research done by their ancient predecessors.[7] The latter remark may have been directed at the Methodists, whose leader Thessalus, physician to Nero, promised to teach medicine in six months and was castigated by Galen as one of the main scorners of Hippocrates.[8]

About half a century after Erotianus, admiration for classical Greek became a fashion; and for Galen, whose readers were not limited to doctors, Hippocrates was "the ancient" par excellence, whose works had only to be interpreted where he had not expressed himself clearly and brought to completion where he had but laid the foundation.[9] Both of these tasks Galen took upon himself.

On the Latin side, Scribonius Largus and Celsus held Hippocrates in the highest esteem. Both wrote for laymen:[10] Scribonius Largus addressed his little pharmacological book to a man influential with the emperor, and Celsus, as an encyclopedist, wrote for an educated public at large. The name of Hippocrates was well known to the philosopher Seneca; Quintilian introduced it in his textbook of rhetoric; and though Plutarch wrote in Greek, his regard for Hippocrates can be assumed to have come to the attention of educated Romans as well.[11]

In the first century, or the second at the latest, the legend of Hippoc-

---

4. Plato (552), *Phaedrus* 270C; p. 548.

5. I agree with Joly (347), p. 419, that the outline was Plato's and that Hippocrates' contribution was limited to supplying authority for the need to understand the nature of the whole in order to investigate any subject.

6. Erotianus (208), p. 4, ll. 8–14. Cf. Edelstein (198), p. 128.

7. Erotianus (208), p. 3, ll. 3–7. The widespread interest in medicine (cf. Nutton [493], p. 38) helps to explain the inclusion of Hippocrates among the classical authors.

8. Galen (241), *Methodus medendi* 1.2; 10:7–8.

9. See Temkin (667), pp. 32–33 and 58.

10. Regarding Scribonius Largus, I believe that the popular fear of drugs was the reason he prefaced a short pharmacological tract with a general essay on professional ethics and the use of drugs. Regarding Celsus, see Harig (284).

11. On Pliny, see below, chap. 5, text to n. 20, and chap. 6.B.1.

rates, in the form of fictionalized letters, also had reached substantially the form in which it is known today.[12] But as far as it is possible, the legend had best be considered separately from what his works had to tell educated pagans about his character.

The fame of Hippocrates was solidly based on his greatness as a physician and as the founder of medicine as a discipline. Before him, Celsus thought, the science of medicine had been in the hands of the philosophers because the strain of thinking and the lack of sleep had weakened their bodies. Hippocrates (as some people believed, a pupil of Democritus)[13] "a man first and foremost worthy to be remembered, notable both for professional skill and for eloquence . . . separated this discipline from the study of philosophy."[14] The fact that very little is known about Greek medicine before the Hippocratic writings has helped to put Hippocrates at the head of the tradition of Western medicine. But for ancient physicians and the educated pagan public, he was much more than "the greatest physician and the founder of [medicine]."[15] As a classical author, he was one of the pillars of their culture, and his works proved him to be a model of honesty and courage, an educator who led physicians to humane behavior, and a very wise person.

Epidemics describes the case of a man who was hit by a stone in the region of the bregma and died after developing convulsions in both hands. The author admitted having mistaken the fissures caused by the injury for the sutures of the skull, with the result that the patient's head was not trephined in time.[16] This frank confession of a fatal mistake appeared to Celsus as an example of a "great man's love of truth in great matters." His own "regard for the memory of a great teacher" prompted Celsus to observe,

> Such a sincere confession of the truth befits a great mind which will still be ready to accept many responsibilities, and especially in performing the task of handing down knowledge for the advantage of posterity, that no one else may be deceived again by what has deceived him.[17]

Celsus recognized in Hippocrates a man whose greatness extended beyond the confines of medicine. For the orator Quintilian and for Plutarch, both about the end of the first century, Hippocrates was a model

12. See below, chap. 6.B.
13. Celsus (137), *De medicina*, prooemium, art. 8; 1:4. It is hard to tell whether this reflects influences of Democritean science (cf. Diller [179], chaps. 2 and 3) and the legend (see below, chap. 5, text to n. 19; and chap. 6.B.2, text to n. 79).
14. Celsus (137), *De medicina*, pp. 4–5 (Spencer's translation, modified).
15. Seneca (615), *Epistulae* 95.20; 3:70.
16. Hippocrates (309), *Epidemics* 5.27; 5:226.
17. Celsus (137), *De medicina* 8.4.3–4; 3:505–7 (Spencer's translation).

of honesty toward others as well as oneself. Since his textbook of rhetoric was intended for young people, Quintilian felt that he too must follow Hippocrates and not give the impression of concealing the truth and hiding his opinion.[18] The moralist Plutarch saw in Hippocrates' honesty a challenge to anybody who aspired to true moral improvement. How could a man, bent on saving himself, lack the courage to confess his shortcomings and accept the blame, seeing that Hippocrates had admitted his error to save others from suffering?[19] Emperor Julian also was acquainted with the story, and used it to excuse a mistake he had made in judging a certain person's character. He cited other great men's mistakes, quoted Hippocrates and the passage in question, and concluded, "Now if those famous men were deceived about persons whom they know and the physician was mistaken in his professional diagnosis, is it surprising that Julian was deceived?"[20] Julian did not dwell on Hippocrates' moral greatness; for him the story was a testimony to human fallibility, from which even the most famous and the most experienced were not exempt.

Methods of higher criticism, though not always the same as ours, had been well developed in Antiquity. They were used in the study of Homer and other classical authors, where it seemed important to separate the genuine from the spurious and to have a reliable text. Physicians had a practical interest in reviewing the books ascribed to Hippocrates critically, so as to be sure to take the genuine Hippocrates as their authority.

Anxious to avoid using spurious religious texts for the establishment of orthodox doctrine, Christian authors adopted critical methods from pagan scholars. To Augustine, the criteria used by physicians regarding Hippocratic texts seemed paradigmatic: "Have not certain writings published as belonging to the most renowned physician Hippocrates failed to be acknowledged by the physicians?" A certain similarity of context and words did not suffice unless they could stand comparison with works well established as Hippocratic, and unless the precedent for considering them to be Hippocratic dated from the time of the established works.

---

18. Quintilian (577), *Institutio oratorica* 3.6.64; 1:441. Quintilian cites Cicero as another example of an author who did not hesitate to condemn what he had published previously.

19. Plutarch (562), *Quomodo quis suos in virtute sentiat profectus* 82D–E; 1:438–40. Babbit (562), p. 438, note b, refers to Celsus, Quintilian, and Julian, and I have not been able to add further testimonies. The renown of Quintilian and Plutarch assured that the story would be well known.

20. Julian (353), *Epistulae* 50; 3:163–64 (Wright's translation).

But where does the certainty come from that those books are by Hippocrates by comparison with which the irregularly published are rejected? Where—and if somebody denies it he is not only refuted but also laughed at—if not because from the very time of Hippocrates until the present, the continuous chain of succession has wanted it so, so that henceforth doubt is the mark of a fool.[21]

This is not without significance for Augustine's interest in Hippocrates.[22] It also helps to understand some of the eagerness with which commentators have searched for Plato's method in the Hippocratic books as a guarantee of their genuineness.

Modern scholarship is more skeptical than that of the ancients, and modern doubt extends to two of the most important works of the Collection: the oath, and *Aphorisms*. Scribonius Largus is the first extant ancient author to mention the oath, and he obviously counted on its being well known. According to him, "Hippocrates, the founder of our profession," placed the oath at the beginning of medical education, and by prohibiting abortion, he early turned the minds of his pupils toward humaneness (*ad humanitatem*). Taught to consider it wicked to harm a potential human life, a physician would judge injuring a fully developed one to be all the more criminal. "Thus he valued it highly that whoever conducted himself according to his principle with a devoted and consecrated heart[23] would preserve the reputation and dignity of medicine, for medicine is the science of healing, not of doing harm."[24]

About half a century later, Soranus, a Methodist, reported the existence of two factions regarding the use of abortives. One allowed abortion, but only if it was to avert harm to the mother. The other faction "banishes abortives, citing the testimony of Hippocrates who

21. Augustine (61), *Contra Faustum* 33.6; pp. 791–92. Speyer (641), pp. 126 and 189–90, suggested that Augustine had in mind Galen's rejection of *De glandulis;* see Galen (241), *De articulis commentarius* 1.45; 18A: 379.

22. However, Augustine's interest in criticism did not prevent him from relating the story of a woman to be punished for adultery because she had given birth to a beautiful boy who resembled neither of his parents nor his family. Hippocrates suggested that a picture resembling the child be looked for in the bedroom. The picture was found and the woman freed from suspicion. Augustine asserted that the story "is handed down and found written in the books of the very ancient and experienced physician Hippocrates" (Augustine [63], *Quaestiones in Heptateuchum* 1.93; p. 35, ll. 1159–64; I owe the reference to the editors of the *Reallexikon für Antike und Christentum*). The extant works of Hippocrates do not contain the story.

23. *Pio sanctoque animo.* This probably is a vision of the oath's ἀγνῶς δὲ καὶ ὁσίως; cf. above, chap. 3, n. 26.

24. Scribonius Largus (614), *Compositiones,* epistula dedicatoria, art. 5: pp. 2(l. 20)–3(l. 2).

says, 'I will give to no one an abortive';[25] moreover, because it is the specific task of medicine to guard and preserve what has been engendered by nature." [26]

Aphorisms provided ready proof that Hippocrates, the courageous and humane doctor for whom medicine was the guardian of life, was also a wise man. This collection of pithy diagnostic, prognostic, and therapeutic pronouncements, whose truth was little doubted, aroused great admiration for its reputed author. A very late commentator listed the names of the most eminent doctors of the first and second centuries (including Galen) as being among those who had declared it genuine and had used it to gauge the authenticity of the other writings. "Besides, the form of presentation, the sagacity of the contents, and the attractive style prove that it is a work of the lofty mind of Hippocrates." [27]

Nowhere was such loftiness more evident than in the first words of the first aphorism, "Life is short, but the art is long," which have become an epigram of enduring vitality. It is now best known in the Latin version, *Vita brevis ars longa*, and through the exclamation in Goethe's *Faust*, "Ach Gott! die Kunst ist lang, und kurz ist unser Leben." In Antiquity, this apophthegm placed Hippocrates in the company of outstanding philosophers, and its relevance was thought to extend far beyond the medical art.[28] "The greatest of physicians," Seneca thought, was voicing most people's complaint about the short life nature had given them.[29] Other philosophers accentuated the length of the art. Zeno of Citium, the founder of the Stoic school, substituted philosophy for medicine:[30] "There is nothing of which we are in greater need than time. For indeed, life is short, but the art is long, especially that capable of healing the diseases of the soul." [31] Similarly, in one of Lucian's satires, an idealized philosopher quoted the saying of "the Coan physician" and insisted that philosophy, because it needed intensive and constant effort, was much more difficult to learn than medicine.[32]

Philo's manner of quoting the apophthegm again confirms how ir-

25. See Edelstein (198), p. 5, l. 15, and p. 6, for the text and translation of the oath.

26. Soranus (637), *Gynecology* 1.19; p. 53. See also Temkin (671), p. 3.

27. Stephanus (646), *Commentary on Hippocrates' Aphorisms*, preface; p. 30, ll. 14–16 (Westerink's translation, modified).

28. Nachmanson (476), lists more references than are cited in the following.

29. Seneca (616), *De brevitate vitae* 1.1; 2:286.

30. But did Zeno substitute philosophy for medicine, or was it the other way around, and had *Aphorisms* borrowed the apophthegm from philosophy?

31. Arnim (50), frag. 323; 1:70. Cf. Nachmanson (476), p. 95.

32. Lucian (432), *Hermotimus* 1; 6:261.

relevant the omission of Hippocrates' name may be. Philo reminds his readers of the time consumed in caring for riches and possessions, and observes that "it is well to be sparing of time, seeing that according to the physician Hippocrates life is short but the art is long." [33] In context, this is an admonition not to waste time on inessentials. When Philo quotes this saying again, this time attributing it to "somebody," he suggests that the magnitude of the art "is best understood by him who immerses himself deeply in it and digs it like a well." [34] The art of which Philo speaks is philosophical study, especially such as he observed among the Therapeutae, the Jewish sect who, dedicated to the contemplative life, interpreted Biblical texts allegorically[35] and thus gained insight into the nature of all things.[36] Philo was an orthodox Jew, but he was also strongly influenced by Stoicism, and what he said about the first aphorism was in harmony with Zeno's remarks.

Other aphorisms besides the first also lent themselves to allegorical use, as we learn from the anonymous preface to a collection of "Problems" of late but unspecified date.[37] The aphorisms are allowed three levels of meaning. Each aphorism has a precise, limited significance, and when taken all together, the aphorisms form a system of medicine wherein one aphorism supports the other.[38] But the extraordinary thing about Hippocrates is that his aphorisms

> are adapted not only to medicine but to all life in general. For they are universal laws foretelling and regulating events. Thus when Hippocrates says, "In athletes, a good [bodily] condition if at its summit is

33. Philo (541), *De vita contemplativa* 2.16; 9:122. According to Clement of Alexandria (151), *Stromata* 5.4; col. 41A, the apophthegms "of those who are called wise among the Greeks [i.e., the pagans]" indicate the significance of an important matter in a few words. "An obvious example [Clement says] is 'be sparing of time [χρόνου φείδου]' either because life is short and one must not spend this time vainly," or, on the contrary, because one must economize with one's private means so that one may not lack the necessities even if one lived many years. Cf. Nachmanson (476), p. 95, on the provenance of the expression.

34. Philo (541), *De somniis* 1.10; 5:298–300. Cf. Nachmanson (476), p. 94, n. 3, for the irrelevance of the omitted name.

35. Philo (541), *De vita contemplativa* 3.28; 9:128, and passim.

36. Ibid. 90; 9:168, says of the Therapeutae that they embrace a view "of nature and what is in it." I believe that this is Philo's translation into Stoic language of an allegorical Biblical interpretation of the world. See idem 2; p. 114, l. 9: ἐκ φύσεως καὶ τῶν ἱερῶν νόμων; and idem 70; p. 156, where the ownership of slaves is called "contrary to nature [παρὰ φύσιν]."

37. The Greek text of the preface has been reedited, translated into German, and interpreted by Flashar (227); I follow Flashar's edition of this difficult and often corrupt text.

38. Flashar (227), p. 405, ll. 22–28.

treacherous,"³⁹ and "All excess is hostile to nature,"⁴⁰ and "Sleep and wakefulness beyond measure are bad,"⁴¹ he gives us as a universal rule and law that in everything due measure is best. Again, [when he says,] "The more you nourish bodies that are not free from impurities, the more you harm [them],"⁴² this can also be transferred to the soul. For the divine Plato said, "The more you educate the souls that are not pure the more you harm them, since in the incorporeal soul education is the incorporeal nourishment."⁴³

Plato did not say this, at least not in these words.⁴⁴ But the comparison with Plato helped to enhance the stature of Hippocrates, for whom the anonymous author was full of enthusiasm. Hippocrates the Asclepiad, he explained, united medicine, which up till then had been floundering, into a complete and perfect whole by putting a head on it.⁴⁵ "And nobody is likely to err who says that the provident god, taking pity on mankind, which was being destroyed by successive diseases,⁴⁶ made nature herself into flesh⁴⁷ and led Hippocrates to the perfect transmission of this [art]."⁴⁸ As the editor remarks, "incarnation" suggests Christian terminology,⁴⁹ so that Christian influences or even authorship cannot be excluded and the date of the preface must be correspondingly late.⁵⁰ Christian influence is all the more likely because of the parallel between God's merciful mission in incarnating nature and His sending Jesus, "the word made flesh" (John 1:14).⁵¹

39. Hippocrates (302), *Aphorisms* 1.3; 4:98. For the citation of this aphorism by Plutarch and Olympiodorus, see Nachmanson (476), p. 98.
40. Hippocrates (302), *Aphorisms* 2.51; 4:120. I follow Jones in translating τὸ πολύ by "excess."
41. Ibid. 2.3; 4:108.
42. Ibid. 2.10; 4:110. For the citation of this aphorism by Olympiodorus and Elias, see Nachmanson (476), pp. 101–3.
43. Flashar (227), p. 405, ll. 18–22.
44. As Flashar (227), p. 405, n. 7, remarks, this alleged quotation cannot be found in Plato. However, Olympiodorus (502), p. 10, ll. 5–8, relates the aphorism to Plato's [552], *Phaedo* 67B; pp. 232–33) "For it cannot be that the impure attain the pure" (Fowler's translation).
45. Flashar (227), p. 404, l. 5: κεφαλὴν ἐπιΘείς, which may refer to *Aphorisms*.
46. This may refer to the Hippocratic *Epidemics* or to the plague (see below, chap. 6).
47. Flashar (227), p. 404, ll. 6–7: αὐτὴν τὴν φύσιν σαρκώσας.
48. Ibid. p. 404, ll. 5–7.
49. Ibid. p. 406, n. 1, and p. 417.
50. On the question of dating, see Flashar (227), pp. 412–15.
51. See also below, Epilogue, text to n. 12.

5

GALEN'S IDEAL
PHILOSOPHER

Galen was a severe moral critic of his contemporaries in general and of most of his fellow physicians in particular. According to him, the age was poor in great men. "It stands to reason that because of the wretched food which people nowadays consume, and because wealth is more valued than virtue, there is nobody any more like Phidias among sculptors, Apelles among painters, and Hippocrates among physicians."[1]

The coupling of right diet and virtue was an essential part of Galenic philosophy. Proper regimen balanced the temperament of the body and its parts, and with them the psychic functions. Correct and incorrect diet could determine health and disease, and because it was under human control, the choice of diet gave a moral dimension to health and sickness.[2] Correct diet and a life of virtue were preconditions for the search for truth[3] and for excellence as physician and philosopher. Hippocrates served as the model. His moral virtue shone forth in his disrespect for Artaxerxes, the king of Persia, in his preference for treating the poor of various small cities rather than taking up residence at the court of Perdiccas, the king of Macedon, and in his delegating the care

---

1. Galen (242), *Quod optimus medicus sit quoque philosophus* 2; 2:4, ll. 3–7.
2. See above, chap. 2.
3. See Temkin (667), pp. 36–38.

of his fellow citizens of Cos to Polybus and to his other pupils while himself traveling about Greece to gather experience.[4]

Whoever wished to emulate Hippocrates must not only despise money; he must also be extremely industrious, and therefore must avoid drunkenness, gluttony, and lechery. "The true physician will prove to be a friend of moderation and a comrade of truth."[5] He must practice the logical method, in order to identify diseases according to their species and genera and hence to determine the therapeutic indications. Also he must know the nature of the body, with respect to its elements, its tissues,[6] and its organs, and the use and activity of each. This knowledge must rely on proof so that it can be taught by the logical method.[7]

"What then is lacking," Galen asks, "that the physician who practices the art in a manner worthy of Hippocrates be a philosopher?"[8] The unspoken answer to this rhetorical question obviously is: nothing. Since skill in the logical method is a prerequisite for such a physician, and since for the steadfast pursuit of his objectives a contempt for money and the cultivation of moderation are indispensible, "all the parts of philosophy will already be in his possession: logic, natural philosophy, and ethics."[9] No fear then that such a man will do any wrong! "For whatever people dare to do wrongfully, they do when love of money seduces [them] or pleasure beguiles [them]."[10]

Galen did not look at medicine and philosophy as two fundamentally independent disciplines that might profitably be allied. A healthy regimen was a moral duty for all, and a physician could not be great without becoming a philosopher. Being a philosopher did not mean finding fulfillment in a contemplative life, which Galen held in low esteem.[11] Ethics, in particular, was not mere speculation about virtue, but virtue lived. A great physician was a philosopher because he was skilled in logic, he engaged in scientific research, and he lived virtuously. He

4. Galen (242), *Quod optimus medicus* 3; 2:5(l. 6)–6(l. 4). For Hippocrates' relations with Artaxerxes and Perdiccas, see below, chap. 6. For Polybus as the alleged son-in-law of Hippocrates, see Hippocrates (309), Pseudepigrapha 27; 9:420.

5. Galen (242), *Quod optimus medicus* 3; 2:6, ll. 4–9.

6. What I here anachronistically call tissues, Galen called "similar parts" (ὁμοιομερῆ, also ἁπλᾶ, or πρῶτα); see Temkin (667), pp. 12–13.

7. Galen (242), *Quod optimus medicus* 3; p. 6, ll. 10–22. This is, of course, essentially a summary of Galen's teaching, but since he claimed to follow the method of Hippocrates, its seeds were imputed to Hippocrates. For a description of Galen's method, for which geometry was the main model, see Temkin (667), p. 28–30.

8. Galen (242), *Quod optimus medicus* 3; pp. 6(l. 23)–7(l. 2).

9. Ibid.; p. 7, ll. 6–8.

10. Ibid.; p. 7, ll. 10–12.

11. See Temkin (667), pp. 45–46.

possessed all three parts of philosophy by practicing them, and he practiced medicine for the love of man (philanthropy), itself a moral motive.[12]

It is not possible to tell to what degree Hippocrates shaped Galen's medical and scientific ideas, to what degree Hippocrates gave Galen authoritative support for his own ideas, and to what degree the two influences were intertwined in Galen's development. Whatever Galen's relationship to Hippocrates may have been, it does not follow that his analysis of Hippocratic methods and principles was not based on the desire to find truth objectively.[13] Galen's undeniable idealization of Hippocrates[14] does not negate his scientific dedication, but the latter does not suffice to explain the idealization. For example, in proving that the hand was built in the best thinkable way, Galen quoted the Hippocratic statements about fingernails and the advantage of having widely interspaced fingers and a thumb opposing the index finger.[15] But to introduce this with the words "And now again let us begin with the words of Hippocrates as with a voice from a god"[16] exceeds the usual tribute paid by a scientist to a great predecessor.

Natural philosophy and ethics were integral parts of Galen's philosophy, and his idealization of Hippocrates correspondingly rested not solely on his views of the latter's medical and scientific works but also on his views of the man. Works such as *Epidemics* and *On Airs, Waters, Localities,* which revealed their author as a traveler studying disease in individuals, many of low social status, and among many peoples, could impress Galen as Hippocratic philanthropy. But in mentioning Polybus as Hippocrates' son-in-law,[17] as well as recounting Hippocrates' disrespect for Artaxerxes and his refusal to settle at the court of Perdiccas, Galen drew on the legendary tradition. In whole or in part, taken as a "historically reliable source,"[18] the tradition furnished biographical details; even more than the works, it made the moral character and the

12. Galen (248), *De placitis Hippocratis et Platonis* 9.5.6; 2:565, ll. 26–30.

13. See Harig and Kollesch (286), pp. 257–74.

14. Deichgräber (165), p. 23: "Für [Galen] ist Hippocrates das menschgewordene Ideal seiner philosophischen und medizinischen Überzeugungen."

15. See Hippocrates (302), *In the Surgery* 4; 3:62–63. I am paraphrasing E. T. Withington's translation.

16. Galen (244), *De usu partium* 1.9; 1:16, ll. 1–3.

17. See above, n. 4.

18. Deichgräber (167), p. 90. Diller (178), pp. 14–15, emphasized the influence of the legend on Galen's notion of Hippocrates. According to Smith (629), p. 222, "After Erotian the pseudepigrapha were in the [Hippocratic] tradition but accorded only selective credence such as turns up in conjectures about authorship of the Corpus and in Galen's use of Hippocrates as the ideally unselfish doctor, and also . . . Hippocrates' apostleship to Democritus which Celsus repeats."

exalted nature of Hippocrates shine forth with a strong light.

Galen certainly was not the first or the only learned author on whom the legend exerted its influence. It can be traced in the works of Celsus[19] and Pliny,[20] and if it is true, as Galen maintained, that the mass of physicians in his day "praise[d] Hippocrates and deem[ed] him the foremost of all," [21] the admiration may well have been enhanced by the legendary reputation of the man. Legends rarely form around nonentities, but as they sprout and grow they create a predisposition to find greatness in their hero's words and deeds. It may well be asked whether Celsus, Quintilian, Plutarch, and Julian would have been quite as strongly impressed by Hippocrates' admission of a mistake had they not been convinced that they were dealing with a great man,[22] and whether *Aphorisms,* known under another author's name, would have been labeled a work "transcending human intelligence." [23]

Various factors may have contributed to Galen's idealization of Hippocrates,[24] the archaizing tendency of the second century among them, although this descriptive designation is of limited explanatory value. Whatever other influences there were, the legend—as a predisposing factor, and as an early imprint—helps us to understand Galen's preoccupation with Hippocrates in subjects where, otherwise, purely historical interest would have to be invoked.[25] It also explains the discrepancy between Galen's exhortation to study the works of the ancients critically,[26] and his lack of substantive criticism regarding Hippocrates. Failure to imitate Hippocrates thus appeared as a severe fault, for which he could blame his contemporaries,[27] whereas following Hippocrates and bringing his work to perfection became a feat on which he, Galen, might well pride himself.

19. See above, chap. 4, n. 13.

20. Pliny (556), *Natural History* 7.37.123; 2:588.

21. Galen (242), *Quod optimus medicus* 1; 2:1, ll. 4–5.

22. See above, chap. 4

23. Souda (653), 2:663, l. 2.

24. See Harig and Kollesch (286), pp. 257–58 and 273–74.

25. According to ibid., p. 261, Hippocratic anatomy was of mere historical value to Galen.

26. Galen (249), *On the Natural Faculties* 3.10; p. 278.

27. Ibid.; and Galen (242), *Quod optimus medicus* 1; 2:1, ll. 4–7.

6

THE LEGEND

The word "legend" has been defined as "a story coming down from the past; especially one popularly regarded as historical although not verifiable."[1] Stories, mingling possible truth with outright fiction, began to form around Hippocrates no later than the third century B.C.[2] By the first or the second century of the Christian era, they had been given literary form in two Greek works that have come down to us: the Pseudepigrapha, which deal with Hippocrates in a novelistic fashion, and a biography. The biography and the Pseudepigrapha, supplemented by comments made by authors such as Varro, Celsus, Pliny, and Galen, provide an approximate idea of how the life and personality of Hippocrates were seen in the second century.[3] There exists other biograph-

1. *Webster's New Collegiate Dictionary* (711).
2. In Soranus's (636) biography, p. 175, l. 6, Pherecydes (fifth century B.C.) and Eratosthenes (third century B.C.) head the list of those who recounted Hippocrates' genealogy. Müri (474), p. 465, thinks it likely that Eratosthenes transmitted what Pherecydes might have had to say in connection with Asclepius and his progeny.
3. The article "Hippokrates von Kos" by Edelstein (200) is still fundamental for the analysis of the Hippocratic legendary material. H. De Ley, "De Samenstelling van de pseudo-Hippokretsche Brievenversameling en haar plaats en de tradite," *Handelingen der Züidernederlandse Maatschapping vor Tael- en Letterkunde en Geschiedenis* 23 (1969): 47–80, was not available to me. For the historical significance of the legendary material, see Smith (629), pp. 215–22; Pigeaud (546), pp. 452–53; and Gourevitch (267), p. 323.

ical material, which reveals different traditions,[4] but since this latter material is of a later date, it is indicative of the Christian survival of Hippocrates' fame rather than of his significance for the pagan world of the second century.

A. The *Vita*

Family and Life of Hippocrates according to Soranus was the title given to the biography (the *Vita*).[5] Whether this Soranus was identical with Soranus of Ephesus, the famous Methodist, or whether he was an otherwise unknown Soranus of Cos, mentioned in the *Vita*, is a moot question.[6] According to the *Vita*, Hippocrates was the son of Heracleides and of Phaenarete and traced his descent back to Asclepius and to Hercules.[7] Several scholars (cited by name, beginning with the famous Alexandrian scholar Eratosthenes of the third century B.C.) occupied themselves with his genealogy. His teachers were his father, then Herodicus, and also, according to some people, the orator Gorgias and the philosopher Democritus.[8]

This genealogy connected Hippocrates with dietetic medicine (via Herodicus), explained (via Gorgias), his style, which was sufficiently well known to allow Epictetus to allude to it,[9] and associated him with Democritus. It also substantiated the notion that Hippocrates was "trained in medicine and the general studies,"[10] that is, that he had received a medical as well as a liberal education. Hippocrates

> flourished at the time of the Peloponnesian war, having been born in the first year of the eightieth Olympiad[11] as Ischomachus . . . says, and as Soranus the Coan, who examined the archives in Cos, adds, during the rule of Abrias, on the twenty-seventh of the month Agrianus. There-

4. See below, chap. 18.
5. In the following notes, the Greek text of the *Vita* will be cited after Ilberg's edition of Soranus (636), pp. 175–78. A good German translation of the *Vita* can be found in Müri (474), pp. 45–51. The Greek text of items 1–24 of the Pseudepigrapha (hereafter abbreviated Pseudep.) will be cited after Putzger's (307) edition (hereafter P.), the remaining items (25–27) after Littré's ([309], 9:400–429) edition (hereafter L.) of the Hippocratic works.
6. I do not think that postulating the existence of a third, otherwise unknown, Soranus would be helpful.
7. *Vita*, p. 175, l. 3.
8. Ibid., p. 175, ll. 5–9.
9. Epictetus (206), *Discourses* 1.8.11–12; 1:62. However, *Vita*, p. 177, ll. 15–16, refers to obscurities in his language.
10. *Vita*, p. 175, ll. 15–16.
11. I.e., 460 B.C.

fore, [Soranus] says, until the present time the Coans bring offerings to Hippocrates[12] on that day.[13]

The citing of sources and the claim to research in the archives of Cos lent a note of credibility to the *Vita,* and 460 B.C. has remained a likely year for the birth of Hippocrates.[14]

After his parents' death, Hippocrates

> left his fatherland because, as Andreas in *On Medical Genealogy* maliciously says, he had burned the archives in Cnidos. However, as others say, [it was] because of his resolve to see the accomplishments in [other] places and to acquire a more varied training.[15] But as Soranus of Cos narrates, he had a dream commanding him to settle in the country of the Thessalians.[16]

The hypothesis that Hippocrates left Cos in search of knowledge and self-improvement was consistent with his authorship of such works as *Epidemics* and *On Airs, Waters, Localities* and would, moreover, not exclude his later return to Cos. In the Pseudepigrapha, Hippocrates, now a famous physician, was a highly esteemed citizen of his native Cos, whom his fellow citizens refused to extradite to the king of Persia.[17]

The *Vita* said nothing of any return and asserted that Hippocrates had died in Larissa (a city in Thessaly) and that his tombstone was still being pointed out between Larissa and nearby Gyrton; for a long time, the *Vita* added, bees used to produce a honey there which nurses applied at the grave in order to heal little children quickly of small ulcers in their mouths (aphthae)[18] Obviously, there was no consensus about the course of Hippocrates' life, just as there was none about the number of years he reached: eighty-five, ninety, one hundred, and one hundred and four were reported, and it was also said that he died at the same time as Democritus[19]—whose life-span is equally uncertain.

12. *Vita,* p. 175, ll. 14–15: ἐναγίζειν ἐν αὐτῇ μέχρι νῦν Ἱπποκράτει φησὶ τοὺς Κῴους. Offerings on the birthday of a great man were nothing extraordinary; see Rohde (589), 1:231–43, especially p. 235, n. 1.

13. *Vita,* p. 175, ll. 9–15. None of these men is known otherwise.

14. See Deichgräber (164), p. 148.

15. This agrees with Galen's version; see above, chap. 5, text to n. 4.

16. *Vita,* pp. 175(l. 16)–76(l. 3). Müri (474), p. 465, and Grensemann (277), p. 4, identify Andreas with the body physician of Ptolemy IV, which places him in the third century B.C.

17. Pseudep. 8 and 9 obviously presuppose that Hippocrates, very famous, was residing in Cos; cf. below, text to n. 53.

18. *Vita,* p. 177, ll. 8–10.

19. Ibid., p. 177, ll. 4–7.

Soranus's belief that a dream directed Hippocrates to Thessaly seems to have been inspired by the existence of the tombstone. The hypothesis that Hippocrates was an arsonist, on the other hand, connected him with other rumors, not all of them flattering. The story of his burning the archives of Cnidos may have been associated with an alleged early rivalry between the Cnidian Asclepiads and those of Cos, though Galen denied that the rivalry was evil.[20] According to others, however,[21] Hippocrates burned the old medical books and the library of Cos, a more likely motive for leaving the island. Moreover, the latter story associated Hippocrates with the temple of Asclepius in Cos and with its inscriptions, which told of the help sick people had received from the god. Hippocrates allegedly copied these inscriptions to benefit from them in similar cases[22] and, Varro believed, he "established so-called bedside medicine after the temple had been burnt" (or "after he had burned the temple," as the clause also has been rendered, and as it probably was to be understood).[23] The existence of a temple of Asclepius in Cos by the mid–fifth century B.C. is highly questionable.[24] But the fable of the development of clinical medicine from temple medicine survived and has not yet been put to eternal rest.

The *Vita* named Hippocrates' two sons, Thessalus and Dracon, who were the most brilliant of his pupils.[25] It does not name his other pupils, but it says that he "ungrudgingly taught the art to suitable people, [combining it] with the appropriate oath."[26] The oath was the only work of Hippocrates to which the *Vita* referred. Concerning the genuineness of his works in general, it contended that the wide variations in the opinions of the works making up the Collection made any pronouncement difficult. The obstacles were "first, [doubtful] ascription; second, ability to keep an eye on the individual style; third, [the fact]

20. Galen (241), *Methodus medendi* 1.1; 10:5. See also Grensemann (277), pp. 2–3.

21. Tzetzes (695), *Historiae* 7.155.955–57; p. 293. Cf. Edelstein (200), col. 1292.

22. Strabo (650), *Geography* 14.2.19; 6:288; also Pliny (556), *Natural History* 29.2; 8:184.

23. Pliny (556), *Natural History,* 29.2; 8:184: "atque ut Varro apud nos credit, templo cremato instituisse medicinam hanc quae clinica vocatur." W. H. S. Jones ([556], p. 185) translates "after the temple had been burnt," which leaves the cause of the fire open. Grensemann (277), p. 4, calls this "the understandable and probably the original version"; Edelstein (200), cols. 1302–3, suggests that the purpose of the story was to associate Hippocrates with the temple, and that by making him the arsonist, it also explained the lack of early records. On the rivalry between Cos and Cnidos in the Pseudepigrapha, cf. Sakalis (599).

24. See Sherwin-White (621), p. 341.

25. *Vita,* p. 178, ll. 4–5.

26. Ibid., p. 177, ll. 3–4.

that one and the same person at one period writes more powerfully and at another, with less vigor, because of his age. Other causes can also be named."[27]

Here skepticism regarding the possibility of identifying the true works of Hippocrates is combined with indifference about the character of Hippocratic medicine. It is hard to decide whether the difficulty of choosing among the purported works was the real reason for not mentioning titles[28] and discussing contents, or whether a lack of interest caused the existing uncertainty to be used as an excuse for not acquainting the reader with the kind of medicine Hippocrates taught. This indifference stands out if compared with the pains taken over the biographical data and the zest with which the Vita reported Hippocrates' exploits, beginning with his curing King Perdiccas of Macedon of lovesickness.[29]

The story is essentially another version of the one told about Erasistratus, though now it is a king who pines for his late father's concubine.[30] It seems that the author of the Vita felt that Hippocrates too should be credited with this kind of impressive feat,[31] made all the more impressive because, as Soranus tells, he was summoned together with the older Euryphon, a famous Cnidian physician.[32] Hippocrates' superiority over Euryphon may also have been an allusion to the rivalry between Cos and Cnidos.

The invitation to take a position at the court of Perdiccas had come when all of Greece resounded with admiration for the healer Hippocrates. The Vita has more stories to tell. The people of Abdera asked him to cure their fellow citizen Democritus, whom they believed to be insane, and to free their city from the plague. When a pestilence reached the barbarian countries of Illyria and Paeonia,[33] their kings summoned Hippocrates, but he did not accept. Instead, he extracted information from the envoys about the winds that predominated in their region.

27. Ibid., p. 177, ll. 19–25.
28. In contrast, the late Latin fragmentary biography did provide lists of titles; see below chap. 18, n. 9.
29. Vita, pp. 176(l. 4)–77(l. 4).
30. Cf. above, chap. 2. The various stories have been discussed by Amundsen (20), pp. 323–25. Mesulam and Perry (454) analyze the stories, including the one told by Galen (250), On Prognosis 6.2–10; pp. 100–2, from his own practice. Cf. also Grensemann (277), p. 5.
31. For the transfer of the story from other versions to the one involving Hippocrates, cf. Edelstein (200), cols. 1296–97.
32. Vita, p. 176, ll. 6–7.
33. Albania and southern Yugoslavia. The Vita, p. 176, l. 14, only speaks of "a pestilence [λοιμοῦ κατασκήψαντος]," which does not point to any specific epidemic.

This enabled him to predict the coming of the plague to Attica, and its consequences, and to take charge of the various cities,[34] which, as the Pseudepigrapha made clear, were Greek cities, which Hippocrates was able to protect by means of written prescriptions or by sending his pupils to them, while he himself went to Athens and told its people what to do.[35]

"So fond of the Greeks was he that dignity, lack of avarice and love for home made him reject" a splendid offer from Artaxerxes to go to the Persian court, "as is also shown by [his] letter to him." [36] This letter and other pertinent correspondence form part of the Pseudepigrapha, as do the stories of Hippocrates' saving his native Cos from the Athenians by appealing for help to the Thessalians, and of the honors paid him by the Athenians. The *Vita* also mentions the latter, together with honors conferred by the Coans, the Thessalians, and the Argives.[37]

Both the *Vita* and the "Decree of the Athenians" (which is part of the Pseudepigrapha) merely speak of "a pestilence [λοιμός]"—from which, moreover, the Greek cities had been saved. Attempts to relate this example of patriotism and medical sagacity to any historical epidemic are not promising.[38]

The *Vita*'s interest in Hippocrates' personality extended to the interpretation of his portraits.[39] Why, it asks, do most of them depict him with his head covered? It reports no fewer than eight answers: According to some people, his head is covered by a felt hat as a sign of noble birth. According to others, his head is covered by his cloak:[40] for the sake of comeliness, for he was bald; because of the frailty of the head; to emphasize the need for guarding the seat of reason; as a symbol of his fondness for travel; as a symbol of the obscurity occurring in his writings; to emphasize the need for protecting oneself from harmful things even when healthy. According to still others, he threw the loose parts of his cloak[41] over his head in order to have his hands free when operating.[42]

34. *Vita*, p. 176, ll. 11–18.
35. Pseudep. (L.) 27; 9:418(l. 2)–20(l. 10).
36. *Vita*, p. 176, ll. 18–23.
37. Ibid., pp. 176(l. 23)–77(l. 3).
38. See above, n. 33; and Pseudep. (L.), 9:400, l. 18. For a discussion of the question, see Pinault (548), pp. 61–68.
39. *Vita*, p. 177, ll. 10–19.
40. Apparently the author of the *Vita* had seen none, or at least not all, of the portraits.
41. According to the Latin fragment, Schöne (611), p. 58, l. 29, this means the sleeves: *hoc est manicas*.
42. The Souda (653), 2:662, ll. 17–20, adds still another possible reason, "or because this was his custom [*ethos*]."

No esthetic comments accompanied the account of the pictures; not a word was said about whether they were true likenesses of Hippocrates, whether they all showed the same physiognomy, or even whether they portrayed him bearded or clean-shaven. The headgear and what the artists wished to convey by it was all that mattered. Yet the very number of interpretations discloses that a lively interest in Hippocrates existed on the part of a public less interested in medical writings and theories than in the life of a great man:[43] a Greek patriot who had become a hero to whom offerings were brought, and whose grave was a place of miraculous healing.

B. The Pseudepigrapha

The Hippocratic corpus contains a collection of twenty-seven pieces, of which twenty-four are letters, two are speeches, and one is an official Athenian decree.[44] The collection has been dubbed the Pseudepigrapha, indicating that the pieces are now believed to be "falsely inscribed." Indeed, the whole reads like a somewhat disjointed novel. In Antiquity, however, it was considered to be not a piece of fiction but a collection of documents of historical value.[45] The pieces deal with three main themes, also touched upon in the *Vita:* the invitation by King Artaxerxes (letters 1–9); the invitation from the Abderites, leading to the meeting with Democritus (letters 10–23);[46] and the fate of Cos as related to Hippocrates and his family. The "decree of the Athenians" praises Hippocrates as a Greek patriot and a deliverer from the plague, and thus supplements the first theme.

1. The Patriot

A devastating pestilence in the Persian army causes King Artaxerxes to write to a certain physician, Paetus,[47] urgently asking him for appropriate remedies or a message from "another physician"[48] capable of effecting a cure. "Without [our] waging war, war is waged against us,"[49] says the despairing king; the enemy is like a wild beast destroying the flock. Paetus's reply is glowing in its praise of Hippocrates, whom,

43. See Edelstein (200), col. 1294.
44. See above, n. 5
45. Cf. above, chap. 5, n. 18.
46. Regarding the disposition of these letters, see Temkin (670), especially pp. 455 and pp. 462–63, nn. 3 and 4.
47. On Paetus (Παῖτος), see Kudlien (394); also Sakalis (599), p. 503, n. 23, and pp. 504–5, who believes that the name was Petos (Πέτος) and not Παῖτος.
48. Pseudep. (P.) 1; p. 1, l. 5. Paetus obviously was a physician.
49. Ibid.; p. 1, l. 7.

he suggests, the king should ask to come.[50] Thereupon the King, in a letter to Hystanes, his satrap of the Hellespont, expresses the wish to have Hippocrates in his service, promising all the gold he might want, anything he might need, and honor equal to that of the foremost Persians.[51] After the King's wish has been duly transmitted to him, Hippocrates sends the following reply:

> Hippocrates the physician to Hystanes, governor of the Hellespont: Greetings. Regarding the letter you sent me saying that it came from the King, convey to the King what I say and write to him as quickly as possible that we enjoy food, garments, housing, and everything essential for life. I have no right to share the wealth of the Persians or to liberate from disease barbarians who are the enemies of the Greeks. Fare thee well.[52]

The King feels insulted and with dire threats demands that the Coans extradite Hippocrates. They, however, refuse.[53]

Elsewhere in the letters, Hippocrates boasts that his refusal to free the enemy from an evil disease was equal to victory in a sea battle.[54] But in the letters as in the *Vita*, Hippocrates' Panhellenism is combined with his local patriotism. The *Vita*, relates that Hippocrates urged the Thessalians to come to the help of Cos when the Athenians were about to wage war against his native city. The Pseudepigrapha contains the speech, and supplements it with an address by Hippocrates' son Thessalus, who was sent to Athens to dissuade the Athenians from their undertaking.[55]

The *Vita* also mentions the honors Hippocrates received from the Athenians.[56] The alleged Athenian decree[57] included in the Pseudepigrapha cites the help he had provided during the advancing plague by sending out his pupils and prescribing the measures by which the plague could be stopped. It also mentions his merits as a physician and a teacher, and it praises his patriotism in refusing the invitation of the king of Persia. To acknowledge and to reward the services Hippocrates

50. This letter will be discussed below, in section C of this chapter.
51. Pseudep. 3.
52. Pseudep. (P) 5; p. 3.
53. Pseudep. 8 and 9.
54. Pseudep. (P.) 11; p. 7, ll. 5–6.
55. *Vita*, p. 176, ll. 22–24; and Pseudep. 26 and 27.
56. *Vita*, p. 177, ll. 1–3
57. Pseudep. (L) 25; 9:400–403. An English translation of the decree can be found in Henry E. Sigerist's *A History of Medicine*, 2 vols. (New York: Oxford University Press, 1951–61), 2:269–70.

had rendered to Greece, the decree continues, he shall, like Hercules, be initiated into the great mysteries, he shall be crowned with a golden wreath worth a thousand pieces of gold—this to be proclaimed at the gymnastic contests at the great Panathenian festival—and all Coan children shall be admitted to ephebic training in Athens "because their land has produced such a man."[58] Moreover, Hippocrates is to be given citizenship and life-long board in the Prytaneum.[59]

Although there are some differences of content, the *Vita* probably referred to this decree. A statement in the decree adds an appreciation of Hippocrates as an author. In addition to enabling the Greek cities to escape the plague, he showed

> how the medical art of Apollo, passed on to the Greeks, unfalteringly saves the sick among them. And he published what he had ungrudgingly written about medicine in the desire that there be many physicians bringing salvation.[60]

This praise of Hippocrates as an author parallels the *Vita*'s praise of him as "ungrudgingly teaching qualified pupils the art in line with the pertinent oath."[61]

The *Vita* characterized Hippocrates as "honorable, no lover of money, [and] fond of [his] kindred," that is, the Greeks.[62] Panhallenic sentiments grew strong after the Greek cities had lost their political independence, and the expression of such sentiments assigns the *Vita* and the Pseudepigrapha to the Hellenistic period.[63] But the outspoken hostility of these writings to barbarians became politically dangerous when Greece, after the defeat of Macedon, entered the orbit of Rome. Conservative Romans, anxious to protect their ancient customs and simplicity from the sophistication of the Greeklings, the *Graeculi,* also turned against Greek medicine,[64] and Hippocrates' reply to Artaxerxes

58. Pseudep (L) 25; 9:400–403. This award, given to a whole city for the merits of one of its citizens, exemplifies the strong feeling of communal unity. Similarly, the decline of one citizen (Democritus) became the misfortune of his whole city (Abdera); see below, section B.2 of this chapter.

59. *Vita*, p. 177, ll. 2–3.

60. Pseudep. (L.) 25; 9:400, ll. 5–2 up.

61. *Vita*, p. 177, ll. 3–4. "Ungrudgingly [ἀφΘόνως]," i.e., free of envy in view of possible competition.

62. Ibid., p. 176, ll. 21–22: διὰ τὸ σεμνὸν καὶ ἀφιλάργυρον καὶ φιλοίκειον.

63. See Philippson (538) and Edelstein (205), cols. 1300–1305, for the layers of the legend and its far-from-homogeneous character.

64. The antagonism of Cato and other Roman conservatives has been discussed in detail by Gourevitch (267), especially in pt. 2, pp. 289–414. Gourevitch has underlined the distinction between Greek medicine and Greek medicine in Rome.

now took on a sinister significance. According to Plutarch, Cato (the Elder) hated Greek philosophers and suspected the practitioners of medicine in Rome.

> He had heard, it would seem, of Hippocrates' reply when the Great King of Persia consulted him, with the promise of a fee of many talents, namely, that he would never put his skill at the service of Barbarians who were enemies of Greece. He said all Greek physicians had taken a similar oath, and urged his son to beware of them all.[65]

Cato had written a book on the diet he used for himself and his household, which excluded any treatment by starvation. He was one of the many Romans down to the end of Antiquity who published collections of recipes intended to make their fellow citizens independent of the services of physicians.[66]

Varro's insinuation that Hippocrates had burnt the Coan temple of Asclepius to use its inscriptions for establishing his own clinical medicine may have stemmed from the same conservative bent of mind seen in Cato. Cato found a sympathetic successor in Pliny, who elaborated on the Greek doctors' exploitation of the sick, and claimed that their learning was derived from the testing of remedies at the expense of human lives.[67] Some accusations of poisoning also were tinged by Roman xenophobia.[68]

Although the notion that there was a conspiracy of Greek doctors against the barbarians, including the Romans, was unfounded, not all suspicions lacked substance. Individual cases of wrongdoing aside, the Empiricists demanded that therapeutic rules be established by the repeated application of treatments that might have been inspired by dreams or incidental observations.[69] Explaining the words of the first Hippocratic aphorism, "Experiment is perilous,"[70] Galen warned that "in the human body, to try out what has not been tested is not without peril in case a bad experiment leads to the destruction of the whole organism."[71]

---

65. Plutarch (561), *Marcus Cato* 23.3–4; 2:373 (Perrin's translation). Cf. Gourevitch (267), pp. 323–414.

66. See for instance pseudo-Pliny, above, chap. 3, text to n. 22.

67. Pliny (556), *Natural History* 29.18; 8:194.

68. For the doctor as poisoner, see Kudlien (390). Roman xenophobia against doctors and the accusation that they were guilty of poisoning and other crimes are elaborated in great detail by Gourevitch (267) in pt. 2, chaps. 3 and 4, of her work.

69. Galen (242), *De sectis ad introducendos* 2; 3:2–4.

70. The Greek *peira* means both "experiment" and "experience," so that the words can also be translated "experience is treacherous," i.e., unreliable.

71. Galen (241), *In Hippocratis aphorismos* 1; 17B:353(l. 12)–54(l. 4). See Temkin (671), p. 4. Galen's warning is as valid today as it was then.

But even Pliny was not consistent in his condemnation of Greek doctors, and Romans as thoroughly imbued with Greek culture as Cicero did not lose their feeling for national identity and political superiority. Vergil's *Tu regere imperio populos Romane memento*[72] did not exempt the Greeks. Celsus clearly demonstrates that among the Romans, antagonism to Greek medicine was counterbalanced by acceptance, and by admiration for Hippocrates in particular.[73] Celsus admired Hippocrates' great mind, and he as well as Seneca thought that a physician ought to be his patient's friend.[74] The little pharmacological text by Scribonius Largus is best understood as written for laymen, with a preface on the ethics of medicine and the use of drugs intended to dispel Roman fears of poisoning and of physicians' experimenting on the patient:

> A man lawfully bound to medicine by an oath[75] will not give a bad drug even to enemies (though as a soldier and a good citizen he will pursue them by any means when the state [so] demands). For medicine does not evaluate people by [their] fortune or character but promises to bring help to all equally and vows never to harm anybody.[76]

It is in this context that Hippocrates is praised for having educated physicians in humanity.[77] Philanthropy limited only by civic and military obligations was a step above the philanthropy of the *Vita* and of the Pseudepigrapha, which did not extend beyond national boundaries. The stress put on medicine as a philanthropic art and on Hippocrates as a teacher of humanity may well have been intended to meet accusations such as Cato's.

2. The Meeting with Democritus

In the Pseudepigrapha, the correspondence dealing with the invitation by the King of Persia is followed abruptly by correspondence that

72. "You, Roman, remember to rule nations by [your] empire" (*Aeneid* 6.851). This contrasts the Roman's task to the accomplishments of other nations.

73. However, Edelstein (198), pp. 308–9, claimed (with a view to Celsus [137], *De medicina* 1.1; 1: 42) that even Celsus rejected the complicated rules of Greek medicine for healthy people as needless for Romans.

74. Celsus (137), *De medicina*, prooemium, art. 73; 1:40; for Seneca, see below, chap. 16B.

75. *Sacramento medicinae*, probably "by the medical oath," i.e., the Hippocratic oath, with which Scribonius Largus assumed the reader to be acquainted.

76. Scribonius Largus (614), *Compositiones*, epistula dedicatoria, art. 4; p. 2, ll. 13–16. For a summary of Scribonius Largus's ethical principles, see Hamilton (282), p. 212; and below, text following n. 77.

77. Scribonius Largus (614), *Compositiones*, epistula dedicatoria, art. 5; p. 2, ll. 20–23.

begins with an invitation to Hippocrates by the senate and the people
of Abdera to come to Abdera, cure its native son Democritus, and save
the city. The Abderites were the laughing stock of Antiquity; like the
Schildbürger of German folk tales, they had a reputation for doing foolish things. An invitation by the Abderites thus carried the promise of
inherent silliness. Democritus, on the other hand, was the founder (with
Leucippus) of ancient atomism, a believer in a plurality of worlds, and
one of the foremost pre-Socratic philosophers, a man who could more
properly be termed a scientist than could the others. His methods of
research seem to have influenced some Hippocratic writings.[78]

He was reported to have been a teacher of Hippocrates, who was
his contemporary,[79] and Hippocrates was said to have intervened when
an Abderian law threatened to deny burial to the impoverished Democritus.[80] In other stories, Democritus impressed Hippocrates by his
scientific acumen. To the latter's amazement, the philosopher was able
to discern that milk shown to him came from a black goat that was a
primipara. Again, Democritus greeted a girl who was accompanying
Hippocrates with "Hail, maiden!" on one day, but with "Hail,
woman!" on the next day, for he recognized her loss of virginity during
the night.[81] Essentially the same story survived in Cos into the twentieth
century, except that it cast Hippocrates as the man of near-miraculous
perception.[82]

Yet there was also another side to Democritus. He was or was seen
as a forerunner of Cynicism, the philosophy that paired a regard for
virtue with contempt for everything that went beyond the bare necessities of life. "The revolt of the civilized against civilization," it has been
called,[83] and Diogenes of Sinope has become the best-known Cynic. By
Cicero's time, Democritus was referred to as an expert on laughter:[84]
"the sides of Democritus shook with unceasing laughter," wrote Juvenal, and Seneca preferred to laugh about human folly with Democri-

78. See Diller (179), chap. 3.

79. Cf. above, chap. 4, n. 13.

80. Diels (174), Democritus, frag. A14; 2:15. The source is Philo, who, according to Philippson (538), pp. 320–21, introduced Hippocrates into the story because
he was influenced by the Pseudepigrapha. Philo thought that their common interest
in philosophy moved Hippocrates to help Democritus in his financial troubles.

81. Diels (174), Democritus, frag. A1, no. 42; 2:12–13.

82. Meyer-Steineg (459), pp. 4–5. For medieval legends about Hippocrates, see
Wickersheimer (719).

83. I must have read this in one of Ludwig Edelstein's publications but cannot
remember the reference.

84. Cicero (144), *De oratore* 2.58; p. 235. See also Horace (316), *Epistolae*
2.1.194; p. 565: *rideret Democritus*.

tus rather than to weep about it with Heraclitus.[85] Democritus had become the laughing philosopher.

In view of the uncertain chronology, it would be difficult to decide how far the Pseudepigrapha inspired legends and rumors about Democritus and how far they reflected them. At any rate, legends and rumors entered into the Pseudepigrapha, together with a modicum of genuine Democritean opinions, all seen from the perspective of the Abderites.[86] The Abderites offered Hippocrates money and honor, though they were aware that the opportunity to acquire knowledge would count more with him. His power in the city, which was in an upheaval, would be unlimited. In their own name and in that of Greece, of culture, and of the future, they urged him to come to Abdera, bringing the proper remedies, and save Democritus and the city.

This is their description of Democritus's condition:

> He carries on, forgetful of all and foremost of himself, awake day and night, laughing at everything great and small, and counting all of life for nothing. One [person] marries, others trade, make public speeches, assume command, or serve as ambassadors, are voted into office, are sick, wounded, die—but he laughs at it all, at those whom he sees downcast and sullen as well as those full of joy.
>
> He also inquires into and writes about the things in the nether world, and he says that the air is full of images and that he listens attentively to the voices of birds. Moreover, often getting up at night, alone he seems to sing songs softly, and he claims sometimes to go off into infinity and that there are innumerable Democrituses like himself. He lives on, his complexion having deteriorated together with his mind.[87]

The Abderites had an explanation for Democritus's strange behavior: Too much wisdom had made him ill, and it was the uneducated mass of the people, *hoi polloi,* who had been looked down upon as fools, who had retained their common sense and realized that the sage had become sick. This hints that there was an element of social strife over the condition of their famous citizen and that this strife was responsible for the turmoil of the city. *Hoi polloi* prevailed: Hippocrates was invited.

This example of genius judged and misunderstood by the incompetent has given this section of the Pseudepigrapha a prominent place in literature. For the French fabulist La Fontaine (1621–95), the Abderites

---

85. Juvenal (357), *Satires* 10.33–34; p. 195 (Ramsay's translation). Seneca (616), *On Tranquility of Mind* 15.2; 2:272.

86. Pseudep. 10. For some additional details and references, see Temkin (670).

87. Pseudep. (P.) 10; pp. 4(l. 24)–5(l. 8).

are "le vulgaire." And the opening line of his "Democritus and the Abderites" reads, "Oh, how I have always hated the thoughts of the vulgar!" He draws the moral that "the people are a doubtful judge and
that the truth of Vox populi vox dei may well be doubted." [88] The German novelist Wieland (1733–1813), in his History of the Abderites,
sees them as the provincial philistines, who lack any understanding of
men of genius such as Democritus and Hippocrates. [89]

In the Pseudepigrapha, matters are more complicated. More than
one issue is involved. Hippocrates accepts the invitation, [90] but not in
the spirit in which it was extended. He accepts in obedience to the gods,
to whose favor he says the arts owe their existence, and to Nature, who
wishes him to mend this endangered piece of her workmanship, man.
He deeply resents the Abderites' offer of money, and objects to being
treated as if he were a hireling rather than a physician. [91] He insists that
medicine must remain free (i.e., independent), and he condemns the lust
for money, which makes life miserable. [92]

Hippocrates' insistence on the freedom of medicine was a defense
of medicine as a liberal art, an art worthy of a free man. By accepting
a fee, a physician becomes a workman, in the service of and hence subject to the orders of his employer, which leads to all kinds of unethical
behavior. [93] Hippocrates had previously written to a friend that the Persian king did not know that "words of wisdom have greater power with
me than gold." [94] The Abderites also conceded that the desire for learning might be more attractive than their material offer. [95] This hinted at
the connection with philosophy and with the knowledge to be gained
by accepting new patients. Both motives, not entirely unrelated, were
also mentioned outside the Pseudepigrapha. The desirability of "wisdom" was stressed in the deontological works, and the desire for additional training and self-improvement was listed among the possible reasons for Hippocrates' leaving Cos. [96] Contempt for money was one of

88. La Fontaine (406), Fables 8.26; pp. 298–300. My attention was drawn to
this fable by Professor Jean Starobinski.

89. Wieland (720), Geschichte der Abderiten, bk. 2 ("Hippokrates in Abdera");
pp. 82–116. Wieland was one of the foremost representatives of "enlightenment"
in Germany.

90. Pseudep. 11.

91. Pseudep (P.) 16; p. 11, ll. 19–20.

92. Ibid. 11; p. 6. See also below, Epilogue.

93. Ibid. On medicine as a liberal art, and on the physician's income, see Kudlien
(391).

94. Pseudep. (P.) 6; p. 3, ll. 21–22.

95. Ibid. 10; p. 5, l. 10.

96. See above, text to n. 15.

the requisites Galen named for those who would become perfect philosophers after the manner of Hippocrates.[97] Actually, the preference for wisdom over gold (Prov. 16:16), and the condemnation of "the love of money [as] the root of all evil" (1 Tim. 6:10) were commonplace in the ancient world.

In the Roman empire, free men, freedmen, and slaves could all be doctors.[98] The possession of a liberal education and the practice of medicine in a philosophical spirit, as described in *Decorum*, allowed a physician to aspire to an elevated social rank. But this alone might not be good enough. In Cicero's scheme of the social gradation of occupations, the rank of all wage earners was ignoble and base, because their labor and not their art was purchased. The wage was a guarantee of their servitude. "However, arts that include considerable learning or aim at no mean usefulness, such as medicine, architecture, and the teaching of worthy subjects, are respectable [*honestae*] for those whose status they fit."[99] This is by no means a clear evaluation of the legal position of doctors in Rome,[100] but it is in agreement with Hippocrates' abhorrence of fees. If freed from the invidious position of a wage earner, the doctor could aspire to gentility, an aspiration furthered by a liberal education and by practicing in a philosophical spirit, as was demanded of the Hippocratic practitioners.

Cicero himself was a barrister, a practitioner of rhetoric, one of the liberal arts, which promised a forensic and a political career. The bar was an occupation worthy of a Roman gentleman. But barristers were not supposed to demand a fee; within certain limits they were allowed to accept an honorarium after the case was closed, as an expression of appreciation by the grateful client. Possibly inspired by the Platonic tradition of the nature of the liberal arts, by the example of Hippocrates, and by desire to imitate the barrister, Galen claimed never to have asked for a fee; yet he was proud of having been given four hundred pieces of gold by a grateful husband whose wife he had cured.[101]

97. See above, chap. 5.
98. See Kudlien (397).
99. Cicero (143), *De officiis* 1.42; p. 154. For a senator, for instance, the practice of medicine would not have been fitting.
100. See Below (88), pp. 57–60, on the quoted passage. The whole complex problem of the social position of doctors in Rome, and of individual practitioners, has been reexamined by Kudlien (401).
101. Galen (250), *On Prognosis* 8.20; p. 116, ll. 16–19; also Temkin (672), pp. 9 and 12. On the Platonic tradition of the definition of liberal arts and its influence on the physician's remuneration, see Kudlien (391), who also includes the model of the barrister. On the assured social position of the barrister in Rome in contrast to the doubtful position of the physician, see Finley (225), p. 57.

In his reply to the Abderites and in subsequent letters written to his friends, Hippocrates acted very much the great and wise physician who expressed opinions on sundry medical and nonmedical subjects. He also elaborated on the lust for money as a madness for the cure of which all doctors should unite.[102] He compared it to a plant from the root of which sprang other vices, and these—together with incorrect opinions and imaginings—formed madnesses that affected reason and needed to be cured by virtue. If only the lust for money could be cut off at its root, the other vices would disappear. An ailing soul would then suffer from madness concomitant with bodily disease, and would be healed with the purging of the latter.[103]

However, Hippocrates' ideas about insanity, as construed from passing remarks provoked by the Abderites' offer of money,[104] are not strictly relevant to the main question confronting Hippocrates: Is Democritus mad and in need of medical help, or is his insanity a baseless allegation of the Abderites, who are incapable of comprehending a great man?[105] From the very beginning, Hippocrates inclines to the latter view. But he is not sure, and he remains uncertain until his arrival in Abdera and his interview with Democritus.

The uncertainty arises from the fact that melancholics and men of great mind can behave similarly, especially as regards the craving for solitude and remoteness from family and social life. A man with a powerful mind may be intent on concentrating upon himself and may therefore live alone "mostly in caves and isolated places, under the shadow of trees, on soft grass or by gently flowing waters."[106] This kind of behavior is more usual in melancholics, yet those dedicated to study are also likely to seek to leave behind distracting thoughts. Finally, in the quest for tranquillity, the body is allowed to rest while the mind surges upwards and "beholds a country of truth" from which all troublesome matters keep away, a realm inhabited by virtues, gods, arts, principles, and plans, and where "the large vault of heaven is decked out with the restless stars." Wisdom may have transported Democritus into this region.[107] The Abderites, with their minds on money, do not understand Democritus. Their belief that an excess of wisdom can cause madness

102. Pseudep. (P.) 11; pp. 6(l. 20)–7(l. 2).

103. Ibid. 16; p. 11, ll. 20–23. To express it in modern terms: psychiatry would then dissolve into neurology; cf. above, chap. 2, n. 5.

104. See Temkin (670), pp. 456 and 459.

105. This either/or contrasts with the pseudo-Aristotelian (49) *Problems* 30.1; 2:154, which raises the question of why all great men are melancholics.

106. Pseudep. (P.) 12; p. 7, ll. 20–21.

107. Ibid.; p. 8, ll. 5–11. See Flashar (228), pp. 68–72.

is an error typical of laymen, who see all excess as morbid. In Hippocrates' view, an excess of virtue never does any harm.[108]

When the ship carrying him is approaching Abdera, Hippocrates
has a dream in which Truth in the form of a beautiful woman promises
to join him at Democritus's house. Another woman whom he sees approaching him is Opinion; she lives with the Abderites. Hippocrates
interprets this dream as meaning that the truth was with Democritus's
being well, and that his insanity existed only in the opinion of the Abderites.[109] Hippocrates does not esteem the Abderites highly. But in spite
of his strong belief in Democritus's sanity, he orders a large supply of
drugs—probably hellebore, a strong cathartic that was used for insanity.[110] He wants to be prepared for any eventuality.[111]

If the issue had merely been one of Democritus's genius against the
Abderites' silliness, as it appeared in both La Fontaine and Wieland,
Hippocrates would have been the astute doctor who guessed the truth.
Even his order of cathartic drugs and his postponement of the final
decision till he had seen the patient[112] would have fitted the picture of a
conscientious and cautious practitioner. But the Abderites had also
complained about Democritus's immoderate laughter at everything that
was done, whether joyous or sad. Hippocrates comments on it in one
of his letters. To him this kind of laughter is not just immoderate, nor
does he take it for meaningless, insane laughter. Rather, he judges it as
morally reprehensible to take delight in sickness and death, and other
misfortunes. Addressing Democritus as if he were present, Hippocrates
tells him: "How very wicked you are, Democritus, and far from wisdom. Or do you think that this is not evil? You are crazy, Democritus,
and in danger of yourself being an Abderite, whereas the city is the
more reasonable." [113]

A person with whom one can argue rationally and whom one judges
morally is not insane in the sense hitherto given to the term. The crazi-
ness of the laughing Democritus is on a different level; it is a lack of
moral sense. It would put the Abderites in the right and would make
Democritus the fool.

In the letter that concludes the story,[114] Hippocrates relates what
took place between him and Democritus after the ship had reached

108. Pseudep. (P.) 13; p. 8.
109. Pseudep. 15.
110. See Starobinski (643), pp. 16–18.
111. Pseudep. 16.
112. Pseudep. (P.) 14; p. 10, l. 7.
113. Ibid.; p. 10, ll. 5–7.
114. Pseudep. 17. For my use of the word "story," see Temkin (670), p. 455.

Abdera. He found Democritus (who looked neglected and far from well) sitting on a bench amidst books and dissected animal corpses. Democritus was now writing, now meditating, now consulting the dissected animals. Asked what he was working on, he answered, "On madness." The irony of the situation did not fail to strike Hippocrates. He was delighted to hear that Democritus was investigating the nature of madness, its origin in man, and its therapy, and that he was dissecting animals to study the bile, the increase of which caused insanity. Hippocrates congratulated Democritus on speaking "truly and reasonably" (there is no longer any question of Democritus's being insane)[115] and on having the leisure that Hippocrates himself lacked because matters such as his country house, children, money matters, diseases, deaths, slaves, and weddings kept him busy. These being just the kind of things said to cause his mirth, Democritus laughed and then kept silent. From this point on, Democritus is the Cynic, the laughing philosopher, who explains the reasons for his laughter and converts Hippocrates to Cynicism.

Hippocrates wants to know whether Democritus's laughter is directed at the happy or the unhappy preoccupations he has mentioned, and when Democritus only laughs more, he insists on hearing the reasons, for he considers it to be absurd to laugh at things like weddings and festivals, as well as sickness and death. Democritus explains that he does not make this distinction, and that his laughter is directed at the human beings who waste their lives in a senseless way. He gives example after example of the folly and baseness of man. Hippocrates admits the truth of all this, yet he sees it as rooted in the conditions of life, in ambition, and in unfulfilled expectations. But Democritus remains the misanthrope. From birth to death, human life is but a disease, he claims, and he again holds forth, condemning the ways of mankind.

He actually succeeds in convincing Hippocrates that he (Democritus) has fathomed human nature and that Hippocrates' own mind has been healed by his conversion. Hippocrates will return to Cos as Democritus's herald, and to the Abderites he declares that Democritus is a very wise man, quite capable of setting people straight.

The encounter between Hippocrates and Democritus was of little interest to both La Fontaine and Wieland. La Fontaine noted that after having argued much about man and his mind, they came to ethics, and he commented, "There is no need for me to relate all that the one said

---

115. Pseudep. (P.) 17; p. 15, l. 14. Hippocrates had previously (idem; p. 15, ll. 2–5) assured himself that Democritus was well oriented.

to the other." [116] Wieland was equally brief; he gave no inkling of what the two great men discussed. [117] For Robert Burton, however, who first published his *Anatomy of Melancholy* under the pseudonym Democritus Junior, this episode was of great significance. He cited the letter "verbatim almost as it is delivered by Hippocrates himself, with all the circumstances belonging unto it." At the end of the paraphrase, Burton added, "Thus Democritus esteemed of the world in his time, and this was the cause of his laughter: and good cause he had." [118] The engraved frontispiece of the editions since 1628 depicted Democritus according to the description in the letter, and its caption read:

> Old Democritus under a tree,
> Sits on a stone with book on knee;
> About him hang there many features,
> Of Cats, Dogs, and such-like creatures,
> Of which he makes Anatomy,
> The seat of black choler to see,
> Over his head appears the skie,
> And Saturn, Lord of Melancholy.

To Burton, Democritus was anything but mad, yet he put him under the symbol of melancholy, which was his great theme, whereas La Fontaine and Wieland were interested in the superiority of genius over the common crowd and the philistines.

The story does not tell what happened after Hippocrates' meeting with Democritus. Yet it poses some intriguing questions. Democritus had suggested that Hippocrates teach him medicine in exchange for the cure he was to undergo, a cure that would make him realize how eager people were to do the most worthless things, spending their life on pursuits that were merely laughable. [119] (Indeed, in the course of their conversation, Democritus had accused himself of foolishness in seeking the cause of madness by killing and dissecting animals rather than pursuing his investigations in human beings.) [120] It may be asked what kind of

116. See above, n. 88.

117. Wieland (720), *Geschichte der Abderiten* 2.6; p. 108: "All we have to say about it [i.e., the conference between Democritus and Hippocrates] is that our cosmopolitans spent the whole evening and the better part of the night in a conversation."

118. Burton (127), pp. 47–52. The following stanza is quoted from the edition of 1676 (idem. [126]).

119. Pseudep. (P.) 17; p. 16, ll. 9–11.

120. Ibid., p. 20, ll. 6–7.

medicine the converted Hippocrates would practice and teach to Democritus. Was he now first to become a moral healer of the Greeks before again attending to their bodies? This is a perturbing question because it raises doubts about the value of Hippocratic medicine and of its modern heir. Is ordinary human life worth treating and saving, only to be left to its follies and crimes? In somewhat different form, the same question will be asked by the Christian theologian Gregory of Nazianzus.

As the story tells it, the meeting with Democritus was a triumph for Cynicism and a defeat for Hippocrates, who proved no match for the philosopher. Whoever invented this letter was not much interested in medicine. The story has to be read and interpreted as it stands, but it is not unreasonable to argue that two themes have been fused together.[121] This assumption is all the more likely since there existed at least one different version of the encounter, documented by an interchange of letters between the two men.[122]

Here Democritus reproached Hippocrates for having allowed himself to be persuaded by foolish people that he, Democritus, was mad, and having arrived all ready to administer hellebore to him. This idea had been dismissed because, fortunately, Hippocrates had found him writing a cosmology and occupied with subjects that ruled out insanity. Hippocrates really ought not to associate with men of superficial and unreliable intelligence. The administration of hellebore would have driven Democritus mad, and how easily that could have happened if Hippocrates had come upon him sunk in contemplation and paying no attention to the people he knew. Diseases, therefore, must not be judged merely on the basis of how they appear to the eye! The physician must take all the circumstances into account.[123]

Hippocrates replied[124] by admitting his error; full of praise for Democritus, he expressed a wish to remain in touch with him, and asked for his writings. There is one more letter to Hippocrates,[125] in which Democritus declares medicine to be a beautiful and useful art, with which everybody, and above all, people of culture, ought to be conversant. Wisdom is the sister of medicine: the one rescues the soul from passions, the other alleviates the diseases of the body. The mind benefits from health, whereas ill health dampens the desire for virtue, and illness blinds the soul. The letter adds a brief, popular outline of the human

121. Edelstein (200), cols. 1303–4.
122. See Philippson (538).
123. Pseudep. 18.
124. Ibid. 20.
125. Ibid. 23.

organs and their functions. This version of the story presents Democritus as a great natural philosopher. Both versions share a contempt for the Abderites, whose invitation to Hippocrates is at their core. In both versions, Democritus is a great man from whom Hippocrates has something to learn. The alleged invitation, and the tradition that Democritus was Hippocrates' teacher, appear to be the seeds from which both versions grew. These were combined with some related pieces: a dissertation on hellebore put together from excerpts of Hippocratic writings and addressed by Hippocrates to Democritus,[126] and a letter on hygiene from Hippocrates to King Demetrius.[127] At some time (or times), and with editorial changes of one kind or another,[128] this material found its way into the Hippocratic Collection to become an important piece of world literature.

C. A Divine Man, but Neither a God nor a Magician

The Pseudepigrapha present Hippocrates in a variety of roles. In his dealings with Artaxerxes, he is the Greek patriot, but in his encounter with Democritus, the great physician of the body is not much more than a foil for the philosopher, the great physician of the soul. In the letter from Paetus to Artaxerxes,[129] however, he is a benefactor of the whole world, a savior, and a godlike man.

"The divine Hippocrates," Paetus wrote, "is the descendant of gods": Asclepius on the paternal side, and Hercules on the maternal. His father and grandfather taught him the rudiments of medicine, "but he taught himself the entire art, for he possesses a divine nature and surpasses his ancestors as much by the good natural endowment of his soul as by the excellence of his art." [130] When Paetus recommended Hippocrates to the Persian king, he did not anticipate any patriotic limitations of the doctor's philanthropy. "He purges the wide earth and the sea of beastly and fierce diseases, from all sides he spreads Asclepius's remedies as Triptolemus once spread those of Demeter.[131] Therefore, in many places of the earth he very justly is an object of veneration, and the Athenians have deemed him worthy of the same gifts as Hercules

126. Ibid. 21.
127. Ibid. 24.
128. For a detailed discussion, see Philippson (538).
129. Pseudep. 2.
130. Pseudep. (P.) 2; pp. 1(l. 17)–2(l. 4).
131. The legendary king Triptolemus brought agriculture and civilization to mankind. He rode over the earth in a winged chariot with sacks full of seed wheat given to him by Demeter.

and Asclepius." [132] Paetus urged the king to send for Hippocrates, "for he knows not [just] one way to cure the affliction, he [the] father of health, [the] savior, [the] mitigator of pain, in short [the] leader of the science befitting a god." [133]

Others called Hippocrates "most divine" and "most holy," [134] which in the context may be rendered as "most worshipful," and Galen compared Hippocrates' words to the "voice of a god." [135] Such attitudes were in harmony with a Greek poem, "On the Ethical Duties of the Physician," in which its author, the Stoic philosopher Sarapion (c. A.D. 100) said, "Like a savior god, let [the physician] make himself the equal of slaves and of paupers, of the rich and of rulers of men, and to all let him minister like a brother; for we are all children of the same blood." [136] The original restorer of the poem thought its tone "Epictetean, if not Christian." [137] The Hellenistic inscriptions previously cited [138] praised individual doctors in similar terms. One passage in the poem [139] sounds like an allusion to the Hippocratic oath, and no doctor fitted the simile of the "savior god" better than the legendary Hippocrates.

This Hippocrates was a divine man and a hero, to whom the Coans made offerings on his birthday; he was "an object of veneration" in many places, as Paetus's letter said. [140] In our own century, stories were

132. Pseudep. (P.) 2; p. 2, ll. 4–7.

133. Ibid., ll. 8–10.

134. For instance, Apollonius of Citium (31), p. 10, l. 5: Ἱπποκράτου τοῦ Θειοτάτου; and Athenaeus (56), Deipnosophists 9.399; 4:307: Ἱπποκράτης ὁ ἱερώτατος.

135. See above, chap. 5, n. 16.

136. Quoted from Oliver (498), p. 246. A first (incomplete) reconstruction of the poem was published by Oliver and Maas (499). In the identification of Sarapion, I am following Oliver (498). For further discussion, see Edelstein (198), pp. 344 and 347; also Kudlien (390), p. 96.

137. Maas (499), p. 323. See also Oliver (498), p. 246.

138. See above, chap. 3.

139. The poem commands the physician "not to look upon [his patient] or make approaches in a manner contrary to divine laws and to the oath" (quoted from Oliver [498], p. 246). In view of the fact that the Hippocratic oath was well known in the first century, it is likely that this oath is meant here. Treatment of all men alike without consideration of wealth or rank can easily be read into the oath, which makes no reference to the patient's economic or social status; see also Temkin (672), pp. 10–11 and pp. 22–23, nn. 29 and 30.

140. See Bieler (97), p. 16, n. 16; p. 121, n. 39; and p. 135. Bieler tried to show that "Antiquity, especially later Antiquity, and early Christianity know the same image of the divine human being" (idem, p. 145). I owe the reference to Bieler to the editors of the Reallexikon für Antike und Christentum.

still current in Cos of the Great Hippocrates who appeared to some pious people as a messenger of God, bringing healing to man.[141] Memories of Asclepius, in Christianized form, had thus become interwoven with those of the Coans' great compatriot. All this raises the question of whether Hippocrates was also venerated as a god. A story by that irreverent wit Lucian illuminates the difference between a hero and a god: A physician has a small bronze statue of Hippocrates that makes a nuisance of itself at night, "especially when we omit the sacrifice that we render [him] every year." It walks all over the house, upsets the medicine boxes, mixing up the medicines, and overturns the oil press. This causes a skeptical listener to ask: "Has it gone so far that even Hippocrates the physician demands sacrifice in his honor and gets angry if he is not feasted on time with full-fledged sacrifices? He ought to be pleased if somebody brings him offerings, or makes a libation of melicret,[142] or puts a wreath around his gravestone." [143]

It was said that remarkable things had taken place at Hippocrates' grave. Other great men, like Sophocles and Plato, were also heroized, and the graves of such men were places where minor miracles might take place.[144] The veneration felt for Hippocrates was well expressed in the epigraph to a portrait of his: "This is he who opened the secret paths of medicine, the divine healer [Παιήων] of men, Hippocrates of Cos." [145] Paeon (Παιήων) was the physician of the gods; the name was used as a title for Apollo and Asclepius. Applied to men, the word covered a range of meanings from physician to savior. It did not elevate Hippocrates to the ranks of the immortals, however; he remained a human being. "Having healed many people, Hippocrates himself fell ill and died," wrote the emperor Marcus Aurelius.[146]

Hippocrates neither ascended to the realm of the immortals, as had Asclepius, nor descended to the sphere of miracle workers, as had Apollonius of Tyana, a neo-Pythagorean philosopher who flourished in the first century. Apollonius, according to his biographer Philostratus, was a sage imbued with the wisdom of the Indian Brahmans, a divine man,

141. See Meyer-Steineg (459).

142. Honey mixed with milk.

143. Lucian (432), *Philopseudēs* 21; 3:353–54 (Harmon's translation, modified). The story brings out the terminological difference between Θύεσθαι (to sacrifice) and ἐναγίζειν (to bring offerings), the verb used by the *Vita*, p. 175, l. 14.

144. According to Leisegang (415), col. 2344, the biography by Apuleius was structured by the notion of Plato as a "divine man."

145. *Greek Anthology* (269), 16.269; 5:320–21 (Paton's translation).

146. Marcus Aurelius (444), *Communings with Himself* 3.3; p. 48.

a worker of miracles whom many of his contemporaries unjustly accused of sorcery.[147] His most prominent pupil believed him to be of a divine nature superior to that of human beings.[148] However, when the Emperor Domitian accused him of claiming divinity, Apollonius denied it. He distinguished between the universe that rested on god the creator and embraced all things in heaven, on earth, and in the sea; and the universe of erring souls.[149] This latter universe depended on a good man who had the likeness of a god, who was "a god sent down by wisdom."[150] His mission was to lead human souls away from their passions and senseless practices.[151] On his own testimony, Apollonius was such a good man, as the Spartan lawgiver Lycurgus had been, whom Apollo had called a god.[152]

To lead people away from their passions and senseless doings was the acknowledged task of the philosopher, the physician of the soul, and perhaps the historical Apollonius claimed no higher status than this. But as depicted by Philostratus, he was not only godlike but transcended the boundaries between god and man. Apollonius claimed to know all languages, and to be able to discern men's thoughts[153] and what the future held for them.[154] He could at will free himself from fetters.[155] When the hearing before the Emperor Domitian in Rome had ended—shortly before noon—Apollonius freed himself, disappeared, and around evening reappeared in Puteoli, near Naples.[156]

His medical feats were no less astonishing. He made a lame man walk by stroking the man's buttocks with his hands; he cured a blind man, and another whose hand was palsied; he helped a woman in difficult labor,[157] and he healed hydrophobia in a boy as well as in the dog that had bitten him.[158] Allegedly, Asclepius recommended Apollonius

147. Philostratus (543), *Life of Apollonius of Tyana* 2.17; 1:162.
148. Ibid. 7.38 and 8.13; 2:256 and 366. His pupils almost worship Apollonius and believe him to be a divine man (idem 8.15; 2:372). See also idem 3.50; 1:334.
149. Ibid. 8.7; 2:314–17.
150. Ibid. 8.7; 2:317 (Conybear's translation). In this sense, Apollonius claimed divinity both for himself and for the Indian sages (idem 3.13; 1:266–67).
151. Ibid. 8.7; 2:316. In accordance with this, Apollonius praises Democritus's laughter (idem 8.7; 2:340).
152. Ibid. 8.7; 2:314.
153. Ibid. 1.19; 1:52.
154. Ibid. 5.12; 1:488. Apollonius prophesied not by sorcery but by divine revelation.
155. Ibid. 7.38; 2:256. This made his pupil realize his divine and superhuman nature.
156. Ibid. 8.10–12; 2:358–62. See also idem 8.5; 2:282–84.
157. Ibid. 3.39; 1:316–18.
158. Ibid. 6.43; 2:140–42

to many supplicants.[159] Apollonius foresaw an outbreak of the plague in Ephesus, and when it struck he saved the city. He assembled all its inhabitants in the theater and ordered them to stone an old man who was there in the guise of a blind beggar but in reality was a demon hateful to the gods. After the stones had been removed, instead of the blind beggar a dog was found, the size of a lion, frothing with rage.[160] Apollonius also drove away hobgoblins[161] and freed people from demons.[162]

In Apollonius the pagan opposition to Christianity found valuable support by putting him on a par with Jesus. To meet this attack and in response to a heathen author who had compared the life of Apollonius to that of Jesus, Eusebius, the historian of the church, denounced Apollonius (as presented by Philostratus) as a wizard and a fraud, who had pretended to be a god. According to Eusebius, Apollonius's alleged miracles had been performed with the help of demons.[163] But this did not silence the anti-Christian opposition. Eunapius, one of its leaders in the late fourth century, gave a glowing account of Apollonius—who, he said, was worshiped by some people.[164] Apollonius "was no longer a philosopher but something between the gods and man. Emulating the philosophy of Pythagoras he fully displayed its more divine and active [side] . . . Philostratus ought to have given his biography the title 'Visit of a God to Men'."[165]

The healing god Asclepius, whose miracles were part of his official cult,[166] became the main rival of the Christ. Opponents of Christianity tried to demote Jesus by declaring Apollonius of Tyana his equal. In contrast to both, Hippocrates did not become the Christ's competitor. A hero, a sage, a divine man, he remained the human head of a secular art.

159. Ibid. 4.1; 1:348.

160. Ibid. 4.10; 1:362–66.

161. Ibid. 2.4.1; 1:124.

162. Ibid. 3.28; 2:314–16. It concerns the case of a young man of sixteen.

163. Eusebius (212), *Treatise* 1; 2:496 and 600–604, allows that in reality, if the myths surrounding him were discarded, Apollonius may have been a philosopher.

164. Eunapius (209), *Lives;* p. 542, l. 11.

165. Ibid., p. 346, ll. 14–20.

166. See below, chap. 7.

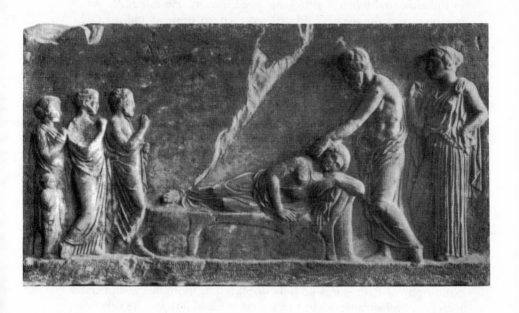

Incubation scene. Asclepius, accompanied by Hygeia, healing a sleeping
woman (family members are on the left), ca. 400 B.C. Piraeus Museum.
From Ulrich Hausmann, *Kunst und Heiltum*. Potsdam: Eduard Stich-
note, 1958. Table 1 and pp. 44–48.

III

Religious Healing and Secular Healing

Hippocratic medicine originated and developed in a pagan culture and had religious associations, the nature of which will be explored below. But in contrast to religious healing—attributed to the Greek god Asclepius, the God of the Jews, and Jesus Christ—Hippocratic medicine was secular, insofar as it promised to heal by the physician's knowledge and skill, and the use of natural means. What, then, was the relationship of these religious forms of healing, all three of which coexisted in the first century, to Hippocratic medicine or, where sufficient specific information is lacking, to secular healing in general?

7

THE CULT OF ASCLEPIUS

The syncretistic paganism of the Roman empire[1] had room for many healing gods, such as the Egyptian Serapis, probably the most renowned healer next to the Greek Asclepius, whose cult had spread vigorously during Hippocrates' lifetime. The legend of Asclepius, current by the first century A.D., combined two traditions: the saga of the hero and the myth of the god.[2] The saga, as sung by Pindar,[3] related that Asclepius was the son of Apollo and Coronis, a princess whom Apollo killed because she consorted with a mortal. However, Apollo saved his unborn child and turned him over to the centaur Cheiron, who taught him how to cure man of disease. Asclepius became a great physician but, yielding to the lure of gold, he brought a dead man back to life and was slain by Zeus with his thunderbolt. This saga was then fused with the myth of the god Asclepius (a chthonic deity or an Epi-

1. On paganism and its syncretism, cf. Fox (230), chap. 2 ("Pagans and Their Cities").

2. In this outline of the legend of Asclepius, I have largely followed Edelstein and Edelstein (197), 2:1–138, which is based on the testimonies collected in vol. 1 (hereafter abbreviated T). Although the Edelsteins' view of the genesis of the Asclepius cult has not met with general approval (see below, n. 4), I have found it acceptable in those points that pertain to my understanding of the relationship of the Hippocratic physicians to Asclepius (see below, chap. 14.A).

3. Pindar (549), *Pythian Odes* 3; also T 1.

daurian invention).[4] Divine will elevated Asclepius to the realm of the gods. Immortal now, he still remained the great physician, revered in cults that spread from Epidaurus to other places, of which Pergamum, in the second century, was the most famous.

In the sanctuary, a place resembling a modern spa, sick people would spend a night in the *abaton,* where Asclepius was expected to appear in their dreams and give them directions for treatment, unless he cured the disease by an instantaneous miracle, which might take the form of dreams in which the god applied remedies or performed surgical operations. Grateful patients donated votive offerings representing the diseased organs, and inscriptions on tablets told of successful cures by the god.[5] The inscriptions covered cures of a great variety of ailments, ranging from baldness and infestation with lice[6] to a case of blindness in which the whole eyeball was missing.[7] Asclepius was also helpful in calamities other than diseases. He assisted a widow to discover a hidden treasure, and in another case, he was responsible for the recovery of a cache of gold.[8]

Long before Asclepius had become the generally accepted god of healing, he was already filling two closely related roles. He was a "culture hero—extolled as the progenitor of all his fellow craftsmen"[9]— and he was "the patron saint" of the physicians.[10]

In Homer's time, physicians were known as descendants of Paeon, the ancient physician of the gods.[11] The *Iliad* also told of a prince Asclepius, a mortal and a great physician, who was the father of Podalirius and Machaon, physician-warriors in the Greek army before Troy.[12] Paeon came to be replaced by Apollo and Asclepius, and the "sons of Paeon" became the "sons of Asclepius" or the "Asclepiads," who claimed descent from Asclepius. The original meaning of the term "Asclepiads" is not quite clear. They may have been a closed clan among

---

4. Edelstein and Edelstein (197), 2:76, reject the theory that Asclepius was an aboriginal deity. Their hypothesis (idem, p. 91) "that Asclepius was a 'special god,' created by men to be in charge of one task alone, that of healing" has met with considerable resistance. For the thesis that he had been a god, see, for instance, Benedum (90). For the theme of this book, this question is of little relevance.

5. The inscriptions have been collected and interpreted by Herzog (300); and by Edelstein and Edelstein (197), 1:209–64 (T 414–62).

6. T 423.19 and T 423.28.

7. T 423.9.

8. Herzog (300), p. 27, n. 46, and p. 32, n. 63.

9. Edelstein and Edelstein (197), 2:54.

10. Ibid., p. 56.

11. *Odyssey* 4.232; *Iliad* 5.889–900. See Edelstein and Edelstein (197), 2:56.

12. *Iliad* 11.518 (T 165), 11.833–36 (T 136), and 2.731–32 (T 10).

whom the practice of medicine was hereditary.[13] Later on they opened their ranks,[14] so that "Asclepiads" or "sons of Asclepius" became synonymous with "physicians." Be that as it may, it was the hero Asclepius, "half human, half divine," [15] the patron saint of physicians, not the healing god, from whom the Asclepiads derived their name.[16]

For some time, father and son were associated as healing gods. The inscriptions found at Epidaurus are entitled "Cures of Apollo and of Asclepius," [17] and the Hippocratic oath swears by "Apollo Physician and Asclepius, and Hygeia, and Panacea and all the gods and goddesses." [18] Asclepius eventually became the leading healing deity, and from healer and helper he grew to a universal savior and thus became the most tenacious competitor of Jesus.

The inscriptions tended to record memorable cases in which the god succeeded where physicians had failed. The motive for consulting the god was clearly stated by the Athenian orator Aeschines:

> Having despaired of the skill of mortals, but with every hope in the divine, forsaking Athens . . . coming to your sacred grove, Asclepius, I was healed in three months of a festering wound which I had had on my head for a whole year.[19]

The frustration felt after a year's unsuccessful treatment is understandable, yet not only is three months a long time, but it is long enough to allow the wound to heal without Asclepius's help. In the inscriptions, examples of healing that we admit to be miraculous because medically impossible, such as the restitution of sight where the eyeball was missing,[20] were balanced by other examples of a trivial kind, or in which a natural explanation is not too farfetched.[21]

Generally speaking, when assessing cures attributed to miracles, superstitious remedies,[22] and treatments by which we nowadays set little

13. So Speyer (640), p. 1179. See also Lichtenthaeler (421), p. 63, who speaks of the Asclepiads as "noble clans of physicians."

14. Galen (241), *De anatomicis administrationibus* 2.1; 2:281–82; also T 229. This theory is contrary to Edelstein and Edelstein (197), 2:57–59, who suggest that the term "Asclepiads" originally designated physicians, and that the clan was a later invention.

15. Edelstein and Edelstein (197), 2:56.

16. Ibid., p. 55; Koelbing (368), p. 60; Lichtenthaeler (421), p. 63.

17. T 423.

18. T 337 and Edelstein (198), p. 6 (Edelstein's translation).

19. T 404 (the Edelsteins' translation).

20. T 423.9.

21. Herzog (300) goes too far in this direction.

22. Unless paraphrasing ancient sources, I use the pejorative words "superstitious" and "superstition" reluctantly and only *faute de mieux*.

store, it has to be remembered that therapeutic criteria have undergone a change during the last hundred and fifty years. We are increasingly skeptical of *post hoc ergo propter hoc* judgments and of crediting doctors with improvements that follow immediately after consultation, and we ask for large-scale statistical studies, controlled trials, and prolonged observation of the patient. The idea that a complaint may have a psychogenic origin or that improvement may be due to autosuggestion comes more easily to mind than it did in the past.

The inscriptions at Epidaurus have a popular character.[23] The tone of the inscriptions was factual rather than solemn, sometimes even marked by a certain levity. A boy suffering from stone of the bladder dreamed that Asclepius asked what he would give him for being cured. " 'Ten dice,' [the boy] answered. The god laughed and said to him that he would cure him. When day came he walked out sound." [24] Asclepius punished those who scoffed at his powers. A man who called Asclepius a liar for boasting to cure lame people was crippled by the horse he was riding but was healed by the god after many entreaties.[25] Another man came to the temple incapable of moving all but one of his fingers. He disbelieved the inscriptions and made fun of them. The god restored his power over his fingers and then asked him whether he still disbelieved the inscriptions. When he denied it, the god ordered that because of his former disbelief his name should forthwith be "Unbeliever." [26]

In most of the inscriptions, a belief in Asclepius was taken for granted; indeed, it would be astonishing if disbelievers had sought his help. Disbelief, where mentioned, concerned his ability to do things that seemed impossible, and Asclepius punished those who offended his medical honor. But his métier was healing; not for him the infliction of pestilences and defiling diseases whose victims required purification. In the *Iliad,* the infliction of disease was left to Apollo, whereas Asclepius's sons tended to the wounds of the warriors.

An inscription at Epidaurus read: "Pure must be he who enters the fragrant temple. Purity means to think holy thoughts." [27] This dictum corresponds to the pledge of the Hippocratic oath, "In purity and holiness I shall guard my life and my art." [28] It was said that Asclepius had

23. See MacMullen (437), pp. 32–34 and pp. 158–60, nn. 70–83.
24. T 423.8 (the Edelsteins' translation).
25. T 423.36.
26. T 423.3. See also T 423.4, the case of a woman who had to donate a silver pig for having laughed at the possibility that lame and blind persons could be cured simply by having a dream.
27. T 318 and T 336 (the Edelsteins' translation, modified).
28. Edelstein (198), p. 6 (Edelstein's translation).

denied help to a youth whose self-indulgent life had ruined his health, but that otherwise "he gives [health] to those who desire it." [29] It was recorded that his temple in Epidaurus was always full of sick people;[30] he healed the poor and was satisfied with small sacrifices.[31] The philanthropy of the gods did not allow them to accept money, but they exacted some sacrifices, because "they wish [people] to be neither ungrateful nor forgetful, even in such matters making us better." [32] Of Asclepius, Emperor Julian wrote, he "does not heal mankind in the hope of repayment, but everywhere fulfills his own function of beneficence to mankind." [33] If, then, it is true that Asclepius was "believed to cure diseases of every kind," [34] even those that defied the doctors, and if, moreover, he was satisfied with very little—less than doctors were likely to have demanded—why did a secular medical art exist at all?

The inscriptions themselves prove the existence of unbelievers, but however large their number may have been in a time when skeptical Epicureanism was fashionable, it would at most have included a fraction of the educated Greeks and Romans. Reasons other than unbelief may have impelled people to seek aid from physicians rather than from the gods. In the cities doctors were at hand; moreover, rich Romans had doctors in their households. Travel to a sanctuary could be expensive and was not always feasible or advisable. Wounds, dislocations, and fractures, as well as acute diseases, needed immediate attention.

The god's help was also more remote than the doctor's in another sense than the geographical. What the doctor could do and would do was limited, but it was calculable, whereas it was uncertain whether the god would do anything at all. He might not appear in the dream, and though the inscriptions recorded successful cures, they did not prove that all who came to the sanctuary were cured. Complete reliance on the god demanded more than belief in his power, it demanded that the petitioner have unquestioning faith that he would be secure in the god's hands and that the god would never desert him. This was a faith that even Asclepius himself did not demand of his supplicants.

Even if the god seemed not to react, his philanthropy might still

29. T 397 (the Edelsteins from F. C. Conybeare's (543) translation of Philostratus's *Life of Apollonius of Tyana*).

30. T 382.

31. T 321 and T 482.14–16. Cf. also Edelstein and Edelstein (197), 2:116.

32. T 455 (the Edelsteins' translation from the fragments of Aelianus).

33. T 320 (the Edelsteins from W. C. Wright's translation of the letters of Julian).

34. T 382 (the Edelsteins from H. L. Jones's translation of Strabo's *Geographica*).

seem credible, as can be seen from a letter by Libanius, friend and follower of Julian the Apostate:

> I have the olive shoot from the sanctuary, but nothing more has come
> to me from it unless the work of the physicians must be considered the
> god's. Thus let it be considered and so be it. For this belief is both fair
> and safe.[35]

In spite of Libanius's hostility to Christianity, it is not impossible that
by the late fourth century, Judaeo-Christian thought influenced his idea
that physicians were instruments of the god.

It is misleading to view the relationship of secular medicine and the
cult of Asclepius as mutually exclusive. As a Hippocratic author stated,
"prayer indeed is good, but while calling on the gods a man should
himself lend a hand."[36] The patient could thus reap the benefits of both
secular and divine care.

The genealogy of Hippocrates traced him to the Homeric physician
Asclepius, who became a god but remained a physician. The legend saw
no rift between the healing god and the Hippocratic doctors.[37] The legend represented the views of even those Hippocratic authors who
fought the notion of the gods as responsible agents of defilement and
disease.

> I, at any rate [wrote the author of On the Sacred Disease], do not be-
> lieve that the human body is defiled by a god, the most perishable by
> the most holy. Even if it happens to have been defiled by another
> [agency] or suffered some harm, it is purified by the god and freed from
> blemish rather than defiled.

The author was thinking primarily of the sacred disease and its treatment by cathartic remedies. The bulk of the book was dedicated to
propounding a natural explanation of the disease in refutation of a
god's responsibility. But he also thought of the gods in positive terms,
for the quotation continues, "It is the divine [ὑπὸ τοῦ θεοῦ] that ex-
purgates the greatest and unholiest of sins, removes the blemish and
washes us clean."[38]

The author's attitude toward the cult of the gods and their power
was positive. He accused the magicians and cathartic healers of disres-

35. T 503 (the Edelsteins' translation from the letters of Libanius).

36. Hippocrates (302), *On Regimen* 4.87; 4:423 (Jones's translation).

37. Amundsen and Ferngren (25), pp. 70–80, have pointed out the lack of conflict between the legend of Asclepius and the secular practice of medicine.

38. *On the Sacred Disease,* chap. 1, art. 44–45, according to Grensemann
(276); chap. 4 according to Jones's edition (302), 2:148.

pect for the gods and of disbelief in their existence.[39] As a secular physician, however, it was his aim to convince people that all diseases, even "the so-called sacred disease," were curable by a dietetic regimen. He categorically denied that the gods defile the human body; rather, they purify men, removing sin and guilt. But in contrast to his painstaking refutation of the gods as agents of disease, he was silent about their power to heal.[40]

Generally speaking, Hippocratic physicians may even have welcomed the cult of Asclepius because it allowed them to refer to him patients they were unable to treat.[41] Nor did the pagan god claim a healing monopoly as the Jewish God did. Asclepius might put the doctors to shame, but he evinced no jealousy toward them. Everybody was free to seek the treatment he preferred.[42]

39. "To me their talk seems to amount not to piety [εὐσεβείης] as they believe, but rather to impiety [ἀσεβείης] and [the implication] that gods do not exist. What with them is pious and divine is impious and unholy, as I shall explain"; chap. 1, art. 28 according to Grensemann (276); chap. 3 according to Jones (302), 2:144.

40. See Edelstein (198), pp. 378–79. I cannot agree with Lloyd's ([426], p. 57) contention that according to the Hippocratic physicians, "appeals to the gods are arbitrary and superfluous."

41. See Edelstein (198), pp. 244–46.

42. For additional discussion of the doctors' relation to the cult of Asclepius, see below, ch. 14.A.

8

THE ALMIGHTY GOD

To turn from a healing god, be he Apollo or Asclepius, to the Biblical God as He was conceived by the Jews around the time of Jesus is to turn from a god who could cure to a universal god who was the source of all healing: "I kill, and I make alive; I smite,[1] and I heal: neither is any that can deliver out of my hand" (Deut. 32:39).

Unlike the monotheistic theories professed by pagan philosophers, and their wavering assertions of the gods' unlimited power,[2] the Jews' belief in the one God was firmly rooted in a national tradition. The recognition of this belief as a national religion made the Romans exempt the Jews from observing the cult of the emperors. The Jews also had their "Epicureans," as they called the skeptics in their midst. But for the rest of the Jews, belief in God as the creator of the world by His pure will, the giver of a law that included all that was good and just, and the omniscient judge who punished evildoers was a matter of course. The Jews believed that their God was the only divine being, and that they had a special relationship to Him. All the gods of the other nations (the gentiles) were mere idols whose very names were not to be mentioned.

---

1. "I smite" for the Hebrew *maḥaṣtī* seems preferable to "I wound," which is the translation found in the Authorized Version.

2. See above, Preface.

Persian influences had led the Jews to invest Satan and his cohort of demons with some power. The belief in evil demons was widespread in the world of the first century; how widespread it was among the Jews is abundantly documented by the Gospels. None of these beings had any power before God, whose will and providence ruled events. Human beings, however, were free to obey His will or to sin. Healing was closely connected with the forgiveness of sins. "[The Lord] pardons all my guilt and heals all my diseases,"[3] sang the Psalmist (103:3).[4] God might inflict disease as punishment and then remove it in response to prayer. Thus Miriam was punished with zara'ath[5] and then healed by God in answer to Moses' prayer (Num. 12:10–15). God could also delegate the power to heal and to transfer diseases. Elisha "the man of God" (2 Kings 5:8), was able to free Namaan, the Syrian, from zara'ath and then to transfer it to Elisha's disobedient servant, Gehazi.[6]

Besides being punishment for sin, disease could also have religious significance as the trial inflicted on a righteous person (Job 2:5–7) or the chastisement of one whom God loved (Prov. 3:12). "Behold, blessed[7] is the man whom God correcteth: therefore despise not thou the chastening of the Almighty: For he maketh sore, and bindeth up: he woundeth, and his hands make whole," said Eliphaz trying to solace Job (Job 5:17–18). Moreover, "through suffering men attain to life in the world to come,"[8] as Rav Huna put it in the later, rabbinical age.

With God as the only healer, there would seem to be little room for the existence of secular medicine. Yet some kind of healer seems to have existed, if perhaps solely for treating wounds and broken limbs.[9] The often-quoted words of Jeremiah (8:22), "Is there no balm in Gilead; is there no healer[10] there?" suggest that medical help was available. On

3. This translation, combining AV and NEB, is closer to the Hebrew text than either of them.

4. See Hempel (296), p. 280.

5. I follow the customary transcription. On the nature of the disease, see below, chap. 9, text to n. 18.

6. 2 Kings 5:1–19 (the story of Namaan) and idem 5:20–27 (the story of Gehazi).

7. 'Ashrê, literally "hail to." "Blessed" is preferable to "happy" (AV), which may be taken to describe a subjective state.

8. Quoted from Bowker (111), p. 35.

9. Hempel (296), pp. 240–41: "Der altisraelitische Arzt ist also gleich seinen Kollegen Machaon und Podaleirios . . . in erster Linie 'Verbinder' (ḥobeš Jes. 3.5) Wundarzt, dessen Ziel es ist, den Verletzten wieder zu Kräften zu bringen," and idem, p. 243: "die grundlegende Gleichung Arzt = Wundarzt."

10. Rōphē, the participle of "to heal," is better translated by a neutral word than by "physician" (AV), which we connect with professional status.

the other hand, a pious person may have been expected to act as Job did. Smitten with boils all over (Job 2:7), all he did was take "a potsherd to scrape himself withal," and sit down "among the ashes" (Job 2:8).

Religious antagonism against doctors is strongly implied in the report of the sickness and the death of King Asa of Judah (about 900 B.C.). In the thirty-ninth year of his reign, according to 2 Chronicles (16:12–13), the king became "diseased in his feet,"[11] and the condition became increasingly severe. "And in his disease too[12] he sought not to the Lord, but to the physicians." In the opinion of the Chronicler, the king ought to have trusted God rather than secular physicians. Since 1 Kings (chaps. 15–23) does not mention Asa's preference for doctors over God, the antagonism as expressed in the relatively late Chronicles may belong to postexilic times, when the relationship of God and man became a matter for deepened reflection.

Two men, Jesus the Son of Sirach (Ben Sira), and Philo, the Alexandrian Jewish philosopher, approached the problem from opposite sides. Both were pious Jews who believed in God as the ultimate healer of all disease, but whereas Ben Sira rose to the defense of physicians, Philo attacked those who relied on medicine rather than on God.

Ben Sira, living in Palestine, wrote his work in Hebrew around the beginning of the second century B.C.[13] "The Wisdom of Jesus the Son of Sirach" was translated into Greek in Alexandria and became part of the Septuagint. Under the title "Ecclesiasticus," it was then incorporated into the Latin Vulgate and is thus to be found in the Catholic Bible, whereas the Jews, in spite of the attention shown it in the rabbinical literature,[14] did not canonize it; hence it is not found in the Jewish and most Protestant Bibles but is relegated to the Apocrypha.

The wisdom of Ben Sira also extended to matters of hygiene, and included a warning against excessive eating, which led many to their graves, whereas "he that taketh heed prolongeth his life" (Ecclus. 37:31).[15] From here, Ben Sira turned to the doctor and to medicines,

11. NEB translates this as "Asa became gravely affected with gangrene in his feet," which I think to be a gratuitous interpretation.

12. W*gam-beḥolyô (AV has "Yet in his disease he thought not"). Asa had previously turned to the king of Syria rather than to the Lord, for which he was severely taken to task (2 Chron. 16:1–10).

13. The Hebrew text, preserved in a fragmentary condition, has been edited by Lévi (194), from whose edition Noorda (486), pp. 218–19, n. 9, prepared an English translation of chap. 38, lines 1–15. In spelling the name Ben Sira, I follow Lévi (194), p. 1. Ben Sirach is the spelling of the Apocrypha (29), p. 133.

14. See Lévi (194), pp. v–vi; also Schürer (613), 2:319.

15. Apocrypha (29), p. 175 (Authorized Version).

both of which were from God and must not be rejected (Ecclus. 38:1–8): "Honor the physician before he is needed; also him God has appointed. From God the physician gets his wisdom." [16]

This religious legitimization of the doctor was followed by a reminder of the high esteem in which he was held by the king and the nobles. (Since there was no Jewish king at the time of Ben Sira, this is likely to refer to the Egyptian or Syrian courts and to members of the Jewish aristocracy.)

The text then continues, "From the earth God produces medicines, and a sensible man should not reject them" (Ecclus. 38:4).[17] God gave man understanding and sound judgment, and so the physician uses medicines to relieve pain, the apothecary[18] produces ointments, and all this accrues to the glory of the Lord.

The religious justification of doctors, medicines, and apothecaries, together with the appeal to good sense, seems to anticipate resistance against the medical arts. The justification of the use of secular medicine was repeated in the following section (Ecclus. 38:9–15), which taught what to do in case of illness:

> My son, in illness be not negligent:[19]
>   pray to God, for He heals.
> Flee from injustice and partiality
>   and from all sins cleanse your heart.
> Offer incense and a memorial
>   and fat; prepare the best you can. (Ecclus. 38:9–11)[20]

Thus far, Ben Sira reaffirms traditional Jewish teaching: God is the unquestioned healer. "Heal me, O Lord, and I shall be healed," said Jeremiah (17:14). The Lord expected a life free from sin; He had promised, "If my people . . . shall humble themselves, and pray, and seek my face, and turn from their wicked ways; then will I hear from heaven and will forgive their sin, and will heal their land" (2 Chron. 7:14). Sacrifice to God was expected at the time when the Temple and the ritual cult still existed.

Having thus reaffirmed the position of God, Ben Sira gives the doctor his due:

16. Noorda's ([486] p. 218, n. 9) translation.
17. Ibid.
18. Ecclesiasticus (194), 38:8, p. 44: *rōqēaḥ*, "he who mixes ointments."
19. Ecclesiasticus (194), 38:9: *'al tithʿabēr*. "Be not negligent" (Apocrypha [29], p. 175) seems preferable to Noorda's ([486], p. 218, n. 9) "don't let it be."
20. Noorda's ([486] p. 218, n. 9) translation, modified.

And also give a place to the physician;
  and he must not be removed, for him too you need.
For there is a time when in his hand [lies] success.
  For he also supplicates God,
that He may make him succeed in his judgment[21]
  and his remedies in order to save life [?].
He who sins before his creator
  let him be arrogant[22] in the face of the physicians.
(Ecclus. 38:12–15)[23]

The physician is God's instrument, sometimes indispensable for healing. Ben Sira thus turns the tables on uncompromising Jews. It is not
the pious but the sinners who reject the doctor and thus prepare their
own doom.

Ben Sira seems to have been thinking of Jewish doctors, who would
pray to God for success. It is not likely that he was the first to reconcile
secular medicine, practiced by God-fearing doctors,[24] with God's almighty rule. But it was he whose formulation exercised a powerful influence upon Jews and Christians, regardless of whether or not his
name was mentioned. Ben Sira admonished those who set all their trust
in doctors that God was the real healer, and he asked those who wished
to condemn all worldly medicine by what right they rejected doctors
and medicine, God's appointees and His creation.

Yet this reconciliation of religious and secular medicine was a compromise, not a final solution. In spite of all textual uncertainties, it is
clear that Ben Sira took medical successes, however limited, for facts,
and regarded medical interference as sometimes indispensable.[25] Without such beliefs, the mere argument that God's creation must not be
held to be worthless or bad remained weak in the face of different approaches, of which Philo's was one.

21. Lévi and Noorda both have "diagnosis," which, though substantially correct, has too modern a ring. Hempel (296), p. 285, thinks that the physician's prayer
is the reason for his sometimes being successful.

22. Gesenius (258) translates *yithgabēr* (hithpael of *gabar*) as *sich übermütig
betragen*. The Greek text of the Septuagint makes little sense; see Noorda (486), p.
221, n. 18. Lévi (194), p. 45, adds note e to line 15: "i.e. he that sinneth will not be
healed." Hempel (296), p. 285, and Noorda (486), p. 221, paraphrase similarly.

23. I follow Noorda's ([486], pp. 218–19, n. 9) translation with modifications.

24. I doubt that the prayers of heathen doctors (to whom?) would have been
reassuring to a pious Jew. I take the reference to the prayers of the doctors as indicating the existence of secular Jewish physicians and of their clientele, of which Ben
Sira was a member.

25. I do not agree with Hempel (296), p. 285, that Ben Sira, with all his acknowledgment of the medical art, did not get beyond its half-hearted appreciation.
On Ben Sira, see also Seybold and Mueller (619), pp. 60–62, 109.

Whereas Ben Sira was intent upon justifying medicine before pious Jews, Philo, writing about two hundred years later in Alexandria, with its Hellenized Jewry, attacked worldly Jews, who trusted medicine and for whom God had become a doubtful last refuge. Being strongly inclined to Stoic philosophy, Philo was subtle in his approach by comparison with the simplicity of Ecclesiasticus.

Philo distinguishes between ordinary health and health as recovery from sickness. The former has been given to man by God. But in recovery from sickness, health is bestowed "by means of art and of medical care," so that healing appears to be due to human knowledge and to the doctors, although in reality it is God who heals, with or without them.[26] Philo takes it as a matter of course that doctors are consulted, and whereas Ben Sira stressed the possible usefulness of the physician, Philo viewed it with a good deal of indifference. His attention and his scorn were directed against "the waverers" who, like Pharaoh, delayed invoking God's help. A master of allegorical interpretation of the Bible, Philo regarded Pharaoh as a man whose soul was incapable of perceiving incorporeal and eternal goods. Pharaoh asked Moses to entreat God for deliverance from the plague of frogs, promising that he would then let the children of Israel go. But in spite of the pressing need for immediate action, he said "tomorrow" when asked by Moses when he should pray to God (Exod. 8:8–10).

"The waverers"[27] are the people who do not confess godlessness openly. However, most of them,

> when anything befalls them which they would not, since they have never had any firm faith in God their Saviour, they first flee to the help which things created give, to physicians, herbs, drug-mixtures, strict rules of diet, and all the other aids that mortals use. And if one say to them, "Flee, ye fools, to the one and only physician of diseases of the soul[28] and cast away the help, miscalled as such, of the created and the mutable," they laugh and mock, and all their answer is "tomorrow for that," as though, whatever may befall, they would never supplicate God to save them from the ills that beset them. But when no human help avails, and all things, even healing remedies, prove to be but harmful,[29]

26. Philo (541), *Allegorical Interpretation of Laws following the Creation* 3.178; 1:420. Noorda (486), p. 220, n. 17, cites Philo, but only as an illustration of Ben Sira's assertion that God is the healer even when "recovery is [so to speak] in the doctor's hands."

27. Philo (541), *On the Birth of Abel and the Sacrifices Offered by Him and His Brother Cain* 19.70; 2:146, l. 14: τοῖσ ἐπαμφοτεριϲταῖς.

28. Whitaker (541) translates "soul-sickness." Like Pharaoh, the waverers need a physician who will open their eyes to what is behind created things.

29. Whitaker (ibid.) has "mischievous," which is not strong enough for βλαβερά.

then out of the depths of their helplessness, despairing of all other aid, still even in their misery reluctant, at this late hour they betake themselves to the only saviour, God.[30]

Philo condemned "all reasoning that believes everything its property and holds itself in greater honor than God."[31] Seen from a Jewish point of view, Hippocratic medicine might well appear as reflecting that rationalistic attitude. As there are people who "prefer the body before the soul, the slave before the mistress, so there are those who have held the creation in greater honor than God."[32] This theme was to reappear in Christian thought.

A third voice, from about the same time as Ben Sira, comes from Mesopotamia, where the story of God-fearing Tobit originated.[33] He was blinded by "a whiteness" that formed in his eyes as the result of some warm sparrows' dung that had fallen upon them.[34] He went to the physicians, but "they helped [him] not" (Tob. 2:10). After eight years had elapsed (14:2), God ordered the angel Raphael "to scale away the whiteness of Tobit's eyes"(3:17). The angel advised Tobit's son to anoint his father's eyes with the gall from a fish from the Tigris (6:1–3), and to rub them when irritation set in. This would remove the whiteness—and so it happened (11:8 and 13).

The angel had instructed Tobit's son that the heart and liver of the fish, when burnt, would ward off "a devil or an evil spirit" (6:7). "As for the gall," the angel said, "it is good to anoint a man that hath whiteness in his eyes, and he shall be healed" (6:8). That was within the scope of the pharmacological teachings of the time, so that the cure of Tobit's blindness, though divinely planned, was not quite outside the realm of natural means.[35]

If it is permissible to draw conclusions from Ecclesiasticus, Philo, and the story of Tobit, the following picture emerges: Even for pious Jews, there was nothing unusual in consulting physicians. Physicians

30. Philo (541), *On the Birth of Abel* 19.70–71; 2:147 (Whitaker's translation, modified).
31. Ibid. 19.71; p. 148, ll. 3–4.
32. Ibid. 20.72; p. 148, ll. 12–15.
33. Tobit, chaps. 1 and 2. The following translations are quoted from the Apocrypha (29), pp. 70 and 70–71.
34. The description suggests keratoleukoma.
35. Cf. Dioscorides (184), *De materia medica* 2.78; 1:159–60: "All kinds of bile are pungent and heating and differ from one another by the more or less of strength . . . Foremost seems to be that of the sea scorpion and of a fish that is called *kallionumos* . . . That of the wild goat is especially fitting for beginning cataracts and mist over the eyes."

and their medicines were God's creations, and their help could be decisive. It could also fail, in which case God's help, which was the basis of
all healing, remained. Judging by the rabbinical literature, this is an
approximate description of the state of affairs. But though a *modus
vivendi* was established between Judaic religious healing and secular
medicine, the antagonism was not basically eliminated. There remained
those who, like Philo, thought it a matter of no great importance
whether doctors were consulted or not; there were those who condemned doctors[36] and did not want any infringement of God's omnip-
otence by secular interference; and there were those whose trust in secular medicine was greater than their trust in God. The last were more
likely to be found in the thoroughly Hellenized Jewish communities
outside Palestine than in the Jewish homeland. This was the approximate state of affairs at the time of Jesus' appearance in Galilee and
Judaea.

36. Preuss (570), p. 24, cites the view of an anonymous teacher in the Mishna
"that even the best doctor belongs to hell."

9

JESUS

The kingdom of God is close at hand. Repent! Sin no more, and life in God's kingdom will be yours. This was the gospel, the glad tidings, that Jesus brought to the Jews and that the four canonical evangelists, each in his own way, recorded. To be believed, the message required faith in its missionary, Jesus, as a true prophet, as the Messiah (Christ), or as the Son of God. Jesus' solitary appearance, backed by no human authority, gave faith and trust[1] a central position in his life and later in Christianity, the new missionary religion that worshipped him as the Son of God.

"Heal the sick . . . and say unto them, The Kingdom of God is come nigh unto you" (Luke 10:9). This command, which Jesus addressed to the seventy disciples, attests to the close relationship between healing

The literature on Jesus' healing activity is legion. I have tried to present the miracles as related in the Gospels and as accepted in the early Christian centuries. With a few exceptions, no attempt has been made to diagnose the sufferers or to evaluate the effectiveness of the cures.

1. Whereas some miracles were based on religious faith in Jesus, others merely show trust or belief in his capacity to perform miraculous cures. The latter is obvious in the healing done at the request of the pagan centurion who believed in Jesus as a man of authority (Matt. 8:5–13). The Greek πίστις covers either sense. MacMullen's ([436], p. 4 and p. 123, n. 9) warning against always translating it by "faith" is well taken, yet in individual cases it is often all but impossible to make the distinction, and no attempt has been made to do so here; see below, n. 3.

and the spreading of the gospel.[2] One story in particular showed Jesus using healing as the means of legitimizing himself. The bearers of a paralytic lowered him through the roof of the house in order to bring him before Jesus, who was surrounded by a dense crowd (Luke 5:19). When Jesus saw their faith,[3] he told the paralytic, "Son, be of good cheer; thy sins be forgiven thee" (Matt. 9:2). Some Pharisees and scribes thought this blasphemy, because God alone could forgive sins (Luke 5:21). Jesus asked them whether it was easier to say "Thy sins be forgiven thee; or to say, Arise, and walk? But," he said to them, "that ye may know that the Son of man hath power on earth to forgive sins"; he then spoke to the paralytic: "Arise, take up thy bed, and go unto thine house." When the people saw him doing this, "they marvelled, and glorified God, which had given such power unto men" (Matt. 9:5–8).

The absolution from sin and the healing as a proof of power were here two distinct events, separated in time.[4] The absolution from sin did not produce an immediate cure, though the faith that led to the former may have been a precondition for issuing the command to arise. At any rate, throughout much of Jesus' life, preaching the gospel and healing were closely associated. He went about Galilee, the main scene of his activity, "teaching in their synagogues, and preaching the Gospel of the kingdom, and healing all manner of sickness and all manner of disease among the people." His fame had spread beyond the border into Syria, "and they brought unto him all sick people that were taken with divers diseases and torments, and those which were possessed with devils, and those which were lunatick, and those that had the palsy; and he healed them" (Matt. 4:23–24). It was not even necessary for him to exert himself. No sooner had Jesus and his disciples landed at the shore of Gennesaret than he was recognized, and the sick were brought to him in their beds. "And whithersoever he entered . . . they laid the sick in the streets, and besought him that they might touch if it were but the border of his garment: and as many as touched him were made whole" (Mark 6:56).

2. According to Harnack (288), chap. 2, Christianity spread because it promised healing.

3. The Gospel does not tell whether it was faith in him as a man of God or as a miracle worker. Here and in many other stories, faith or trust in Jesus, regardless of the nature of this faith (see above, n. 1), was decisive, though Jesus himself attributed his power to God. John Chrysostom's (322) sermon on the paralytic is an instructive example of the early Christian interpretation of the story.

4. Was the paralytic brought before Jesus to have his sins forgiven or to be cured?

This sounds like magic, and many may have regarded him as a mere magician and miracle worker. Some of his healing acts were accompanied by the laying on of hands and by spitting. For instance, a blind man was brought before Jesus with the request that he touch him. Jesus spat on his eyes[5] and put his hands on him, and when the eyesight had not yet been fully restored, he again put his hands upon the man's eyes (Mark 3:22–25).

In the Gospels, of course, the miracles Jesus performed were not viewed as magic. Jesus valued the faith in himself, even when he may have been regarded as a powerful miracle worker rather than a man of God. The Roman centurion who approached Jesus on behalf of his sick servant took Jesus to be a man of authority whose commands would be obeyed, just as his own were[6]: "Speak the word only, and my servant shall be healed" (Matt. 8:8). "Verily," Jesus exclaimed to those following him, "I say unto you, I have not found so great faith, no, not in Israel." To the centurion he said, "Go thy way; and as thou hast believed, so be it done unto thee." The servant "was healed in the selfsame hour" (Matt. 8:10–13).

The power to heal might emanate from Jesus' garment, but it was the belief in him that activated it. A woman who had suffered for a long time from a bloody flux touched the border of his garment from behind him, and the flux stopped. Jesus could not see her but insisted that somebody had touched him, for, he said, "I perceive that virtue is gone out of me" (Luke 8:46). Trembling and on her knees, the woman told him why she had touched him and "how she was healed immediately." "Daughter," Jesus told her, "be of good comfort: thy faith hath made thee whole; go in peace" (Luke 8:47–48, also Mark 5:25–34).

Faith in Jesus has the power to heal; the faith that heals need not be that of the sick person (it is the centurion rather than his sick servant who expresses belief in Jesus); and it can be activated without Jesus' command (the woman with the flux was healed before Jesus even saw her). But to be effective, the faith must be strong, on the part not only of the supplicant but of the healer as well. This is brought home by the episode of the "lunatick" (Matt. 17:15) boy who had "a dumb spirit" (Mark 9:17). His father had brought him to the disciples, who had been unable to cast the spirit out. Jesus decried the "faithless generation" (Mark 9:19) and asked to see the boy. "If thou canst do any thing, have

5. According to Tacitus (663), *Historiae* 4.81; pp. 603(l. 28)–9(l. 15); and Suetonius (659), *Lives of the Caesars* 8.7.2; 2:298, Vespasian also cured a blind man by spitting upon his cheeks and eyes. This was done as an act of legitimizing himself. Cf. Kee (359), pp. 75 and 130; and Seybold and Mueller (619), p. 104.

6. See above, n. 1. On Jesus' faith in himself, see Meier (451), p. 17.

compassion[7] on us, and help us," the father begged. Jesus replied, "If thou canst believe, all things are possible to him that believeth." With tears the father cried, "Lord, I believe; help thou mine unbelief" (Mark 9:22–24), and Jesus cast out the demon. Asked by the disciples why they had been unable to do so, he told them, according to Matthew (17:20): "Because of your unbelief: for verily I say unto you, if ye have faith as a grain of mustard seed, ye shall say unto this mountain, Remove hence to yonder place; and it shall remove; and nothing shall be impossible unto you."[8] The disciples had lacked the faith that God would act through them.[9]

While the cult of Asclepius presupposed the belief that the god could cure, it did not assume that mere faith in the god would heal; nor did it make healing dependent upon the intensity of this belief. Asclepius did not demand much in return for his services, but the little he did demand was in the form of donations and grateful inscriptions. Jesus, however, made no demands for tangible rewards. The Jewish crowds that expected Jesus to cure their sick probably regarded him as a prophet, a man of God such as Elijah had been,[10] and Jesus himself considered the power given to him to come from God. In a few cases, like that of the centurion, Jesus healed gentiles because of their trust in him. The centurion did not ask where Jesus' authority came from. But to the Jews, Jesus' message of the Kingdom of God was the more credible if it came from an agent of God rather than a mere miracle worker. Altogether there exists an essential difference between Asclepius and Jesus: the Greek god cured because this was his function, whereas Jesus healed in fulfillment of a divine mission.

Jesus likened himself to a physician whose task it was to heal the sick, explaining, "I will have mercy, and not sacrifice: for I am not come to call the righteous, but sinners to repentance" (Matt. 9:13). When performed as a work of mercy, healing springs from motives other than the wish—or the need—to legitimize one's power. It can spring from a very human feeling of pity and compassion, or it can be done as a part of a divine plan that human beings would consider merciful.

7. Mark 9:22: σπλαγχνισθείς. Cf. below, nn. 11 and 23.

8. Matt. 17:21 adds, "Howbeit this kind goeth not out but by prayer and fasting"; see also Mark 9:29.

9. According to Luke 9:1, Jesus had given his disciples "power and authority over all devils, and to cure diseases." In view of the fact that Jesus took trust in himself to be sufficient to effect a cure, it is not impossible that he was thinking of faith as an autonomous power.

10. See Matt. 16:14, as well as Vermes (701), pp. 7–8; and idem, (702), chap. 3, for Jewish charismatic healers in Jesus' time.

In the cases of healing reported in the Gospels, it is by no means always possible to determine whether Jesus' motive was human emotion, a sense of mission, or the need for legitimization. The missionary dedicated to his work of salvation can also be compassionate and use his healing ability to prove himself. Yet there were instances where no motive other than pity seems to have been involved, and there were others where pity was conspicuously absent. When Jesus happened to see the funeral procession of a young man, the only son of a widowed mother, "he had compassion on her,"[11] and said unto her, Weep not" (Luke 7:13). He touched the coffin, restored the young man to life, and returned him to his mother. However, when a gentile woman from the Phoenician coast "cried unto him, saying, Have mercy on me, O Lord, thou son of David; my daughter is grievously vexed with a devil . . . he answered her not a word." To his disciples beseeching him to send her away, he said, "I am not sent but unto the lost sheep of the house of Israel." But the woman "worshipped him, saying, Lord, help me." He, however, told her, "It is not meet to take the children's bread, and to cast it to dogs." Only when she insisted, "Truth, Lord: yet the dogs eat of the crumbs which fall from their master's table," did he accede to her request as he had acceded to that of the Roman centurion, saying, "O woman, great is thy faith: be it unto thee even as thou wilt." Her daughter "was made whole from that very hour" (Matt. 15:22–28).

The woman addressed Jesus as "son of David." Descent from David was a requisite for the Messiah, the Christ. Matthew (1:1–25) recounted all the generations from Abraham through David to Joseph who married Mary, who had conceived "of the Holy Ghost" the child to be called Jesus. If Jesus' work conformed to what the prophets had predicted, he was legitimized as the Messiah. Those who saw the Christ in Jesus, who "shall save[12] his people from their sins" (Matt. 1:21), drew his healing too into the domain of Biblical prophesies and God's design. Matthew (8:16–17) tells of many brought before Jesus who were "possessed with devils: and he cast out the spirits with his word, and healed all that were sick: that it might be fulfilled which was spoken by Esaias the prophet, saying, Himself took our infirmities, and bare our sicknesses."[13] On another occasion, Jesus had healed many, but asked them not to make him known (Matt. 12:15–16). Matthew (12:17–21) adds, "That it might be fulfilled which was spoken by

11. Ἐσπλαγχνίσθη (see above, n. 7, and below, n. 23). The word suggests a visceral feeling.

12. The Hebrew name for Jesus is cognate to the root *shv^c*, for which see Gesenius (258), s.v.

13. Cf. Isa. 53:4–5.

Esaias the prophet,[14] saying, Behold my servant, whom I have chosen
. . . And in his name shall the Gentiles trust."

Healing became even more removed from human emotions and human goals when Jesus was seen as "the true Light" (John 1:9), as God's
"Word . . . made flesh," "the only begotten of the Father" (John 1:14).
It could go so far that disease was declared to have been inflicted in
order to manifest divine purpose, as happened in the case of a man
congenitally blind. Jesus' disciples wondered whether the blindness was
due to the man's own sin or to that of his parents. Jesus answered:
"Neither hath this man sinned, nor his parents: but that the works of
God should be made manifest in him.[15] I must work the works of him
that sent me, while it is day" (John 9:3–4). Having said this, Jesus put
upon the blind man's eyes clay he had soaked with his spittle and told
him to wash in the pool of Siloam. The man did so, and returned able
to see. Brought before the Pharisees, he told them how Jesus had cured
him, and during the ensuing interrogation, sharpened by the fact that
the healing had taken place on the Sabbath, the man called Jesus a
prophet and insisted that unless "he were of God, he could do nothing"
(John 9:33). Thereupon he was thrown out. Then Jesus asked him,
"Dost thou believe on the Son of god?" The man replied, "Who is he,
Lord, that I might believe on him?" Being told that he was looking at
and talking to him, the man said, "Lord, I believe." Then, "he worshipped him" (John 9:35–39).

In this healing process, faith was not involved; faith in Jesus as a
man of God and, subsequently, as the Son of God came only afterwards. The story had a sequel in which Jesus explained his mission to
the Jewish audience, which became divided, one party claiming that
"he hath a devil, and is mad" others objecting that a devil could not
make blind people see (John 10:20–21).

As John relates the miracle of the resurrection of Lazarus (John,
chapter 11), Jesus' task was pitted against human compassion. Jesus
loved Lazarus and his two sisters, Mary and Martha, yet when the sisters asked him to come to Bethany[16] because Lazarus was sick, he delayed and went only after he knew that Lazarus was dead. "And I am
glad for your sakes," he told the disciples, "that I was not there, to the
intent that you may believe" (John 11:15). Lazarus had been in his
grave for four days when Jesus and his disciples arrived in Bethany,

14. Cf. Isa. 42:1–6. Matthew's quotations are very free paraphrases.
15. This particular case does not represent a general denial of sin as a cause of
illness.
16. Bethany was in Judaea, not far from Jerusalem, and dangerous territory for
Jesus (see John 11:8).

where Martha went to meet him. She reproached him for not having come earlier and saved Lazarus's life. Jesus told Martha that her brother would rise again, which she took to mean the resurrection "at the last day" (John 11:24). "I am the resurrection, and the life," said Jesus; "he that believeth in me, though he were dead, yet shall he live: And whosoever liveth and believeth in me shall never die" (John 11:25–26). When Mary, accompanied by the Jews who had come to comfort her, welcomed Jesus, she also reproached him for not having saved her brother in time. Seeing Mary and the Jews weeping "he groaned in the spirit, and was troubled" (John 11:33), and asked where Lazarus had been laid. "Lord, come and see," was the reply. "Jesus wept" (John 11:34–35). Mary warned Jesus of the smell of the dead man, but he reminded her that if she believed, she would see "the glory of God" (John 11:40). After the stone protecting the grave had been removed, Jesus thanked the Father for having heard him. "And I knew that thou hearest me always: but because of the people which stand by I said it, that they may believe that thou hast sent me" (John 11:42). He commanded Lazarus to come forth, and ordered the people to loosen the bandages of the resurrected man and to let him go. Many of the Jews believed in Jesus, but others denounced him to the Pharisees. Lazarus had been allowed to die so that his resurrection would cause the glory of God to shine all the more, and cause faith in Jesus to be confirmed in his disciples and awakened among the Jews. Yet with all this, Jesus could also be troubled in his mind and weep.

Jesus went about curing diseases and throwing out demons, and the synoptic Gospels agree that he instructed the twelve apostles to do likewise. According to Mark (3:15) Jesus gave them "power to heal sicknesses, and to cast out devils" or, as Luke (9:1) puts it, he "gave them power and authority over all devils, and to cure diseases." To the distinction between the curing of diseases and the casting out of devils, Matthew (10:8) added two more categories: cleansing the lepers, and raising the dead.

Demons (devils) were able to recognize Jesus and to communicate with him. The "unclean spirit" that possessed the man of the country of the Gadarenes spoke through the man's mouth. He adjured Jesus not to torment him. He confessed that the spirits were many, and begged Jesus "not [to] send them away out of the country" but to send them into the swine feeding nearby. Jesus "gave them leave," whereupon they entered into the swine, which promptly ran into the sea and drowned (Mark 5:2–13).

The lunatic boy who was possessed by a dumb spirit did not speak, but when he was brought before Jesus, "straightway the spirit tore him;

and he fell on the ground, and wallowed foaming" (Mark 9:20). He and the Gadarene man are examples of intrusive possession, in which the demon seems to have invaded the body and taken command of the individual's personality.[17] These people were the demoniacs proper, usually marked by convulsions and mad behavior.

However, there was also a less dramatic form of possession, in which a disease was attributed to a demon. Luke (13:11–16) tells of a woman "which had a spirit of infirmity eighteen years, and was bowed together, and could in no wise lift up herself." Jesus said to her, "Woman, thou art loosed from thine infirmity." He laid his hand on her, and "she was made straight, and glorified God." Rebuked for having done this on a Sabbath day, Jesus reminded his critics that none of them would hesitate to "loose his ox or his ass from the stall, and lead him away to watering." "And ought not this woman," he asked, "being a daughter of Abraham, whom Satan hath bound, lo, these eighteen years, be loosed from this bond on the sabbath day?"

Nevertheless, the boundary between disease and alleged possession was not fixed. Matthew (8:14–15) relates that Jesus entered Peter's house and found the apostle's mother-in-law "sick of a fever." The fever left her when he touched her hand. According to Luke (4:39), however, Jesus "stood over her, and rebuked the fever; and it left her."

Leprosy had a position of its own. The word leprosy (lepra in Greek) was the Greek rendering of the Hebrew zaraʿath, described in Leviticus (chapter 13) as a condition of the skin that made the individual unclean. If it were healed, it was up to the priest to examine the former sufferer, who had to go through a purification rite before being pronounced clean (Lev. 14:1–7). What Leviticus describes does not look like leprosy as the disease is understood today (Hansen's disease), nor does lepra in the Greek medical literature conform with leprosy. However, it is probable that the Greek term in the Gospels included true leprosy, which came to be widespread in the Orient. If so, then the terminology of the Septuagint and the New Testament is the terminological bridge from zaraʿath and lepra to modern leprosy. At any rate, Jesus observed the Levitic injunction to have a healed leper ritually cleansed by the priest.[18]

If the lepra that Jesus healed was real leprosy, he succeeded where physicians would have failed. The Gospel (Matt. 9:23) tells of Jesus

17. According to Smith (631), possession as the Greeks knew it before their exposure to oriental influences was not intrusive, i.e., the gods and demons took command of a person without, however, invading him or her.

18. See Matt. 8:2–4 and 17:12–19. On zaraʿath and lepra, see the discussion by Grmek (278), chap. 6, especially pp. 160–68.

having cured all kinds of diseases, but certain ailments received special emphasis and were singled out by him. He told the two disciples John the Baptist had sent to him, "Go and shew John again those things which ye do hear and see: The blind receive their sight, and the lame walk, the lepers are cleansed, and the deaf hear, the dead are raised up, and the poor have the gospel preached to them" (Matt. 11:4–5). He could have added more to this list of conditions, most of which (excluding purely psychogenic ailments) doctors could not or did not heal or were not expected to be able to cure. In the case of the woman with the bloody flux, Luke (8:43) noted that she "had spent all her living upon physicians, neither could be healed by any."

Asclepius and Jesus differed radically in the nature of their healing power. Yet both performed miracles, accomplishing what doctors could not do. Both were ready to cure all diseases, but cures of mild, self-limited illnesses were not likely to receive much public attention. It was the extraordinary that caused the multitude to marvel and to praise the Lord.

The comments of Luke (8:43) and Mark (5:26) are remarkable also because they are the only instances where Jesus' cure is contrasted to the unavailing efforts of physicians. In only two more places do the Gospels mention physicians: in quoting the proverb "Physician heal thyself" (Luke 4:23), and in likening Jesus' mission to the physician's task.[19] Otherwise it is as if doctors did not exist. Jesus' acts of healing take place in a world that is outside secular medicine: they are not explicitly said to be superior or preferable. They stand alone as miracles performed by the prophet, the Messiah, the Son of God. They have nothing to do with Hippocratic medicine, nor does Hippocratic medicine have anything to do with them. No Hippocratic doctor attempted to raise the dead; even the god Asclepius had learned his lesson in this regard while still a mortal. As a class, Hippocratic doctors of the Early Empire neither attributed diseases to demons, nor did they engage in exorcising them. A reputable Hippocratic physician was not supposed to undertake the cure of a condition that was, or had become, hopeless.

Doctors were aware of the importance of instilling hope and confidence in their patients; they knew that psychic factors influenced the course of disease and could lead to healing. *Precepts* speaks of some sick people who recovered their health "through their satisfaction with the decency of the physician."[20] Stretching a point (at the risk of stretching it too far), it may be conceded that Hippocratic physicians at least

19. Matt. 9:13.
20. Hippocrates (306) *Precepts* 6; p. 32, l. 11. Cf. above, chap. 3, text to n. 88.

envisaged the possibility that faith in the physician could cure a disease. But they did not set out to cure by faith, which in any case they saw as a general psychological force. For Jesus, on the other hand, it was the faith in him that cured.[21] As the examples showed, many of those who approached him already possessed it; others were cured by his mere command and acquired their faith afterwards, or the question of faith did not arise at all. In spite of the overwhelming importance of faith, it would therefore be wrong to see Jesus as a faith healer pure and simple.

Attempts to diagnose Biblical diseases in terms of current medical categories are very old.[22] The diagnoses largely rely on the alleged cures. Particularly regarding the Gospels, questions as to the nature of the diseases and as to their cures are not promising, because there is no independent support for any unbiased answers. The world of Jesus and the world of secular medicine—including Hippocratic medicine—are not congruent. To the Christians of late Antiquity, the Gospels represented sacred truth, and they saw the cures as historical facts.

Jesus the healer was unique. Only those to whom he had given power and authority to cure could do as he did. Jesus the teacher also was unique, but his message was for all who wished to be worthy of the kingdom of God. They were ordinary people, prone to disease and dependent on others for help. The message that Jesus had for them did not exclude secular healing, but it preached compassion for the sick and attendance upon them.

To explain the Biblical command (Lev. 19:18) "Thou shalt love thy neighbour as thyself," Jesus told the parable of the good Samaritan, who "had compassion"[23] on a man robbed, wounded, and left half dead. The Samaritan "bound up his wounds, pouring in oil and wine, and set him on his own beast, and brought him to an inn, and took care of him." He also gave money to the landlord, telling him, "Take care of him; and whatsoever thou spendest more, when I come again, I will repay thee" (Luke 10:33–35). Acting like the good Samaritan was in accord with Jesus' promise of the kingdom of Heaven to those who had visited "the least of these my brethren" when sick (Matt. 25:36 and 40).[24]

"Blessed are the merciful; for they shall obtain mercy" (Matt. 5:7), Jesus said, and he declared his own work to be one of mercy. He had referred to publicans and sinners who were in need of mercy. Summing

21. However, see above, n. 9.
22. For an example, see Temkin (669).
23. Ἐσπλαγχνίσθη; cf. above, nn. 7 and 11.
24. More on this parable in the Epilogue.

up his accomplishments, he had added to his acts of healing the preaching of the gospel to the poor (Matt. 11:5).[25] His concern was mainly for poor people, for suffering people (Matt. 25:35–45), and for sinners. He left sacrificing to the righteous, and while not excluding rich people from God's kingdom, he wanted them first to divest themselves of their possessions (Matt. 19:21–24; Luke 6:24). Concern for the sick and the poor thus became a special duty for his followers.

The social stratum that supplied most of the clientele of Hippocratic doctors was not of great concern to him. In the parable of the good Samaritan, secular remedies are applied; doctors are not mentioned. Yet the parable does not exclude their use: there is nothing in the story to make it seem implausible that the landlord might have summoned a doctor, if he had deemed it necessary. The Jesus of the Gospels appears to be in no way hostile to secular healing.[26] It is rather a matter of indifference how sick people are cured, as long as there is charity and compassion for them.

The different facets of Jesus' personality—the human being, the Christ, and the divine being, which were to lead to severe Christological struggles—made it difficult to assess his own share of human compassion. But there is no ambiguity about his insistence on compassion among men. This becomes very clear in the episodes of his healing on the sabbath day, which was considered a sin by the Pharisees. It was argued that as a sinner, Jesus could not possibly be a man of God. Jesus' reaction to any such objections was one of indignation. "Thou hypocrite," he called the ruler of the synagogue who censured him for having exorcised a spirit on the sabbath (Luke 13:15). To Jesus it was a question of religious principle whether good and necessary deeds superceded the commandment against working on the sabbath.

"The sabbath was made for man, and not man for the sabbath: Therefore the Son of man is Lord also of the sabbath" (Mark 2:27–28), Jesus said to the Pharisees who had taken exception to his disciples' plucking ears of corn on the sabbath. Then Jesus went into the synagogue, where there was a man with a withered arm.[27] Jesus told the man, "Stand forth," and to the watching Pharisees he put the question whether it was "lawful to do good on the sabbath days, or to do evil? to save life, or to kill?" There was no response. "And when he had

25. On the connection between poverty and sickness, see Agrimi and Crisciani (4), p. 14.

26. The remark regarding the doctors' inability to cure the woman with the bloody flux (Luke 8:43) merely shows Jesus' superiority.

27. The AV translates χεῖρ as "hand." However, the word can also mean "arm," which is preferred by the NEB.

looked round about on them with anger, being grieved for the hardness of their hearts," he commanded the man, "Stretch forth thine arm." The man did as he was told, and his arm was "whole as the other" (Mark 3:1–5). There is no word about faith here, and it is not clear whether compassion for the man or the desire to make a point was Jesus' guiding motive in restoring the withered arm. However that may be, his indignation was for the unfeeling attitude of the Pharisees.

The Gospels show Jesus as he appeared to the mainstream of those who made him the center of a new religion. The Gnostics had their own gospels, and the Jews who refused to accept Jesus saw him and his activity, including healing, in a different light, of which the Gospels allow some glimpses. The Jewish historian Josephus (A.D. 37–c. 100), on the other hand, seems to have thought of him as a "wise man . . . a doer of wonderful work."[28]

What, then, was the place of Hippocratic medicine in the development of the catholic apostolic church, for which the four Gospels became true history, and the other books of the New Testament sources of inspiration?

28. Josephus (352), *Jewish Antiquities* 18.63; 9:48. Cf. Vermes (699), p. 28. Unfortunately, the *Testamentum Flavianum,* Josephus's report on Jesus, has been manipulated so as to make the original text a matter of conjecture.

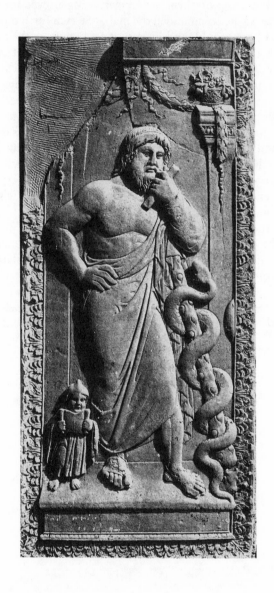

Asclepius, the god of healing, from an ivory diptych, ca. A.D. 400. At his feet stands Telesphorus, the tiny god of convalescence, reading from a scroll. Giraudon/Art Resource, New York.

IV

Early Christianity and
Hippocratic Medicine

10

TO THE TURN OF THE THIRD CENTURY

A. The New Testament

After Jesus' death, his apostles established in Jerusalem a community of believers who held their possessions in common. The primitive Christian church was a Jewish sect similar to that of the Essenes; even Pharisees belonged to it.[1] Jesus had been a missionary of his gospel: the Apostles heeded his command to heal and to preach, and the faith spread.

The events surrounding Peter's cure of a lame beggar at the gate of the Temple illustrate conversion among the Jews. Accompanied by John, Peter told the beggar, "In the name of Jesus Christ of Nazareth rise up and walk" (Acts 3:6). "Walking, and leaping, and praising God," the beggar entered the Temple (Acts 3:8). A large crowd formed, and Peter, addressing them as "ye men of Israel," explained that "the god of our fathers hath glorified his Son Jesus" and that "his name through faith in his name hath made this man strong" (Acts 3:11–16). Peter told them of the crucifixion and the resurrection of Jesus in fulfillment of prophetic predictions and called upon them to "repent" and "be converted" (Acts 3:19). Peter and John were led off to jail, "howbeit many of them which heard the word believed; and the number of the men was about five thousand" (Acts 4:4).

With his last words, as they were reported by the synoptic Gospels,

1. See Acts 15:5.

the resurrected Jesus had told the apostles to "go . . . into all the world, and preach the gospel to every creature" (Mark 16:15). The command "to teach all nations" (Matt. 28:19), though of dubious authenticity, was obeyed after Jesus' death, thus causing the extension of missionary activity to all the Jews outside of Palestine, as well as to the gentiles. The widespread Jewish settlements served as stepping stones; it was in their synagogues that the apostles preached.[2] The drawing of gentiles into the Christian orbit received its strongest impetus after the Pharisee Saul of Tarsus was converted on his way to Damascus (Acts 9:3–6). Paul, as he was now called, had turned from a zealous persecutor to an equally zealous and indefatigable missionary, whose letters, antedating the Gospels, did much to establish Christianity as a new religion. It was mainly at Paul's insistence that gentiles were exempted from circumcision and the strict observance of the Levitic laws (Acts 15:29), a step that made the separation of the Christians from the Jewish people virtually unavoidable. The exodus of the Christians from Jerusalem during the war with Rome, as well as the Jews' concentration on the Law after the destruction of the Temple had put an end to Judaism as a cult religion, intensified this process.

By the beginning of the second century, the abstractions "Judaism" and "Christianity" were already current.[3] Jesus himself had signaled out "the law of Moses," "the prophets," and "the psalms" (Luke 24:44) as the writings that predicted his coming, and these books came to be accepted as authoritative for the Christians. Around the middle of the second century, Justin Martyr estimated that "the Christians from among the Gentiles [were] both more numerous and more true than from the Jews and Samaritans."[4] Christians who were practicing circumcision and observing the Levitic laws gradually found themselves outside the pale of the orthodox apostolic church as defined by Irenaeus.[5] By the end of the second century, the process of separation was virtually complete.[6]

The resurrected Jesus was also reported to have said: "And these

2. See Frend (236) for details, and see idem (237) for a summary. Fox (230), chap. 6 ("The Spread of Christianity"), pp. 263–335, has subjected the whole question of conversion to Christianity to a new analysis.

3. Ignatius (321), *To the Magnesians* 10.2; 1:206. "Paganism" also belongs to these systematizations of doctrine from a Christian point of view; see Fox (230), p. 31.

4. Justin Martyr (355), *First Apology* 53; p. 52 (Dods's translation).

5. See Chadwick (138), pp. 22–23, 42, 66–71, and 80–83.

6. For this sketch of the early spread of Christianity I am greatly indebted to Frend (236) and Daniélou and Marrou (160).

signs shall follow them that believe; In my name shall they cast out devils; they shall speak with new tongues; . . . they shall lay hands on the sick, and they shall recover" (Mark 16:17–18).[7] In the early days, there were already those who spoke in tongues.[8] Charismatic healers must also have existed,[9] though the Epistle of James, which gives explicit directions for what to do in sickness, does not mention them:

> Is any sick among you? let him call for the elders of the church; and let them pray over him, anointing him with oil in the name of the Lord: And the prayer of faith shall save [σώσει] the sick, and the Lord shall raise him up [ἐγερεῖ]; and if he have committed sins, they shall be forgiven him. (James 5:14–15)

The elders were to do as the Apostles did, who "anointed with oil many that were sick, and healed them" (Mark 6:13). And just as the paralytic's sins were forgiven him because of his faith and he was then cured,[10] so here in the case of the Christian who was severely ill.[11] Then James had this advice for all: "Confess your sins[12] one to another, and pray one for another, that ye may be healed [ἰαθῆτε]. The effectual fervent prayer of a righteous man availeth much" (James 5:16). The efficacy of prayer was demonstrated by Elias (Elijah) (James 5:17–18), who prayed that the rain might stop and, later, that it might start again.

The Epistle of James is a sermon preached in the belief that "the coming of the Lord draweth nigh" (James 5:8). It tells the sick Christian what he should do to get well, and it tells it with an eye to his recovery and to his salvation.[13] In the Septuagint, the words that James uses are those used in Jeremiah's prayer: "Heal me [ἴασαί με], O Lord, and I shall be healed; save me [σῶσόν με], and I shall be saved" (Jer. 17:14).

---

7. According to the anonymous reader of my manuscript, "the so-called 'long ending' of Mark, from which these verses are quoted, is widely regarded as a later addition to Mark's Gospel and therefore spurious."

8. See 1 Cor. 14:39.

9. According to Tertullian (673), *Apology* 43.2; pp. 192–94, Christians were famous as exorcists by about A.D. 200.

10. See above, chap. 9.

11. I cannot agree with Cantinat's ([132], p. 247) denial that the patient had to be gravely ill. The elders would hardly have been discommoded in the case of a mild illness.

12. Ἁμαρτίας, which the AV translates as "faults."

13. Cf. *Catholic Encyclopedia* (136), 5:717; also Cantinat (132), pp. 249–52. The citation of Elijah, whose prayers concerned mundane affairs, confirms that James included somatic recovery. I disagree with Dibelius (171), p. 242, who holds that James 5:14 describes a magic ceremony.

James also said: "Is any among you afflicted? let him pray. Is any merry? let him sing psalms" (James 5:13). Here, as in his directions for what to do in case of sickness, James is a single-minded Christian with no thought for whether any nonreligious responses to circumstance are permissible: whether the friends of the afflicted may help him, whether he who is merry may also invite his neighbors to share his joy, and whether relatives, friends, and neighbors may also do for the sick what common sense suggests. It is hard to believe that the sick person's thirst may not be quenched, a bleeding wound not be dressed, and a broken leg not be bandaged or even supplied with a simple splint. Whether summoning a doctor would be compatible with James's vision is indeed problematic; but James does not call on a charismatic healer either. The Epistle of James rivals the Gospels in condemnation of the rich,[14] and for the poor, a doctor may not even have been accessible.

Christian healing as outlined by James disregarded secular medicine instead of demanding its replacement by faith and prayer and showing hostility to it.[15] Similarly, Clement asked God "to heal the sick" in the context of a long list of misfortunes and calamities in which God's help was implored.[16] The first epistle to Timothy advised its recipient to drink a little wine instead of water "for thy stomach's sake and thine often infirmities" (1 Tim. 5:23). It also praised elderly widows who "lodged strangers" and "relieved the afflicted" (1 Tim. 5:10), and among the Apostolic Fathers, Polycarp counted the care of the sick[17] among the presbyter's duties.[18]

Healing was good, and there was no command against secular healing, though some individuals, perhaps even many, might reject having recourse to doctors. This stands out all the more sharply in the face of the unequivocal condemnation of magic and witchcraft, both of which often touched on medicine. They were forbidden by Jewish law,[19] and early Christian sources repeated the ban. "You shall not use magic, you shall not use witchcraft, you shall not murder a child by abortion nor kill it when born," said the *Didache*.[20]

14. See James 5:1–6.
15. I disagree with Angus's ([28], p. 418) generalization (with an eye on the Epistle of James) that for Christians "it would have been a breach of faith to call in a professional physician."
16. Clement (148), *First Epistle to the Corinthians* 59.4; 1:112.
17. Πάντας ἀσθενεῖς, which includes the sick.
18. Polycarp (566), *Epistle to the Philippians* 6.1; 1:290.
19. Deut. 18:10–12; 2 Chron. 33:6. However, the prohibition of the practice of magic seems to have often been disregarded in the Hellenistic and Roman periods; see Stone (649), pp. 82–84.
20. *Didache* (172), 2.2; 1:310–12. See also *Apostolic Constitutions* (33), 7.3; p. 179; as well as above, n. 19.

B. Early Hellenization of Christianity

Jesus spoke Aramaic. The Gospels, however, appeared in Greek, and followed a Hellenistic literary form;[21] they were already part of the Hellenization of Christianity, a process that extended over several centuries. Among the Jews of Palestine, Greek was probably understood by many; among those outside Palestine, it was probably the common language, and Greek culture was probably not unfamiliar to the Jews.

The gradual predominance of gentile converts over Jewish ones compelled a new orientation: the pagan healing god Asclepius was now confronted. The fight to assert Jesus' superiority over his most formidable opponent may go back to the Gospel of John.[22] As long as Christians lived in a Jewish milieu, they shared the idea of the one almighty God and concentrated upon the recognition of Jesus as the Messiah and the Son of God. Pagans, however, needed conversion to monotheism and to all it entailed.

Galen had praised the Christians for their morality, an unusual recognition for his time. But accustomed to having theology treated by philosophers,[23] he looked at Christianity as a philosophy and censured it as grounded on faith rather than on reason.[24] For educated pagans, Christianity had to be defended by rational arguments; they had to be convinced that the Christian faith rested on truth. The plea for understanding was all the more necessary when the hope of an imminent coming of God's kingdom began to pale. Christians had to reconcile themselves to life in a pagan world that despised and ridiculed them and sometimes persecuted them cruelly in outbursts of hatred.

Without taking the trouble to cite any evidence, the Roman aristocrat Tacitus, certainly no friend of Nero, who had caused the persecution of Christians in Rome, branded the Christians as a gang of the worst criminals, fully deserving severe punishment "for their hatred of mankind."[25] There is here an unmistakable social undertone that is still noticeable in the work of Minucius Felix, written around the turn of the third century. In this dialogue, Ciceronian in its urbanity, a participant described Christians as criminals and as people of a low order,

21. Vermes (701), p. 148, n. 28.

22. See Rengstorf (583).

23. For the connection of philosophy and theology from the pre-Socratics to the patristic authors, see Jaeger (335) and idem (337).

24. See Walzer (709), pp. 15, 43, and 53. The Apologist Theophilus of Antioch (681), *Autolycus* 1.8; p. 74, ll. 9–10 and 13–14, pointed out that in all things faith came first. Thus a sick person had to entrust himself to his doctor if he wished to be cured.

25. Tacitus (663), *Annales* 15.44; p. 360, ll. 22–23: *odio humani generis*.

ignoramuses collected from the dregs of society, and credulous women.[26] The eminent role played by women in the rise of Christianity is certain; for the rest, the dialogue itself refuted the alleged social composition of the Christians.

The most savage persecution before the one that occurred under Diocletian took place at Lyons and Vienne (A.D. 179). A certain Alexander, a Phrygian by birth and a physician by profession, had joined the Christian community of the Rhone valley (which had connections with Asia Minor)[27] and had become "known to almost every one for his love toward God and boldness of speech (for he was not without a share of the apostolic gift)."[28] Alexander proved his courage and steadfastness by encouraging his fellow Christians to confess their faith (and thus be doomed to die), which earned him the wrath of the mob and of the governor, and a cruel death. Alexander, like Luke—Paul's "beloved physician" (Col. 4:14)—before him and sundry others after him, confirms the existence of physicians among the early Christians as well as the acceptance of physicians by the Christian communities.[29]

Galen was right in seeing faith as the cornerstone of this religion. Christianity developed in a large number of communities, and Paul's letters to the Corinthians are evidence that there were early disagreements about what to believe. From its very beginning, the unity of Christianity was threatened by beliefs that were heresies from the point of view of a catholic church that was orthodox, the keeper of the only true faith. As Irenaeus, one of its main architects, put it, the church was "the entrance to life; all others are thieves and robbers."[30] Through its bishops and its legitimate priests in succession from the Apostles, the church had received "the certain gift of truth."[31] The church was the guardian of internal unity, and it also supplied an authoritative tradition matching the national religions. It was willing to render unto Caesar that which belonged to Caesar, but by refusing to worship him as divine, it threatened the symbol of the unity of the Roman empire.

The building of the catholic doctrine was the work of the Apostolic

26. Minucius Felix (465), *Octavius* 8.3–4; p. 334. On the social composition of the Christian population of the late second century, see Brown (120), pp. 60–68.

27. Chadwick (138), p. 63.

28. Eusebius (211), *Ecclesiastical History* 5.1.49; 1:431 (Kirsopp Lake's translation).

29. According to ibid. 3.4.6; 1:196, Luke was a physician who, by his association with Paul and the apostles, learned the "healing of souls."

30. Irenaeus (330), *Against Heresies* 3.4; 1:264 (Roberts and Rambaut's translation).

31. Ibid. 4.26.2; p. 462 (Roberts and Rambaut's translation).

Fathers and later theologians. The defense of Christians against their pagan adversaries was carried on by the Apologists. This is by no means a strict distinction: Apostolic Fathers also defended the Christians, and Apologists expounded the faith. Justin Martyr, Athenagoras, Tatian, Tertullian, and Minucius Felix are counted as Apologists because their apologetic works were outstanding and formed the Christian front, so to speak, against paganism. All were philosophers or philosophically trained, and all were themselves pagan converts. "Yes! we too in our day laughed at this. We are from among yourselves. Christians are made, not born." [32]

Apologists asked for justice against unfounded accusations.[33] They also endeavored to minimize the appearance of a willful withdrawal from social and economic life, claiming that Christians participated fully except in spiritual matters and where withdrawal was to their credit:

> While living in Greek and barbarian cities, according as each obtained his lot, and following the local customs, both in clothing and food and in the rest of life, [Christians] show forth the wonderful and confessedly strange character of the constitution of their own citizenship.[34]

This constitution exalted the soul over the body.[35]

Tertullian went into considerable detail about the things Christians shared with their pagan neighbors.[36] Only "procurers, panders, and those who attend lewd women, ... assassins, poisoners, magicians, also diviners, soothsayers, [and] astrologers" could complain of not deriving profit from Christians.[37] Neither the *Epistle to Diognetus* nor Tertullian's remarkable evaluation of Christianity's impact on the private and national economy mentioned medicine and physicians as out of bounds for Christians. Perhaps the practice of medicine was included in the general statement that Christians and pagans were to be found in the crafts.[38] Tertullian praised the advantage that accrued to all from the Christians' famous prowess in exorcising demons and from their

32. Tertullian (673), *Apology* 18.4; p. 91 (Glover's translation). On Theophilus of Antioch, who does not belong to this group, see above, n. 24, and below, chap. 11, n. 1.

33. See the early chapters in Tertullian's *Apology*.

34. *Epistle to Diognetus* (183), 5.4; 2:359 (Lake's translation). According to Lake, this letter belongs to the apologetic literature rather than to the Apostolic Fathers (idem, p. 348).

35. Ibid. 5.5–11; 2:358–61.

36. Tertullian (673), *Apology* 42.1–3 and 8–9.

37. Ibid. 43.1; p. 192.

38. Ibid. 42.3; p. 190: *miscemus artes.*

praying to "the true God."[39] The real damage to the state, which nobody considered or computed, was the waste[40] of so many upright and innocent men.

Irenaeus's great work was entitled *Against Heresies,* and specifically dealt with the Gnostic heresy that flourished during the second century in Alexandria. (Alexandria was a Greek city with a large Hellenized Jewish community, of which Philo is the best-known member.) The Gnostics had created a mystic religion in which pagan, Jewish, and Christian elements were combined. While Gnosticism was rejected by Christians as an aberration, Greek culture and philosophical thinking made their way into the teaching of the two great Alexandrian theologians: Clement, a contemporary of Tertullian; and Origen, the son of a Christian father, a pupil of Clement, and a theologian versed in Platonic philosophy. Clement and Origen represented the incorporation of Greek philosophy into the Christian life, and with them Christian theology began to construct its own, rationally supported doctrines of the nature of God, man, and the world. For this reason, and though Origen's book directed against Celsus was one of the great apologetic works, they will be considered with third-century and later developments.

C. Gods, Demons, and Drugs

In the world of the Gospels, Satan, evil spirits, and demons threatened people on all sides. They possessed them, they caused diseases among them, and they deceived them. The Pharisees said that Jesus cast out devils "through the prince of the devils" (Matt. 9:34). It was Satan who had entered Judas Iscariot (Luke 22:3) and made him betray Jesus; it was Satan again who threatened the work of the Apostles[41] and inspired the heretics. Paul promised the faithful that God would soon "bruise Satan under [their] feet" (Rom. 16:20). Nevertheless, Satan and his host, whom Jesus had rebuked and driven out from so many people, remained in existence to plague the Christians, who saw them trying to thwart God's plans and to seduce them from their faith.

To the traditional demons, Christians now added the pagan gods. The rejection of all these gods was inherited from the Jews, to whom "all the gods of the nations [were] idols" (Ps. 96:5).[42] But whereas Jews

39. Ibid. 43.2; pp. 192–94.
40. Ibid. 44.1; p. 194: *impedimur* and *erogamur* both have an economic meaning.
41. Acts 5:3; 2 Cor. 2:11; 1 Thess. 2:18.
42. The Septuagint translated *'elîlîm* by "demons [δαιμόνια]."

were little concerned with the heathen gods outside their own community, the Christian mission among the gentiles attacked them persistently and publicly. The battle began when Paul caused an uproar among the silversmiths in Ephesus, who felt their craft and their income endangered by Paul's preaching "that they be no gods, which are made with hands" and that the temple of Diana "should be despised, and her magnificence should be destroyed, whom all Asia and the world worshippeth." The irate crowd responded with the cry "Great is Diana of the Ephesians" (Acts 19:26–28).

The Christian opposition to pagan worship was indeed an ever-increasing threat to the cult of the gods, which was expensive and depended on contributions.[43] Tertullian countered the complaint that the income of the temples was diminishing daily, by contending that "our compassion spends more street by street than your religion does temple by temple."[44]

Devils and demons had to be fought mercilessly, yet their existence was needed to explain both the obstacles and the adversities that Christians encountered, and the very existence of evil in a world that was good, as created by God.[45] This may have enhanced the reluctance to declare the heathen gods mere fiction, and the need to demote them to the status of evil demons.[46] For example, Justin told the Roman rulers, "Driven by irrational passion and [the] whip of depraved demons, you punish [Christians] thoughtlessly and without examination."[47] According to Justin, the angels who had mixed with women,[48] and their descendants, the demons, had sown murder, war, adultery, and every evil among men. But in their ignorance, pagan poets and mythologists had adopted the names that these angels had given to themselves and to their offspring and had made them the names of gods.[49] The genealogical accounts of the demons might vary, but there was consensus among the Apologists as to their wickedness and their identity with the Greek gods.

43. See MacMullen (436), pp. 52–55.
44. Tertullian (673), *Apology* 42.8; p. 193 (Glover's translation).
45. See below, text to n. 75; and chap. 13, text to n. 1.
46. Underlying, however, was a reluctance to deny the existence of phenomena whose existence had been asserted. Even the author of *On the Sacred Disease,* with all his distrust of magicians and sorcerers, did not simply declare all magic and sorcery mere fantasy. The Epicureans and Methodists (see Soranus [637], *Gynecology* 1.3 and 4; pp. 5–7 and p. xxxi), on the basis of their atomistic physics, went further in their skepticism, though they did not deny the existence of the gods.
47. Justin (354), *Apology* 1.5.1; p. 14.
48. On fallen angels, cf. Gen. 6:1–4; Kee (358), p. 72; and Stone (649), p. 32.
49. Justin (354), *Apology* 2.4; p. 120. See also idem 1.9, p. 21, where Justin holds forth against the cult of statues.

Asclepius did not escape their condemnation. Justin classed him with other "so-called gods."[50] In addition to mentioning his greed,[51] Tertullian ridiculed the futility of his having medically supported the life of people who were destined to die anyhow on some other day.[52] Minucius Felix thought it laughable that Asclepius, the son of eternally young Apollo, was portrayed full-bearded.[53] Tatian reported that Athene and Asclepius had both used the blood dripping from the decapitated Gorgon: he for saving people; she, the warmonger, for slaying.[54] It was the use of filthy gore, as Tatian referred to the blood,[55] that was reprehensible to him.

Defying and ridiculing Asclepius did not necessarily imply a dismissal of medicine. Arnobius insisted that no pagan god had achieved a cure without having recourse to material means such as drugs, diet, exercise, and so on:

> In this manner, doctors also cure the creature [*animal*] made of earth, [a creature] not entrusted to a science based on truth but founded on an art that is open to doubt and wavers with [its] appraisal of conjectures. There is no virtue in removing with medicaments that which is harmful. These benefits result from the powers of the things and not of the healers.[56]

This criticism did not go much beyond that expressed by Celsus, who had called medicine a conjectural art (*ars coniecturalis*)[57] without, however, dismissing it. But Arnobius's attack was directed at the pagan gods, above all Asclepius,[58] who could do no more than the doctors did with their uncertain art. The doctors' healing was proper for human beings, whereas the true God healed by his own, unassisted power.

> And commendable as it may be [Arnobius continued the above quotation] to know who should be cured by what medicine or [by] what art, this praise is not proper for a god but for man. Indeed for him it is not shameful to have improved the health of a human being by things taken

50. Ibid. 1.25; p. 28.
51. Tertullian (673), *Apology* 14.5; p. 74.
52. Ibid. 23.6; p. 124.
53. Minucius Felix (465), *Octavius* 25.5; p. 385; also Edelstein and Edelstein (197) T 685. Cf. Cicero (142), *De natura deorum* 3.34.83; p. 163; and T 683.
54. Tatian (664), *Oratio* 8.1; pp. 8(l. 27)–9(l. 2). For the underlying legend, see T 92.
55. Tatian (664), *Oratio* 8.3; p. 9, l. 2: λύθρων.
56. Arnobius (51), *Contra gentes* 1.48; cols. 780B.–781A.
57. Celsus (137), *De medicina*, prooemium, art. 48; 1:26.
58. Asclepius is particularly mentioned by Arnobius (51), *Contra gentes* 1.49; col. 781B.

from outside, [while] for a god it is disgraceful not to have the power in himself but to bestow health and freedom from harm with the help of external things.[59]

Previously, the pagan gods had caused diseases and had also cured them. Now that they had become evil demons, their relationship to illness and cure posed questions and complications. In Tertullian's opinion, the demons inflicted diseases and certain dire woes on the body, while on the soul they inflicted "sudden aberrations extraordinary in their violence."[60] Their subtleness and thinness enabled them to act upon the substances of the body and of the soul. The demons were invisible and imperceptible, yet they could be recognized by their actions. As an unknown blemish in the air and in the wind poured out a pestilential breath and also spoiled the crop, so the breath of the demons and the angels[61] corrupted the mind, leading to rages and disgraceful insanities, or savage passions combined with various errors.[62]

Minucius Felix held a similar robust and relatively simple view.[63] The complex relationship of demons to disease, magic, and drugs received a more searching, though one-sided, treatment by Tatian, whose *Address against the Greeks,* published sometime after A.D. 155, gained considerable attention. A Mesopotamian by birth and an orator by profession, Tatian was converted in Rome to Christianity, probably under the influence of Justin, whom he admired and cited.[64] According to Tatian, the demons were the angels who rebelled against God.[65] They were followed by man and, as a consequence, the divine spirit departed from both.[66] The makeup of the demons was wholly material, like that of fire and air. All matter was pervaded by a material spirit, as distinguished from the divine spirit. Man's soul (ψυχή) also was material and hence mortal, but man had retained the ability to know God and to become reunited with the divine spirit.[67] The demons, however, who hated man,

59. Ibid. 1.48; col. 781A.
60. Tertullian (673), *Apology* 22.4; p. 118, ll. 8–12.
61. Presumably the fallen angels, see above, n. 48.
62. Tertullian (673), *Apology* 22.6; p. 118, ll. 18–21. On Tertullian's attitude toward demons, cf. Harnack (289), p. 116.
63. Minucius Felix (465), *Octavius* 27.2; p. 398.
64. See Eusebius (211), *Ecclesiastical History* 4.16; 1:362; idem 4.28; pp. 394–96; and Tatian (664), *Oratio* 18; p. 20, l. 16. I use the Greek text of Whittaker's edition, with its marginal citations of the pages of Schwartz's edition. Cf. below, text to n. 83, for the praise of Justin.
65. See above, n. 48.
66. Tatian (664), *Oratio* 7.2–3; p. 7, ll. 24–31; also idem, 13.2; p. 14, ll. 26–28.
67. Ibid. 13.1–2; p. 14, ll. 10–16 and 21–26.

were trying to bind him to material things and to make him their slave. All that Tatian had to say about disease and healing was seen in the context of the demons' battle to subjugate man by dragging him down deeper and deeper into material things: "If anyone wishes to conquer [the demons], he must reject matter." [68]

Man is subject to diseases as well as to disorders of the matter of which he is made, "but the demons take credit for these whenever they occur, and follow sickness wherever it strikes." [69] It can happen that the demons themselves shake the whole body with the fury of their folly; but when they are smitten by a word of the power of God, they are afraid, they depart, and the sick man is cured.[70]

According to Tatian's general statement, diseases have a material origin. This is supported by his casually mentioning the "change of seasons by which manifold diseases are brought about." [71] The demons do not cause diseases but merely insinuate themselves, through myth, legends, and superstitions, as the cause. Quite logically, Tatian condemns any overt or covert dealing with demons, from the use of antipathetic remedies (as described by Democritus, allegedly a pupil of the magician Ostanes)[72] to the use of drugs: "An affliction is not done away with by antipathy, nor is a maniac cured by pendants of leather." [73] Tatian indicts the use of magic in illness as well as in a spectrum of other conditions. People who are sick or who say they are in love, or who hate, or who long for vengeance take the demons for their helpers. Roots and arrangements of bones and sinews are not active by themselves; they are the material with which the demons' wickedness operates. The demons get hold of the people who use these things and make them their slaves.

Surely, Tatian argues, it can neither be good to assist in hatred of one's neighbor, nor can it be right "to attribute to matter, instead of to God, the aid rendered to maniacs. The demons craftily turn people away from the worship of God and make them trust in herbs and roots." [74] God created all that is good, "but the profligacy of the demons

---

68. Ibid. 16.2; p. 18, ll. 3–4 (Whittaker's translation, modified). The role of the demons in Tatian has been emphasized by Amundsen (16), pp. 345–47.
69. Tatian (664), *Oratio* 16.3; p. 18, ll. 7–9 (Whittaker's translation).
70. Ibid. 16.3; p. 18, ll. 9–12.
71. Ibid. 20.2; p. 22, ll. 21–22.
72. Ibid. 17.1; p. 18, ll. 12–20. This Democritus, whom Tatian identified with the philosopher, was a certain Bolos of Mendes who, under the name of Democritus, wrote a book on sympathies and antipathies; see Whittaker (664), p. 33, note a, and p. 35, note a.
73. Tatian (664), *Oratio* 17.2; p. 18, ll. 23–24.
74. Ibid. 17.3; p. 19, ll. 10–13.

used things in the world for doing evil, and the idea [εἶδος] of evil derives from them and not from the perfect God." [75]

Magic and witchcraft were forbidden to Jews and to Christians, and Tatian's demonology basically followed Justin's, but, not satisfied with rejecting magic arts, he also rejected the use of drugs, declaring that "the use of drugs [φαρμακεία] in any of its forms belongs to the same machinations." [76] The triple meaning of the Greek word *pharmakon* was "poison," "spell" or "magic draught," and "medicament," and Tatian made the medicinal use of drugs subject to the same condemnation as the other uses, "for if somebody is cured by matter, trusting in it, he will be more readily cured by relying on God's power." [77] Indeed, medicinal drugs are of the same substance as pernicious drugs, which are material compositions. [78] We may reject the baser kind of matter, yet "some people" [79] often undertake to heal by associating with evil people and make use of evil means, though for a good end. As a man who is not a robber himself but associates with robbers is punished, so they will be punished by the Lord even though they are not themselves evil and in spite of their good intention. [80]

Having dealt with the associates of evil, Tatian addresses a series of questions to all who make use of drugs: "Why does he who trusts [the working] of matter not wish to trust God? For what reason do you not go to the more powerful ruler but rather cure yourself with grass like the dog, with a snake like the deer, with river crabs like the pig, with monkeys like the lion? Why, I beg of you, do you deify the things in the world? Why do you call yourself a benefactor when healing your neighbor?" [81]

"Follow closely the power of the Word," Tatian continues, "The

75. Ibid. 17.4; p. 19, ll. 16–18 (Whittaker's translation, modified). Evil did not exist before the demons gave it to the world.

76. Ibid. 18.1; p. 19, ll. 25–26.

77. Ibid. 18.1; p. 19, ll. 25–28.

78. Ibid. 18.1; p. 19, ll. 28–30. That which may be pernicious in plants was caused by the Fall (idem 19.4; p. 22, ll. 6–7).

79. Ibid. 18.1; p. 20, l. 2. Tatian uses the indefinite τινες, which may also be rendered by "certain people."

80. Ibid. 18.1–2; pp. 19 (l. 30)–20(l. 8).

81. Ibid. 18.2; p. 20, ll. 8–14. Whittaker translates the last question, "Why if you heal your neighbour are you called a benefactor?"Although outsiders rather than the healer are likely to apply this praise, this translation would shift the guilt away from the addressee. Knowingly or unknowingly, Tatian paraphrased the Wisdom of Solomon 16:12: "For it was neither herb, nor mollifying plaister, that restored them to health: but thy word, O Lord, which healeth all things" (Apocrypha [29], p. 128, [Authorized Version]).

demons do not cure." It is really God's word against the demons, who "by art make prisoners of people."[82] As the "most admirable Justin rightly observed,"[83] the so-called gods resemble bandits who release their prisoners for a ransom. They invade the bodies of "certain people" whose attention they direct to themselves by means of dreams, they command these people to step forward publicly in the sight of all, and having enjoyed the encomia, they fly away, thus terminating the illness they contrived and restoring these people to their former state.[84] This description of "certain people" whom the demons invade, whose praises they enjoy, and whom by leaving they cure of their suggested diseases, sounds like an anticipation of Aristides and his *Sacred Tales*[85] and of Tertullian, who may have been thinking of Asclepius when he declared that demons inflicted diseases, prescribed unheard-of remedies, then ceased doing harm to sufferers, who believed that the demons had cured them.[86]

Tatian is interested in drugs only as used by the demons. He does not believe that drugs cure; however, if this were to be so, the credit should be given to God.[87] Tatian is concerned with theology, not with medicine. The words "medicine" and "physician" do not occur in the *Address against the Greeks* at all. Tatian does not express what he thinks about medicine as a whole, for his criticism does not go beyond pharmacology; neither directly nor indirectly does it touch upon the other two branches of medicine: diet and surgery. Somatic diseases are material processes, as Tatian too believed. Dietetic medicine essentially is a reordering of the way of life; it does not ascribe healing power to any particular remedy. Nor does surgery, as long as it consists of cutting, cauterizing, bandaging, and manipulating the body without the aid of drugs.

Tatian should not be quoted as a witness for early Christian hostility to medicine. More than a hundred years earlier, Philo had gone much further than he. It was Philo who had admonished his readers "to cast away the help, miscalled as such, of the created," and he had included physicians, pharmacy, and dietetics.[88] But although Tatian did not reject

82. Tatian (664), *Oratio* 18.2; p. 20, ll. 14–15.
83. Ibid. 18.2; p. 20; ll. 15–16. See above, text to n. 64.
84. Ibid. 18.2–3; p. 20, ll. 15–24.
85. According to Whittaker (664), p. 37, note d, it was Wilamowitz who suggested an allusion to Aristides. The inscriptions in Epidaurus and Pergamum seem as likely.
86. Tertullian (673), *Apology* 22.11; p. 120.
87. Tatian (664), *Oratio* 20.1; p. 22, ll. 9–10.
88. Philo (541), *On the Birth of Abel* 19.70–71; 2:147 (Whitaker's translation).

medicine, he rejected pharmacology and any entanglement with magic practices. Did Hippocratic doctors also fall under his censure?

In the *Odyssey* (19:487) a wound that Odysseus had received at a boar hunt was bandaged and the blood stilled by an incantation. But antagonism to this kind of magical healing was ancient too. Sophocles warned, "'tis not a skillful leech who mumbles charms o'er ills that need the knife." [89] In principle, Hippocratic doctors rejected magic, purifications, and any association with magicians and sorcerers; the Hippocratic *On the Sacred Disease* gave impressive voice to this attitude. Galen censured Pamphilus, a botanical author, because "he turned to some old wives' tales and certain Egyptian nonsensical sorceries together with some incantations which those add who pick the plants; moreover, he uses [plants] for amulets and other magic practices, all of which are not only superstitious [περιέργους] and outside the medical art, but false as well." [90] As to Galen's reference to Egyptian sorceries, the Greek magical papyri from Egypt offer a plenitude of magic formulae, most of them for nefarious purposes. Medical incantations are not altogether excluded, as, for instance, the adjuration of a spirit who "will tell you about the illness of a man, whether he will live or die, even on what day and at what hour of night. And he will also give [you both] wild herbs and the power to cure, and you will be [worshiped] as a god since you have a god as a friend." [91]

However, principle was one thing and practice another. Besides, it was not always easy to draw the line between legitimate and magical remedies, and there remained the nagging suspicion that the proscribed remedies might be helpful after all. Popular lore did not stop at downright cannibalistic practices, such as drinking human blood, eating of the liver of a fallen gladiator, or drinking from the skull of a dead person. [92] Here Scribonius Largus drew the line: "Whatever is of this kind falls outside professional medicine [*extra medicinae professionem*], although it has apparently helped in some cases." [93] This was in keeping with Roman law, which did not allow a physician to sue for his fee "if he had practiced incantations, invocations, and if, to use the vulgar

89. Sophocles (633), *Ajax* 581–82; 2:51 (Storr's translation).
90. Galen (241), *De simplicium medicamentorum temperamentis ac facultatibus* 6, prooemium; 11:792, ll. 11–16.
91. Quoted from the translation by Betz (91), pp. 7–8 (from Pap. Berlin 5025; for the Greek text see Preisedanz [569], 1:12, ll. 189–92).
92. Celsus (137), *De medicina* 3.23.7; 1:338; and Scribonius Largus (614), *Compositiones* 17; p. 20.
93. Scribonius Largus (614), *Compositiones* 17; p. 20, ll. 29–30. The references are to epilepsy; see Temkin (666), p. 23.

expression of the impostors, he had exorcised. These are not kinds [*genera*] of medicine, though there are people who publicly assert to have benefited from them." [94]

Galen knew "that some of our people have cured epilepsy and arthritis in many cases by prescribing a draught of burned [human] bones, the patients being ignorant of what they drank, lest they be nauseated." [95] And though he, like Scribonius Largus, did not condone such cannibalistic remedies, he and Dioscorides listed human menstrual blood for external use. [96] Galen rationalized the use of remedies proved by mere experience by ascribing their action to their whole substance, rather than to any particular quality. Such remedies were known as empiricals, or *physica* (that is, that in which nature acted by an occult force).

Stoicism—and the central role that Posidonius, its most influential representative in the second and the first centuries B.C., gave to "sympathy" as interconnecting all things in the cosmos—left a strong mark on the so-called Pneumatists, a subdivision of the Hippocratic Dogmatists. Archigenes, one of the later Pneumatists, whom Galen repeatedly mentioned, wrote on antipathetic remedies—occult or empirical prescriptions, many of a downright magic character. The influence of Archigenes extended to the very end of Antiquity, when he was among the authors used by Alexander of Tralles. [97]

According to a late Latin author, some physicians "approved also of amulets and of calling in magicians with their incantations." [98] If this statement is valid for the second century, Bolus of Mendes, the pseudo-Democritus [99] and an alleged pupil of the arch magician Ostanes, had his equals among Hippocratic practitioners of medicine. Moreover, what Lucian says regarding a follower of Alexander of Abonoteichus corroborates the suspicion that even among public physicians, the worst kind of magician-sorcerers could be found. This man was "a sorcerer, one of those who engage in magic practices, wondrous incantations, gratification in love affairs, troubles for [one's] enemies, the

94. Translated from the Latin text of *Corpus iuris civilis, Digesta* 50.13.1, par. 3, as quoted by Edelstein (198), p. 237, n. 109.

95. Galen (241), *De simplicium medicamentorum temperamentis ac facultatibus* 11.18; 12:342. See Temkin (666), p. 23.

96. See Dioscorides (184), *De materia medica* 2.79; 1:161, ll. 15–18.

97. See below, chap. 17.A.

98. Caelius Aurelianus (130), *De morbis chronicis* 1.4.19; p. 516 (Drabkin's translation).

99. See above, n. 72.

excavation of treasures, and succession to estates."[100] Yet this man "professed[101] to be a public physician"; he knew "drugs, many beneficial when compounded yet many baneful," as Homer (Odyssey 4:230) said of the wife of Thon the Egyptian.[102]

At any rate, what Tatian said about the entanglement of "some people" with evil held true even for Hippocratic physicians.[103] As to the substances that animals ate to cure their ills, which Tatian cited in his derisive characterization of medicinal treatment, they were borrowed from the animal lore of the time[104] and had their parallels in medical pharmacology as well. Grass and herbs are covered by the same Greek word, poa, which could stand for herbal drugs in general; the flesh of vipers, as Galen explained,[105] had been found effective in elephantiasis; and river crabs were listed by Dioscorides together with other animal substances, such as the testicles of the hippopotamus and of the beaver.[106]

Tatian's fight was with demons and matter, not with medicine. But if taken out of context, his question "Why do you call yourself a benefactor when healing your neighbor?" and his command "Follow closely the power of the Word" might be extended to physicians in general. Why not, indeed, entrust oneself to God in all disease and give thanks to Him, rather than to doctors? Tatian did not raise these questions; others may have done so without even knowing of him. After all, the questions were very old ones, inherent in Jewish monotheism. They would be raised loudly and insistently when hermits and monks set out to follow Jesus, to give the spirit power over the flesh, and to find the true healer in God and in Christ, the physician.

100. Lucian (432), Alexander the False Prophet 5; 4:180 (Harmon's translation, modified).

101. Δῆθεν, which leaves it open whether he was a public physician or pretended to be one.

102. Lucian (432), Alexander the False Prophet 5; 4:182.

103. On the involvement of physicians in magic, see Edelstein (198), pp. 205–46; also Temkin (666), pp. 21–27.

104. Such as now preserved in Pliny and Aelianus.

105. Galen (252), Subfiguratio emperica 10; pp. 75–80.

106. Dioscorides (184), Materia medica 2.10; 2:125. For additional material, see Riddle (584), pp. 82–88; and Kee (358), pp. 35–47.

THE ADOPTION OF HIPPOCRATIC MEDICINE

A. The Infiltration of Hippocratic Medicine

There is no good evidence that the mass of people, especially educated and well-to-do persons, who had recourse to Hippocratic doctors before their conversion to Christianity shunned Hippocratic medicine thereafter. Rather, the question is when and how Hippocratic medicine moved into the purview of Christian theology, and when and how Christian theologians, starting with the Apologists, began to make use of Hippocratic science, expertise, and wisdom.

The Apologists of the second century, though they attacked the gods and the culture of Greece and Rome, legitimized the use of rhetoric and philosophical argument, and Theophilus of Antioch and Tatian offered a chronology[1] proving that their "philosophy [was] older than the pursuits of the Greeks."[2] If Tatian, with whose *Address* Galen might well have been acquainted, could call Christianity a philosophy, there was nothing remarkable in Galen's doing so. The works of the Apologists were also missionary works, and to assert their religion, to spread it, and to defend orthodoxy against heresy, Christian authors used the

---

1. With the help of his chronological calculations, Theophilus of Antioch (681), *Autolycus* 3.20; p. 246, placed Moses about 900 to 1000 years before the Trojan war. He proved that the prophets and the origins of the Christian faith were old, and far from being recent lies and fables (idem, 3.29).

2. Tatian (664), *Oratio* 31.1; p. 31, ll. 4–5. See also idem 35–41.

concepts and the imagery of the Bible as well as of the culture they and the pagans had in common.

To condemn the pagan gods and to claim moral superiority for the Christian way of life was a part of the Christian's faith, shared by simple folk as well as by the philosophically educated, though it was left to the latter to defend it and make it plain to the heathen. But the Christian religion contained articles that faith might accept, yet at which reason balked, as in the case of the resurrection of Jesus and of human beings. Pagans mocked and Christians disagreed among themselves.

Trouble began with Paul's address to the Athenians. All went well until he spoke of the day on which God would have the world judged by the man whom He had raised from the dead. When Paul's audience "heard of the resurrection of the dead, some mocked: and others said, We will hear thee again on this matter. So Paul departed from among them" (Acts 17:32–33). From Athens, Paul went to Corinth, where he concentrated on the conversion of gentiles.[3] However, the new congregation began to be troubled by dissension (1 Cor. 1:11–13), and in his first letter he tried to answer those among them who said "that there is no resurrection of the dead" (1 Cor. 15:12).

Belief in the pure spirituality of Jesus, coupled with the assumption that his body and the pain he suffered in the crucifixion merely existed in the eyes of the beholders, offered a possible way out. This heresy, which became known as Docetism, may have raised its head in Corinth.[4] However, Docetism found an early adversary in Ignatius, who combined a hatred of heretics with the idea that heretics were sinners, and hence the kind of sick people whom Jesus had come to call to repentance. Warning against those who were to be shunned "as wild beasts, for they are ravening dogs, who bite secretly," Ignatius added: "for they are scarcely to be cured. There is one Physician, who is both flesh and spirit, born and yet not born, who is God in man, true life in death, both of Mary and of God, first passible and then impassible, Jesus Christ our Lord." [5] The acknowledgment of Jesus in all his attributes, including his existence as both flesh and spirit and his ability to feel pain and then become impervious to it, was the only cure for them.

Among Christians, the debate about the resurrection was to involve the relative value of body and soul. But for Christians as for pagans,

3. See Orr and Walther (517), *1 Corinthians;* pp. 82–83.
4. See ibid.
5. Ignatius (321), *To the Ephesians* 7; 1:181 (Lake's translation). For the gnostic interpretation of Jesus' resurrection, see Pagels (521), pp. 3–27 and 82–83.

the possibility of a resurrection of the body was at the bottom of the difficulty. The survival of the soul had been asserted by Plato and was not inconceivable to the pagans. But the resurrection of the body was another matter. For "children of the Church," the exposition of the truth in plain words or with scriptural citations and Apostolic texts could be deemed sufficient, wrote the author of a work on the resurrection (ascribed to Justin, though his authorship is not beyond dispute).[6] But unbelievers, especially pagans, had to be convinced of the very possibility of a resurrection of the flesh. For them, he explained, the resurrection demanded "arguments drawn not from faith, for they are not within its scope, but from their own mother unbelief—I mean, of course from physical reasons."[7] And so Justin adduced Plato, Epicurus, and the Stoics, all of whom in their own ways, he said, agreed that the elements out of which all things were generated were indestructible. Therefore, it was possible for God to reconstruct the body out of its elementary parts.

The book ascribed to Justin, whether genuine or not, shows the direction in which Christian theologians had to look for support, though his relatively simple solution was not enough to rebut the sophisticated objections of pagan doubters: Suppose that a human being had been devoured by an animal and the human flesh assimilated to the animal flesh. Suppose further that a second person ate of this animal and assimilated its flesh to his own flesh. Or, suppose that wittingly or unwittingly a cannibalistic act had taken place, with the same result— the assimilation of one person's flesh to that of another. In either case, the resurrection of one body was possible only at the expense of the other.[8]

Here was a disconcerting argument resting on the physiology of digestion. Athenagoras—if it was he who had written *The Resurrection of the Dead*—took up the challenge and tried to meet it on its own physiological ground. By God's foresight, not everything ingested was utilized. Digestion took place in stages: in the stomach, the liver, and the parts to be nourished, which could accept or reject what was offered to them. Now, every kind of animal depended on food proper for it, and only the portion of its proper food that had been completely purged by digestion and harmonized with the body was assimilated. Everything else must "either pass through the belly before it produces strange raw

6. See Quasten (576), 1:205.
7. Justin (355), *On the Resurrection* 5; p. 346 (Dods's translation).
8. Athenagoras (57), *Resurrection of the Dead* 4; p. 84.

juices or rottenness," or else it will lie there for a long time and cause pain or intractable disease. It will corrupt the proper food or even the flesh, until eventually it may be "dislodged by drugs or by better food, or because it has been mastered by the power of nature," but not without considerable harm.[9]

The dissolution of ingested improper food into its hot, cold, wet, or dry elements had no bearing on the resurrection. The elements would enter into the blood and other humors, but "blood and phlegm, bile and breath no longer make any contribution to life."[10] They will not be needed in the resurrected body that is composed of the organic parts. Even if it were argued that the body takes its nourishment from the humors and therefore must be affected by improper food, such food need not remain in the flesh. Metabolic change (as we would say), and pain, weariness, and all kinds of diseases and distempers would take care of its ejection. In short, human bodies can never be integrated into other human bodies.[11] "Indeed, the creator has not assigned any animal as food for others of its kind"; as for cannibalism, it "is a horrid abomination."[12]

Athenagoras regarded his defense of the resurrection of the body as the extirpation of falsehood which had to precede the seeding of truth, just as the physician cannot "introduce any wholesome medicine into the body that needed his care, if he did not previously remove the disease within or stay that which was approaching."[13]

If *The Resurrection of the Dead* really was written by Athenagoras, it hails from the second century. The physiology of the book not only is broadly Hippocratic[14] but also approaches the physiology of Galen,[15] and the harmony with medical theories of the second century has been cited in defense of Athenagoras's authorship.[16] But even if the book

9. Ibid. 6; p. 87 (Crehan's translation).
10. Ibid. 7; p. 88 (Crehan's translation).
11. Ibid. 7; pp. 88–89.
12. Ibid. 8; pp. 89–90 (Crehan's translation).
13. Athenagoras (355), *On the Resurrection of the Dead* 1; p. 424 (Dods's translation). For additional discussion of the problem of the resurrection among patristic authors, see Grant (268), pp. 251–63, and Brown (115), especially pp. 222–24 and 441–42, on the relationship between ascetic discipline and the resurrection.
14. Cf. Hippocrates (302), *On Regimen* 1.6; 4:240, regarding the elimination of unsuitable food.
15. See Crehan (57), pp. 170–71, nn. 16–23. However, the agreement with Galen is not very specific.
16. Ibid., p. 177, n. 62a.

belongs to a later date, it demonstrates that Hippocratic ideas were needed to meet the objection to the resurrection that Augustine still was to call most difficult.[17]

As a part of Greek philosophical culture, Hippocratic medicine was readily adopted around the turn of the third century by Clement of Alexandria and, in particular, by Origen, who was looking for a synthesis of Christian faith and Greek philosophy. In Origen's opinion, Ecclesiasticus 1:1 ("All wisdom cometh from the Lord") meant that all the skills deemed necessary for human use, as well as man's knowledge of any given subject, should be attributed to God. "And surely there can be no doubt about medical knowledge. For if there is any knowledge [that comes] from God—which will be more so than the knowledge of health,[18] in which the virtues of herbs as well as the qualities and differences of [the] humors are discerned?"[19]

At about the same time, there was in Rome a heretical Christian sect, some of whose members "almost worshiped Galen," that studied Euclid, Aristotle, and Theophrastus, and wished to replace faith by logical proof.[20] Their alleged enthusiasm for Galen may have had its source in his writings or in personal acquaintance; at any rate, it confirms the openness of some Christians to Hippocratic doctrines.

It was not necessary to embrace Hippocratic medicine as a whole to find much in it useful. Where Hippocrates spoke as an expert, as in his *Aphorisms*, his opinions were not open to judgment by the common people. As examples, the pagan Alexander of Aphrodisias quoted the dicta "Spontaneous fatigue indicates disease," and "Liquid diets are good for those with a fever."[21] Hippocratic sayings could, therefore, be used to buttress one's opinions. Christian theologians continued what pagan philosophers had done. For instance, there was the Hippocratic saying "The practice [ἄσκησις] of health [consists in] moderation in

17. Augustine (58), *City of God* 22.20; 2:515. The recourse to Hippocratic physiology in the problem of the resurrection has been mentioned by Schadewaldt (608), p. 18 of the reprint.

18. For medicine as the science of health, see Galen (242), *De sectis ad introducendos* 1; 3:1.

19. Origen (515), *In Numeros homiliae* 18.3; vol. 12, col. 715B: "in qua etiam herbarum vires, et succorum qualitates, ac differentiae dignoscuntur." I take *succorum* to be the human humors rather than juices in general.

20. Walzer (709), p. 77. See Eusebius (211), *Ecclesiastical History* 5.28.14; 1:522. Cf. Temkin (667), p. 55.

21. Alexander of Aphrodisias (6), *In Aristotelis Topicorum libros*, p. 73 (on *Topica* 104a33). Cf. Hippocrates (302), *Aphorisms* 2.5; 4:108; and idem 1.16; 4:106; also Nachmanson (476), p. 99.

food [and in] not shrinking from toil."[22] Plutarch alluded to it, and so did Isidore of Pelusium, both taking it literally.[23] But Clement of Alexandria adapted it to the Christian life, demanding asceticism in everything that aroused passion and promoted luxury and licentiousness. In so doing, he broadened the Hippocratic meaning to include the health of both body and soul.[24]

Direct or indirect acquaintance with the Hippocratic work *On the Number Seven*[25] enabled a patristic author of the early third century, Hippolytus of Rome, to denounce an alleged saying of Jesus as belonging to Hippocrates rather than to Jesus. The Gnostics had improperly used the Hippocratic division of human life into seven ages to put a statement about the date of his appearance into Jesus' mouth.[26] This is an example of the support Hippocrates could offer in debates against opposing philosophical systems and heresies.[27] Hippocrates also gave valuable help to Augustine in his struggle to free himself from a belief in astrology. From Cicero, Augustine borrowed the following story:

Cicero says[28] that Hippocrates, the most renowned physician, left it in writing that he suspected certain brothers to be twins because they fell

22. Hippocrates (309), *Epidemics* 6.4.18; 5:312. See also Hippocrates (302), *On Regimen* 2.60; 4:346.

23. Plutarch (562), *De tuenda sanitate praecepta* 15.129F; 2:254; Isidore of Pelusium (331), *Epistolae* 5.528; col. 1625C. Cf. Nachmanson (475), p. 198, n. 4; and idem (476), p. 106, n. 4.

24. Clement of Alexandria (151), *Stromata* 2.20; vol. 8, col. 1072A: Γίνεται δὲ ἡ ἄσκησις κατὰ τὸν Κῷον Ἱπποκράτην, οὐ μόνον τοῦ σώματος, ἀλλὰ καὶ τῆς ψυχῆς ὑγείας ἀοκνίη πόνων, ἀκορίη τροφῆς. Cf. Nachmanson (476), p. 106, n. 4.

25. On this work, see Roscher (304).

26. "He who looks for me will find me among the children of over seven years; indeed, hidden there, I manifest myself in the fourteenth eon." Hippolytus objected, "This is not [the word] of Christ but of Hippocrates who says: 'a child of seven years is the half of his father.'" The *Philosophoumena* of Hippolytus was formerly ascribed to Origen (see Littré [309], 8:627, who also suggested *On the Number Seven* as the possible source), and I have used the Greek text of Origen (511), *Contra haereses* 5; col. 3134A, for the above translations. Siouville (312), 1:132, the French translator of Hippolytus, explains: "*In the fourteenth eon* here means *in the fourteenth year.* However, there is an allusion to the system of eons."

27. Probably through its Latin version, the Hippocratic work was well known among Latin patristic authors. Ambrose (10), *Letters* 50; p. 269, wrote, "The number seven should be esteemed because the life of man passes through seven stages to old age, as Hippocrates, the master of medicine, has explained in his writings" (Beyenka's translation).

28. Probably in the lost *De fato*.

ill simultaneously, and their disease became worse and was eased at the same time. Posidonius, the Stoic, much given to astrology, used to assert that they were born and conceived under the same constellation. Thus, what the physician believed to be related to a very similar constitution, the philosopher-astrologer related to the power and disposition of the stars at the time they were conceived and born.[29]

The Hippocratic works mention the case of two brothers whose illness started at the same time and took a similar course,[30] and it has been suggested that Cicero and Posidonius had this case in mind.[31] Augustine thought that "in this case the medical conjecture is much more acceptable and more credible because of what is most obvious."[32] The parents' somatic disposition at the time of intercourse could have affected the fetuses in their very origins, and having derived the same nutriment from the maternal body, they could have been born in the same state of health. They were reared in the same house with the same food—and "medicine attests to the power of air, locality, and the strength of waters[33] over the good or bad state of the body. And, having also been accustomed to the same exercise, they would have possessed bodies so similar as to react similarly to the same causes at the same time."[34] The similar dispositions of twins were thus attributed by Augustine to common hereditary, nutritional, and environmental factors; moreover, the dissimilarities in the later fate of twins could also be used as an argument against astrology: "We know that twins not only engage in different activities and travels but also endure diseases that are not similar. On this matter, as far as I can see, Hippocrates would give a very simple explanation: [exposed to] different foods and exercises, which do not depend on the body's constitution but on the soul's will, they could also have presented different states of health."[35]

The likely Hippocratic sources were *On Airs, Waters, Localities* with its strong environmental emphasis, and *On Regimen,* in which the similarity of twins was explained by their developing in the same

29. Augustine (59), *City of God* 5.2; 2:138–40. See also Edelstein and Kidd (205), frag. 111; pp. 109–10.

30. Hippocrates (302), *Epidemics* 1.20; 1:176.

31. Edelstein and Kidd (205), p. 109. However, far from suspecting them to be twins, Hippocrates spoke of the brothers as the older and the younger. The suspicion seems to have been Posidonius's.

32. Augustine (59), *City of God* 5.2; 2:140.

33. An obvious borrowing from the Hippocratic work of that title.

34. Augustine (59), *City of God* 5.2; 2:140. This explanation is not contained in *Epidemics.*

35. Ibid.

uterus, gaining individual existence simultaneously, growing by the same nourishment, and seeing the light of day together.[36] Augustine had become so deeply involved in astrology that even his aged friend the physician Vindicianus, who had studied Hippocrates, could not dissuade him.[37] Vindicianus is a likely source of Augustine's Hippocratic argumentation. Nevertheless, Augustine's distrust of astrology grew, and when he heard that a noble friend of his and a slave were born under the same constellation, his doubts hardened. It was then that he began to pay attention to "those who are born as twins," usually with a minimal interval of time in between.[38] In the final analysis, as Augustine came to realize, astrology absolved man from all sin, for by subjecting all human actions to the stars, it shifted the responsibility to their creator and governor. "And who is he if not our God." [39]

Augustine's argumentation had its pagan counterparts in the use of Hippocratic expertise against a different philosophy. Thus Sextus Empiricus, who wished to confound the Stoic doctrine of the superiority of man's rational capabilities over those of dumb animals, counted among the accomplishments of the dog its observation of Hippocratic rules. Since rest cures the foot, as Hippocrates had taught, the dog "lifts [its foot] if it is injured and keeps it undisturbed as much as possible. And when [the dog] is troubled by strange humors, it eats grass, after which it vomits and becomes healthy." [40]

These examples of the infiltration of Hippocratic medicine into other fields illustrate that there was a need for its scientific aspect in theoretical discussions. On a broader level, Hippocratic medical science was needed for the elaboration of a Christian anthropology, a doctrine of man that accepted those parts of Greek natural philosophy that were useful, without sacrificing Christian beliefs. Hippocratic medical science became part of the building of a Christian universe without neglecting pagan knowledge, but a part that had its particular problems, such as safeguarding the immortality of the soul. God had created man

36. Hippocrates (302), *On Regimen* 1.30; 4:272.

37. Augustine (60), *Confessions* 4.3; 1:152–54; and idem 7.6; 1:350–52. On Augustine's relationship to Vindicianus and his attitude to astrology, see Brown (114), pp. 57–58 and 67. Augustine (60), *Confessions;* 1:156, suggests that, impressed by the names of the authors of astrological works (e.g., Ptolemy), he wanted proof that their predictions were due to chance.

38. See Augustine (60), *Confessions* 7.6; 1:352–58. For his study of twins, see idem (58), *City of God* 5.2–6.

39. Augustine (60), *Confessions* 4.3; 1:152.

40. Sextus Empiricus (618), *Hypotyposes* 1.71; 1:43. Hippocrates (302), *On Fractures* 9; 3:120, advised rest during the twenty days of recovery. The example of the grass-eating dog was probably current folklore.

in His image, and Christians ought to take cognizance of the medical, anatomical, and physiological investigations of the pagans:

> Thousands of things have been studied by them of which none of us has any experience, because no instruction is given in this part of inquiry, and because we do not all of us wish to know who we are. For we are content with knowing heaven better than ourselves. Do not despise the wonder within you![41]

The best-known Christian anthropology is *On the Nature of Man,* by the bishop Nemesius of Emesa. Paraphrased into Latin by the archbishop Alfanus of Salerno in the eleventh century, it became one of the most influential Christian anthropological works. Nemesius built largely on Galen, but rejected his suggested identification of the soul with the temperament of the brain.[42]

Not only was Hippocratic medical science incorporated into learned theology but also, through popular sermons such as those on the six days of creation (the Hexameron), some Hippocratic teachings were passed on to ordinary people. Ambrose of Milan, in a somewhat garbled account, said that "those skilled in the art of medicine maintain, in fact, that the brain is placed in a man's head for the sake of the eyes and that the other senses of our bodies are housed close together on account of the brain. The brain is the source of our nervous system and of all the sensations of voluntary movement." He asserted that the nerves "proceed from the brain like cords and musical strings. They fulfill their individual functions throughout the various parts of the body." But he also made the brain "the starting point of the arteries and of that natural heat which gives life and warmth to the vital parts," though he added that "many are of the opinion that their starting point is the heart."[43]

B. Soul and Body

Hippocratic doctors were not banished from Christian life, and Hippocratic medical science gained entry into Christian theology. But

41. In a previous book (Temkin [667], p. 81), I assigned this passage to Gregory of Nyssa (275), *In Scripturae verba: Faciamus hominem ad imaginem et similitudinem nostram,* oratio 1; col. 257B–C. Frings (239), p. 95, n. 38, adds, "ebenso Pseudo-Basil. 30, 57." However, Smets and van Esbroeck (85) have shown that this is probably a paraphrase from Basil's work; see below, chap. 13, n. 28. Brown (115), pp. 293–94, reveals a different view of Gregory's ideas of the human body: whereas Adam originally was created in the image of God, the body after the Fall "'is now plain to view in all its wretchedness'" (idem, p. 294, Brown quoting Gregory).

42. See below, chap. 15.B.

43. Ambrose (11), *Hexameron* 6.61; p. 273 (Savage's translation).

the usefulness of the medicine of the body, both for the healing of the body and for theological dispute and teaching, did not assure it a place with the Christian medicine of the soul comparable to its pagan appreciation. To be sure, Plato had made the dying Socrates console his friends with the idea that in death the philosopher's soul was freed from the prison of the body.[44] Plotinus had viewed his body with shame rather than with pride.[45] Galen had thought the philosopher's task in shaping the health of the soul superior to the physician's concern with the relationship between the soul and the body.[46] Cynics might neglect the body[47] and Stoics value virtue higher than health. But bodily health held its place not only in the lives of men but also in their thoughts. The healthy body was beautiful, and the gods—with some exceptions— were represented in the shape of beautiful human beings. To Homer, a healthy, beautiful human being was godlike, and the misshapen Thersites was an object of contempt.

For Christians, however, the body became a problem. On the one hand, the flesh was despised and its desires, especially its sexual desire, severely repressed. On the other hand, the body housed the soul, and for that reason, if for no other, it deserved respect. Origen, who inclined toward a spiritual understanding of man's resurrection, conceded that the dead body might as well be thrown away were it not that "respect for the soul that [had] dwelt within" induced us to give the body honorable burial.[48]

Indeed, the discussion over the resurrection revealed the difficulty very clearly. In his dispute with the Corinthians, Paul insisted that without the resurrection of Jesus and of the dead, Christian preaching and Christian faith were in vain (1 Cor. 15:14–15). He answered the question "How are the dead raised up? and with what body do they come?" (1 Cor. 15:35) by declaring that the natural body is corruptible, it is seed sown in dishonor and weakness, yet like wheat grown from seed, it is raised in incorruption and in power as a spiritual body. "Flesh and blood cannot inherit the kingdom of God," but at the last trumpet "we shall all be changed, in a moment, in the twinkling of an eye . . . For

44. Plato (552), *Phaedo* 28–32.
45. Porphyry, *Life of Plotinus*, in Plotinus (560), 1:2.
46. See above, chap. 2.
47. See, for instance, the description of Democritus above, chap. 6.B.2.
48. Origen (510), *Contra Celsum* 5.24; p. 282 (Chadwick's translation); see also idem 5.14; pp. 274–75 (Chadwick's translation). The problem that the body and its relationship to the soul presented to the early Christians has been made the subject of Brown's (115) *The Body and Society: Men, Women, and Sexual Renunciation in Early Christianity.* Its subtitle indicates the aspect under which Brown approaches the problem. I regret that this book appeared too late for me to give it the full consideration it deserves.

this corruptible must put on incorruption, and this mortal must put on immortality" (1 Cor. 15:50–53).[49]

Heretics contended that in denying the kingdom of God to flesh and blood, Paul denied the resurrection of the body. Yet the resurrection of the body became Christian doctrine, and Irenaeus made Paul's denial of the kingdom of God to flesh and blood the cornerstone of his orthodox argument. What was impossible for mere flesh and blood was possible for the complete human being, formed in the image of God, in whom the soul "that accepts the spirit of the Father" is commingled and joined with the flesh.[50]

This was not just a continuation of the debate about the physiological possibility of the resurrection. At issue was the value of the mortal body. As a letter antecedent to or contemporary with Irenaeus put it:

> Let none of you say that this flesh is not judged and does not rise again. Understand: in what state you receive salvation, in what state did you receive your sight, except in this flesh? We must therefore guard the flesh as a temple of God, for as you were called in the flesh, you shall also come in the flesh. If Christ, the Lord who saved us, though he was originally spirit, became flesh and so called us, so also we shall receive our reward in this flesh.[51]

Jesus was believed to have referred to his body as a temple (John 2:19–21), and the comparison of the body to a temple of God occurred repeatedly in the early Christian literature.[52] In defense of the resurrection, Irenaeus could even cite Paul: "Know ye not that ye are the temple of God, and that the Spirit of God dwelleth in you? If any man defile the temple of God, him shall God destroy; for the temple of God is holy, which temple ye are" (1 Cor. 3:16–18).

Defenders of the resurrection tried to show that the resurrected body would be free from diseases, disabilities, and base desires. At any rate, the body that God had formed in His likeness was not a vile

49. See also 1 Thess. 4:14–17.

50. Irenaeus (328), *Against Heresies* 5.6.1; col. 1137A. On the *imago Dei* doctrine (that "God created man in his own image" [Gen. 1:27]), which plays a great role in Irenaeus's work, see Ferngren (217). For Irenaeus, cf. also Grant (268), pp. 248–49. It was, however, also contended that only before the Fall was man the *imago Dei*; cf. above, n. 41. Flesh (σάρξ) and body are not identical, insofar as the flesh is embodied earthly desire. Matt. 26:41 (quoted below) opposes the spirit to the flesh, and the body rather than the flesh is a temple. This distinction, however, is not consistently drawn.

51. Clement (149), *Second Epistle to the Corinthians* 9.1–5; 1:141–43 (Lake's translation).

52. For instance, Ignatius (321), *To the Philadelphians* 7.2; 1:246.

thing.[53] If it was true that the flesh led the soul to sin, it was also true that the flesh did not sin unless it be incited by the soul.[54] Body and soul, as partners in good and bad deeds, must both be rewarded and punished.[55]

Regard for the body was not easily reconciled with Jesus' remark "The spirit indeed is willing, but the flesh is weak" (Matt. 26:41), and with Paul's exhortation "If ye live after the flesh, ye shall die: but if ye through the Spirit do mortify the deeds of the body, ye shall live" (Rom. 8:13). There remained the question of how much care in health and disease to give to the body, and how far to go in mortifying the flesh.

In different form, the problem was inherent in the Jewish belief in disease as a trial inflicted by God (as in the Book of Job) or as the castigation of those whom the Lord loved (Prov. 3:12). Smitten by Satan "with sore boils from the sole of his foot unto his crown," Job did nothing but take "a potsherd to scrape himself withal" and sit down "among the ashes" (Job 2:7–8). Job's passivity[56] accentuated his submissiveness to the will of God, but it did not mean that he was insensitive to suffering or had Stoic contempt for the disease. Paul all but gloried in the thorn in his flesh (2 Cor. 12:7–10)—whatever it may have been. In his last prayer before being burnt alive, the bishop Polycarp of Smyrna praised God for having thought him worthy of partaking of the cup of Christ as one of the martyrs. The letter by the Church of Smyrna describing the persecution affords an insight into the thoughts and feelings that inspired early Christians to endure torture and death:[57] "And fear not them which kill the body, but are not able to kill the soul; but rather fear him which is able to destroy both soul and body in hell" (Matt. 10:28). The flesh was despised and yet it was not. By comparison, the fear of eternal fire made the fire of the torturers seem cold.[58] Polycarp met the threats of the imperial official by comparing the fire that would burn him now with the eternal fire reserved for the impious at the day of judgment.[59] In contrast to Stoics and Epicureans, who

53. Justin (355), *On the Resurrection* 3–4; pp. 343–45. Cf. Ferngren (217), pp. 39–40. According to Harnack (289), *Medicinisches aus der ältesten Kirchenge-schichte*, p. 78, n. 2, Tertullian, in opposition to the Manichaeans and to Origen, also defended the body.

54. Justin (355), *On the Resurrection* 8; p. 349.

55. Athenagoras (57), *Resurrection of the Dead* 20–21; pp. 109–11. On the questionable genuineness of the books by Justin and Athenagoras on the resurrection, see above, section A of this chapter.

56. He made no attempt to seek a cure.

57. *Martyrdom of Polycarp* (567), 14.2; 2:330.

58. Ibid. 2.3; 2:314.

59. Ibid. 11.2; 2:326.

minimized the importance of bodily pain, Christians tended to maximize it, so that suffering endured in obedience to God and Christ made the victory of the spirit over the flesh stand out all the more.

In all such disputes, the supreme value of the immortal soul was not questioned. At best, the body was thought to be the partner of the soul, and at worst it was despised as its degrading vehicle. The dogma of the resurrection of the body triumphed, yet both ways of viewing the body persisted, the positive in secular Christian life, the negative in the tendency to asceticism. Both were reflected in the attitudes toward healing and the healer.

C. Medicine and Christian Ministry

"Error resembles a disease or insanity that, for a time, renders a person sick or insane," wrote a bishop of the late second century.[60] Heresies were errors and hence resembled diseases. Irenaeus ended his detailed discussion of heretical doctrines by asserting the impossibility of healing the sick without a knowledge of the patient's diseases.[61] Theodoretus, who wrote a book exposing the errors of pagan philosophy and expounding their cure by the truth of God's word, called it *Cure of the Greek Diseases*.[62] It may well have been intended as a reply to Emperor Julian's comparison of Christians to sick people who deserved compassion rather than hatred.[63]

Such variations on the ancient theme of the medicine of the body and the medicine of the soul went a long way to make religious matters understandable. *The Apostolic Constitutions,* written about the late fourth century, admonished the bishop "as a compassionate physician[64] [to] heal all that have sinned, making use of saving methods of cure; not only cutting and searing, or using corrosives, but binding up and putting in tents, and using gentle medicines, and sprinkling comfortable words."[65]

Step by step, the proper remedy for the wound is stated, so that the whole becomes a veritable summary of wound healing of the time:

60. Melito (453), col. 1225A. The English translation (from the Syriac) by Cureton, *Specilegium Syriacum* (London, 1855), of which Migne's is a Latin version, was not available to me.
61. Irenaeus (330), *Against Heresies* 4, preface, art. 2; 1:375.
62. Theodoretus (677), *Curatio,* preface, art. 16–17; p. 103.
63. See Carnivet's introduction to Theodoretus (675), pp. 42–46.
64. An allusion to Matt. 9:12–13.
65. *Apostolic Constitutions* (33), p. 70 (Donaldson's translation).

But if, after all that thou hast done, thou perceivest that from the foot to the head there is no room for fomentation, or oil, or bandage, but that the malady spreads and prevents all cure, as a gangrene which corrupts the entire member; then, with a great deal of consideration, and the advice of other skilful [sic] physicians, cut off the putrified member, that the whole body of the church be not corrupted.[66]

Giving up a hopeless case could be justified by the Hippocratic rule that it was an essential part of the medical art "not to take in hand those overpowered by the disease." [67] Shortly before his death, and despairing of the political situation in Rome, Cicero wrote to a friend, "Hippocrates too forbids employing medicine in hopeless [cases]." [68] Apuleius, the author of The Golden Ass, also extended the meaning of the maxim from the body and somatic disease to disorders of the soul, and to those "whose souls are saturated with vice." John Chrysostom deemed it "folly and utter madness to treat those suffering from incurable [diseases]." To him, as a Christian, incorrigible heretics were hopeless patients.[69] But Chrysostom's admirer (and perhaps his pupil) Isidore of Pelusium thought differently. In defense of his own attitude toward a certain reprobate, Maron, he wrote that some people agreed with the physician Hippocrates and had despaired of Maron. Yet ridicule notwithstanding, Isidore thought he had acted rightly in correcting Maron: "I have heard of many changes that have taken place in people; I see them happen and I expect them to happen." [70] In another letter, Isidore criticized a bishop for doing nothing and "obeying Hippocrates" by handling a certain priest as a hopeless case:

Even if [the Hippocratic rule] has seemed correct to some people regarding bodies (although it has often proved wrong, for many physicians have successfully treated persons who had been overpowered), it has yet definitely proved false with regard to souls. Indeed, we know people who from the depth of evil have risen to the peak of virtue. For [our] bodies have been given over to natural necessity, whereas [our] souls have been honored with the power of purposeful choice. To the same extent to which choice is more agile than is nature, it is also easier to restore the soul.[71]

66. Ibid. (Donaldson's translation).
67. Hippocrates (306), On the Art 3; p. 10, ll. 21–22.
68. Cicero (146), Letters to Atticus 16.15; 3:424.
69. For the references to Apuleius and John Chrysostom, see Isidore of Pelusium (331), Epistolae 2.16; col. 468B, apparatus.
70. Ibid. 2.16; col. 468B.
71. Ibid. 2.79; cols. 520C–521A.

To contradict Hippocrates on his own ground was even more remarkable than to reject the inference from body to soul.

The Christians' adoption of the pagan analogy between the medicine of the body and the medicine of the soul had its limits in that the soul took priority over the body, however great the value of the latter might be, and the care of the soul took priority over that of the body, however desirable the latter might be. The pagan analogy could be supplemented or replaced by the Biblical analogy between sickness and wounds of the body and those of the soul. God, the creator, Origen wrote,

> knew that the frailty of the human body would be such that it could incur diverse diseases and would be liable to wounds and other infirmities. For this reason, providing for the afflictions to come, He also produced medicaments from the earth and assigned the discipline of medicine, so that if sickness befell the body, a cure would not be lacking.

What sounds like another justification of medicine turns out to be a preface to Origen's interpretation of the Thirty-eighth[72] Psalm, with its rich imagery of arrows, wounds, disease, and failing strength. "Where does this preface lead us?" Origen asks. And he answers that it is applicable to the soul. "Because when the creator of all things made it also, He knew that it would be capable of faults, and therefore subject to, and burdened with, sins. Thus, as He made provision for medicines that are artfully compounded from herbs, so he also made provisions for medicaments for the soul in utterances that He sowed and dispersed through the divine Scriptures," so that people perceiving an injury to their soul might seek a science (*disciplinam*) that would cure them on the basis of God's precepts.[73]

It was but one step from here to Basil's belief that one of God's reasons for granting medicine to man was that it might serve as a model for the therapy of the soul.[74] Moreover, while it was admitted that "the adversaries," that is, the pagans, had discovered much that was good, it was pointed out that "many remedies for somatic diseases had also been discovered by the God-fearing[75] and by King Solomon.[76] None of

---

72. The thirty-seventh in the numeration of the Septuagint and hence of Origen.

73. Origen (513), *Explanatio super psalmum tricesimum septimum*, homily 1; col. 1369A–C. For the continuation, see below, text to n. 96. On Origen's interpretation of this psalm, cf. Barnes (76), pp. 95–97.

74. See below, chap. 13.

75. This included the Jews.

76. Cf. 1 Kings 4:33; and Stone (649), p. 82.

the unbelievers, however, understood how to cure the souls." [77]

One Hippocratic characterization of the medical art, already famous among pagans, was especially apt to apply to both the doctor and the Christian physician of the soul. No other Hippocratic dictum, not even the first Hippocratic aphorism, obtained such widespread attention throughout Antiquity as did the complaint that "the physician sees terrible things, touches what is loathsome, and from others' misfortunes harvests troubles of his own." [78] In its original context, it substantiated the claim that medicine was an art that benefited those who used it, but was a hardship for those who practiced it.

Lucian had Zeus bewail the fate of Asclepius, who was importuned by the sick and who "sees terrible things" and so on. [79] Plutarch, and others after him, substituted the political ruler for the physician. [80] Sometimes quoted in full and sometimes only alluded to, the Hippocratic saying was accorded a prominent place by Christian authors. Gregory of Nazianzus wrote:

> We know of the toil, sleeplessness, and worries endured by those who treat the body, and it is theirs to harvest grief for themselves from others' misfortunes, as said one of their sages. To those who need it, they will offer the result of their own labor and discoveries, as well as what others have inquired into and contributed. For them, nothing that is found or left out, be it ever so small, is too insignificant to be considered important for health or, on the other hand, as a threat. And all this to what purpose? That a human being may live more days on this earth. Perchance, this person is not good but very bad, and for him, being bad, it might perhaps have been better to have died much earlier, so that he might be relieved of the greatest of diseases: evil. But even if we suppose him to be good, how long will he live? For ever? What profit accrues [to him] from a life the release from which is the highest and safest good to be striven after by a man who is truly healthy and intelligent? [81]

High regard for the physician is here mixed with a low regard for human life. A Platonist or a Cynic philosopher might have accepted

---

77. Pseudo-Justin (356), *Responsiones ad orthodoxos*, quaestio 55. I follow the Latin translation in adding "the souls."

78. Hippocrates (306), *On Breaths* 1; p. 91, ll. 5–7. The afterlife of this passage has been covered by Nachmanson (475), pp. 186–89; Frings (239), pp. 45–46 and nn. 291–97; idem (238); Schubring (612), pp. 451–55; and Kudlien (382), pp. 14–15. I am restricting myself to a few examples and to the metamorphosis the meaning underwent.

79. Lucian (432), *Bis accusatus* 2; 3:86.

80. Plutarch (562), *Quaestiones Romanae* 113; 4:168–70.

81. Gregory of Nazianzus (271), *Oratio apologetica* 27; cols. 436B–437A.

Gregory of Nazianzus's pessimistic outlook. Had not Aristotle said that not to be was better than to be? But medicine then, as today, had a positive outlook on life, and held that life was to be respected and maintained. Hippocratic doctors did not consider whether their patients were good or evil. Whatever the physician thought about his patient, it would hardly be allowed to influence his therapy. For Gregory, however, the moral considerations served to bring into relief the heavy, yet rewarding, responsibility of the priest, whose concern was the soul destined for eternal glory or eternal punishment. How great was the struggle at hand, how great the art needed for correct treatment, so that we may turn life to the better "and give this heap of earth over to the spirit!" [82]

Gregory's praise of the physicians' dedication to their work actually throws doubt on the meaningfulness of their work. This passage illuminates the conflict between the acceptance of the mundane life as supported by Hippocratic medicine, and life's spiritual Christian interpretation. [83]

The patient's attitude could make the doctor's task very arduous. Patients who suffer from mental disorders, so we read in some late deontological medical texts, [84] are not responsible for what they do; their insults have to be borne. [85] The doctor served as a model for the physician of the soul. As the doctor healed the disease but remained unruffled in the face of the patient's anger, so the ideal philosopher would assail wrongdoing yet forgive the wrongdoer. To do wrong was human, but to restore that which had gone wrong was worthy of a god

82. Ibid. 28; col. 437.

83. See also below, chaps. 12, 13, 15, 17.B, and the Epilogue, for the discrepancy between Hippocratic naturalism and Christian spirituality.

84. Regarding these late texts, the name "'testament' or 'instruction' of Hippocrates [waṣīyaṭu ʾabuqrāṭ]" occurs in Ibn abī Uṣaibiʿah (320), p. 26, ll. 14–15. For the translated Arabic version, see Rosenthal (592), pp. 253–54, for the Arabic version of the Hippocratic Law, see idem, pp. 252–53. For the Greek versions of what he calls "The Testament of Hippocrates," see Deichgräber (167), pp. 97 and 100. For early medieval Latin versions, see Hirschfeld (313) and Laux (412). The introduction to the Quaestiones medicinales of pseudo-Soranus in Rose (590), 2:243–47, also should be classified among these texts. The Latin material has been presented in English translations by MacKinney (435). Deichgräber (167), p. 107, suggests that the composition of the Testament of Hippocrates may date as far back as the first century. I am using this title in a wider sense, to include descriptions of the perfect doctor, which goes beyond the rules for "how to learn medicine" (idem, p. 88).

85. See Deichgräber (167), pp. 95 and 97–98; also MacKinney (435), pp. 18–19 (text K).

or a godlike man.[86] Plutarch spelled out the difference in behavior in bodily and mental disease. People suffering from pain went to the physician, and those with a fever called him to their house, but not so people who had become mentally deranged: "Sometimes they cannot bear having the physician visit them but chase [him] away or flee, not even being aware that they are suffering from a violent disease. So also with wrongdoers."[87] On the Christian side, the theme was treated similarly. Deranged persons resisted being treated as if they were ill, but they had to be tolerated even if they struck with their fist, and kicked. Those who suffered from "the leprosy of unbelief" were their spiritual counterparts, and thought they enjoyed the best of health. Thus the expert in the treatment of the soul was much worse off than the specialist in the medical treatment of the body, to whom his patients submitted, however disagreeable or painful the cure, and to whom they paid an honorarium when restored to health, because, unlike the sick in soul, they longed for health.[88]

Christian authors appropriated the Hippocratic saying regarding the physician's toilsome life, applying it not only to the pastor of his flock but also to a hierarchy of physicians of the soul. Origen described at length the life of the physician, spent "among injuries, among patients with spreading ulcers, patients full of discharging matter, fevers, and various diseases. And if a man wishes to be fit for medicine, he must not be angry nor neglectful of the demand of the art that he has taken upon [himself] when among such people as I mentioned."[89] This description was intended to emphasize the labor of the prophets, whom God had sent to the people as their physicians. The prophets suffered from those who were unwilling to be cured, as doctors suffered from undisciplined patients. And there was Jesus, who took so much suffering upon himself for the sake of mankind's salvation.[90] However, there was a difference between the doctors—human beings who did not entirely escape being affected by the terrible things they saw and the loath-

86. Lucian (432), *Demonax* 7; 1:146. Lucian was speaking of the idealized philosopher.

87. Plutarch (562), *Quomodo quis suos in virtute sentiat profectus* 11.81F–82A; 1:434–36.

88. Theodoretus (677), *Curatio* 1.1–5; pp. 104–5. The original order of the argument, which I have somewhat changed, is as follows: There exists medical treatment of the body and of the soul, both being subject to many afflictions. But whereas those of the body are involuntary, those of the soul usually are self-inflicted.

89. Origen (514), *In Jeremiam homiliae* 14; col. 404C.

90. Cf. below, text to n. 97.

some things they touched—and Jesus, "who treated the injuries of our souls by the word of God in him [and] was immune to all evil." [91]

God was the supreme healer of the Old Testament; according to Tatian, man should rely on the power of God's word. [92] God's word, the *logos*, healed man of his sinful passions, said Clement of Alexandria, [93] and Jesus was "the Word . . . made flesh" (John 1:14). And so Clement's pupil Origen spoke of "the word of God" as "the physician of the soul, who uses various fitting and most timely ways of treatment for those who are ill." [94]

To refer to Jesus as a physician seems not to have been unusual by the end of the second century. "But that the Lord came as the physician of the sick, He does Himself declare," wrote Irenaeus, quoting Matthew (9:12). [95] Also with reference to the Gospel, Origen called Jesus "the master physician [ἀρχιατρός] who would be able to cure every disease and every infirmity. His pupils, Peter and Paul, and the prophets, as well as all those who after the Apostles were appointed in the church, were physicians whom God wished to be physicians of the soul in His Church." [96] They served as physicians for sinners. But though Jesus was the master physician, Origen saw him primarily as the physician of the soul, and as such he also appeared in the writings of Eusebius, the great historian of the Church:

> And like some excellent physician, who, to save those who are sick, "though he sees terrible things and touches what is loathsome, and from others' misfortunes harvests troubles of his own," so He by Himself saved from the very abyss of death us, who were not merely sick or oppressed by grievous sores and wounds already putrifying, but even lying among the dead; . . . He, then, it was who alone laid hold upon the grievous suffering of our corruption, alone endured our sorrows, alone took upon Himself the penalty for our wickednesses . . . He who is the Giver of life, the Enlightener, our great Physician and King and Lord, the Christ of God. [97]

91. Origen (509), *Contra Celsum* 4.15; cols. 1045B–1048A.
92. See above, chap. 10.C, text to n. 81.
93. Clement of Alexandria (150), *Paedagogus* 1.1; 1:108.
94. Origen (512), *Comment. in Exodum*, col. 269B.
95. Irenaeus (330), *Against Heresies* 3.5.2; 1:267 (Roberts and Rambaut's translation).
96. Origen (513), *Explanatio super psalmum tricesimum septimum;* col. 1369C–D. This is the continuation of above, text to n. 73.
97. Eusebius (211), *Ecclesiastical History* 10.4.11–12; 2:403–5 (Oulton's translation). I have, however, substituted my translation from Hippocrates' *On Breaths* for Oulton's.

Hippocrates, the metaphorical language of the Thirty-eighth Psalm, and the crucified Jesus who had taken the sins of man upon himself all came together in this praise of Jesus the physician of the soul, the savior of man. Self-sacrifice in the fulfillment of the physician's professional duty and in the fulfillment of the divine mission established a bond between the secular healer and the divine healer, Jesus, "the lamb of God, which taketh away the sin of the world" (John 1:29). To be self-sacrificing was the mark of a good physician; therefore the excellent physician could be defined as one who, in contrast to many who practiced medicine solely for the sake of profit, took his patient's troubles upon himself.[98]

The bond with the divine healer added to the dignity of the secular healer; it added to the respect that the profession of healing bestowed upon him as upon the Christian minister.[99] The physician of the body was a valuable partner for the priest, and the personal union of the two professions was welcomed. Theodoretus wrote letters on behalf of a certain very pious presbyter "adorned by the priesthood and also adorned by the rational [art of] therapy." He had trained in this art while residing in Alexandria, and was capable of "helping the sick and fighting diseases."[100] And the Arian deacon Aetius studied medicine "that he might be able to heal not only the diseases of souls but of bodies as well."[101]

"The rational art of therapy" meant the dominant Hippocratic medicine, which was also studied in Alexandria by Caesarius, the brother of Gregory of Nazianzus and, in its fundamentals at least, in Athens by Basil the Great.[102] But the symbiosis of Hippocratic medicine and patristic theology was by no means accepted generally. The very right of secular medicine to exist among Christians was questioned by the ascetic movement.

98. Isidore of Pelusium (331), *Epistolae* 2.171; col. 621B–C. With reference to Rose (590), 2:244, Schubring (612), pp. 454–55, writes, "aus der Feststellung der hippokratischen Schrift [*On Breaths*] [ist] hier eine sittliche Forderung an den Eleven im Sinne der ärztlichen φιλανθρωπίη geworden." Cf. below, Epilogue.

99. To meet the accusation that Paul had looked for unintelligent persons to instruct, Origen (509), *Contra Celsum* 3.74; col. 1016C–D, used the comparison with the "philanthropic physician [who] looks for the sick that he may bring them the remedies and make them strong."

100. Theodoretus (675), *Epistolae* 1114; col. 1324A.

101. Philostorgius (542), *Kirchengeschichte* 3.15; p. 47, ll. 10–11. Cf. the hateful account of Aetius by Gregory of Nyssa (Keenan [361], pp. 151–52).

102. On Caesarius, see chap. 14, text to n. 8; on Basil, see chap. 12, text to nn. 86–89.

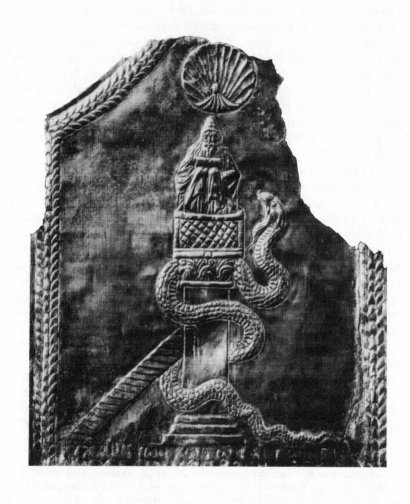

Simeon the Stylite on his pillar. The snake represents the devil. Plaque from a Syrian reliquary, sixth century. From Peter Brown, *The World of Antiquity: From Marcus Aurelius to Muhammad*. London: Thames and Hudson, 1971, p. 99.

V

Asceticism and Spiritual Medicine

12

ASCETICISM

A. The Monastic Movement

The desire to attain a spiritual goal in solitude and at the expense of the body's demands is not bound to any civilization and did not emerge with Christianity. John the Baptist preached in the wilderness of Judaea, and he "had his raiment of camel's hair, and a leathern girdle about his loins; and his meat was locusts and wild honey" (Matt. 1:4). Jesus was driven into the wilderness by the Spirit descending from Heaven (Mark 1:10 and 12). There were the Essenes, a Jewish sect associated with the Dead Sea Scrolls, which flourished from about the late second century B.C. till the Jewish-Roman War (A.D. 66–70). There may have been Christian ascetics in the Egyptian desert before Antony, with whom the history of the Christian monasticism started in A.D. 271. Within about one hundred years, the number of hermits living in isolation or in clusters, and of cenobites living in monasteries, had greatly multiplied; Pachomius had formulated his monastic rules, the movement had spread to Palestine and Syria, and Basil the Great had established a monastery in which communal service was paired with the hermit's concentration on his personal relationship to God and Jesus.[1] The Christian cenobite, ever since Pachomius, was committed to a way of life that imposed a high or moderate degree of asceticism upon him. Saints and holy men were to be found within monasteries as well

---

1. See Knowles (366), pp. 7–24.

as outside them. Monks might be very learned men, like Jerome, who not only became responsible for the Vulgate, the revised Latin version of the Bible, but also possessed a considerable knowledge of secular, including medical, authors.[2] But simple, uneducated, often illiterate people probably predominated among the monks.

It was not mere coincidence that the monastic movement gained momentum at a time when the church was becoming rich and powerful and after it had, in A.D. 313, gained imperial protection. In many respects, the movement was a reaction to the worldliness of the church. Educated Christians were not above feeling contempt for the rustics,[3] and in its beginning the movement was viewed with some suspicion by leaders of the church. It was not an intellectual movement, however many intellectuals might be attracted to the monastic life. The relationship of the ascetic to his body, to its health and disease, was a matter of doctrine, of theological debate, and of his personal experience, and was also determined by his personal feelings and thoughts, described in the narratives of the hagiographic literature (which had its beginning with Athanasius's life of Saint Antony), as well as documented by addresses to his brethren and to other audiences, if the monk functioned as a preacher.

Antony set out in search of perfection and crossed the Nile to spend the next twenty solitary years in an abandoned fort in the Egyptian desert, praying, fasting, and battling the demons. Later in his life, he became more accessible to the monks of the region, to whom he imparted advice and instruction.[4] Paul's warning against living "after the flesh" (Rom. 8:13), his assertion "But I keep under my body, and bring it into subjection" (1 Cor. 9:27), and the command "Put on the whole armour of God, that ye may be able to stand against the wiles of the devil" (Eph. 6:11), may well have guided Antony and other ascetics. Perhaps the greatest inspiration, however, came from the advice Jesus gave to the young man who asked what he lacked to gain eternal life: "If thou wilt be perfect, go and sell that thou hast, and give to the poor, and thou shalt have treasure in heaven: and come and follow me" (Matt. 19:21). To follow Jesus (or imitate him) and to gain perfection meant to master the flesh by the spirit and to combat Satan and the demons who tried to prevent the victory of the Spirit.

No sharp distinction was made between holy men and saints.[5] In the East, holy men came to exercise great influence over the minds of

2. See Pease (535).
3. See MacMullen (437), pp. 7–10.
4. See Athanasius (55), *Life of Saint Antony.*
5. Formal canonization by due process was introduced about the end of the millenium.

the people, an influence with which both ecclesiastical and secular powers had to reckon.[6] If sanctity was achieved, it assured a blessed life hereafter and power to help those who merited it and to defeat the enemies of God and men. In Heaven, holy men joined the prophets, the apostles, and the martyrs[7] to form a group whose intercession with God was eagerly sought.

Demons were experienced as powers that forced themselves upon the ascetic against his will and caused desires and fantasies—especially sexual fantasies—that had to be countered by prayer and an ever stricter control of the flesh. To monks who wished to hear him, Antony delivered a long disquisition on the wiles of the demons and the way to resist them. In the Devil's first assault, as Antony's biographer recounted, he had vainly tried "to incite [Antony] to lust, but Antony, sensing shame, would gird his body with his faith, with his prayers and his fasting";[8] afterwards, knowing that the Devil would try again, he "more and more mortified his body and brought it into subjection."[9] He taught the monks that "by prayers and fasting and confidence in the Lord" the demons were promptly thwarted, yet would return to the attack "with all wickedness and cunning."[10]

The monks should not fear the demons "though they appeared to attack us and to threaten death" because "in reality, they are weak and can do nothing but threaten."[11] Antony's own experience, however, was painful enough. Even before he had crossed the Nile, the devil came "with a great number of demons and lashed him so unmercifully that he lay on the ground speechless from the pain. He maintained that the pain was so severe that the blows could not have been inflicted by any man and cause such agony." The next day he was seen "lying on the ground as though dead," and only regained consciousness about midnight.[12] At another time, the demons made a din as if breaking through the walls; they filled the place "with the phantoms of lions, bears, leopards, bulls, and of serpents, asps, and scorpions, and of wolves . . . The lion roared, ready to spring upon him, the bull appeared about to gore him through," and so on. "Pummelled and goaded by them," Antony "groaned, it is true, because of the pain that racked his body, but his mind was master of the situation."[13]

6. See Brown (118), to which cf. Drijvers (191).
7. See Palladius (524), pp. 167–68, n. 4
8. Athanasius (55), Life 5; p. 23 (Meyer's translation).
9. Ibid. 7; p. 25 (Meyer's translation).
10. Ibid. 23; p. 39 (Meyer's translation).
11. Ibid. 27; p. 42 (Meyer's translation).
12. Ibid. 8; pp. 26–27 (Meyer's translation).
13. Ibid. 9; p. 28 (Meyer's translation).

The extent of the physical power of the Devil and his host was a matter for theological debate until the end of the witchcraft trials in the eighteenth century. However, the people little doubted the Devil's ability to cause sickness, famine, earthquakes, and other disasters. Evil spirits were not a Christian invention, and demonology was a serious topic among the philosophers of late Antiquity.[14] Christian ascetics, more perhaps than others, experienced demoniac power as a reality, reflected in the wondrous world of hagiography and also in the role attributed to demons in historiography.[15] If we look at Grünewald's "Temptation of St. Antony" as a portrayal not of artistic fancies but of an imagined reality, we may obtain a feeling for what the people of late Antiquity and the Middle Ages accepted as fact.

It was one of the ruses of the demons to cause disgust with the ascetic life by continuously rousing the monk to prayer, thus denying him sleep, and by advising him against eating altogether.[16] Ascetic practice obviously had limits beyond which its practitioner risked committing the sin of suicide. Actively seeking martyrdom also was forbidden. Many gradations of ascetic practice could be found, ranging from mere abstemiousness to severe mortification of the flesh. In asceticism, the ambiguous relationship between the body and the soul presented itself in a concrete form and easily led to conflicting thoughts and sentiments. Basil absolved the body of evil (though he asserted that the mind had to keep a firm rein on it)[17] and thought it the abbot's duty to determine the tasks of the monks in proportion to the strength of their bodies.[18] Yet he also reminded a renegade monk of the time when together they had rejoiced over the latter's progress in his ascetic labors:

> Abrading your body with rough cloth of hair and compressing your loin with a hard belt, you bruised your bones with patient endurance. By your abstinence you hollowed your waist so that it sank in as far as the vertebrae of your back. You denied yourself the use of a soft bandage, and whittling down your belly from within like a gourd, you forced it to cleave to the region of your kidneys. Removing all the fat of the flesh, you nobly drained the ducts of the hypogastric region and made the

14. See Geffken (261).
15. Momigliano (468), p. 93: "It is no exaggeration to say that a mass invasion of devils into historiography preceded and accompanied the mass invasion of barbarians into the Roman empire."
16. Athanasius (55), Life 25; pp. 41–42.
17. Basil (80), Constitutiones asceticae 2.2–3; col. 1340C–1344B.
18. Ibid. 31; col. 1420D.

stomach flatten out. You made your ribs overshadow the region of your navel like eaves of a roof.[19]

Paul's joyful profession "I take pleasure in infirmities, in reproaches, in necessities, in persecutions, in distresses for Christ's sake: for when I am weak, then I am strong" (2 Cor. 12:10) was apt to stimulate the zeal of ascetics who exuberated in the self-inflicted torture of their bodies as a pious and God-pleasing deed. Basil was not a fanatic, and certainly not if compared with the holy men such as Simeon the Stylite and other Byzantine pillar saints.

> For forty years [writes Simeon's Syrian biographer] he stood on a pillar which was one ell in breadth. His feet were tied and fettered as in the stock, so that he could not turn either of them to the right or the left, until the bones and sinews of his feet became visible on account of the pain, and his abdomen tore from standing . . . Three of the vertebrae of his back detached themselves because of the constant praying when he bent and straightened up before his lord until he ended his battle.[20]

Simeon "loved to be in pain in this world and wished for it, for the sake of Christ, to attain glory with him in the holy city." [21] The "battle" that ended with Simeon' death was the ascetic's struggle to win glory in heaven. Saints and martyrs were thought of as fighters (ἀθληταί) in an arena.[22]

B. Ascetics and Their Diseases

When Antony came forth from his solitude in the deserted fort after nearly twenty years of ascetic life, his friends and admirers were surprised to find the appearance of his body unchanged, "neither obese from want of exercise, nor emaciated from his fastings and struggles with the demons." He was in full control of himself, "a man guided by reason and stable in his character." [23] He was nearly 105 years old when the time came for him to die.[24] His health was unimpaired, his eyesight was normal, he had retained all his teeth,[25] and there was nothing

19. Basil (81), *Letters* 45; 1:178. I have tried to make some anatomical sense of this difficult passage.

20. Lietzmann (423), *Leben* 83; p. 130 (from Hilgenfeld's German translation).

21. Ibid; p. 129 (from Hilgenfeld's German translation).

22. See Brown (118), pp. 94–95.

23. Athanasius (55), *Life* 114; p. 32 (Meyer's translation).

24. Ibid. 89; p. 93. See also below, n. 30.

25. They were, however, worn down, a condition probably due to particles of sand or to "the slow, steady way people chew food of a certain firm or rubbery consistency" (Grmek [278], pp. 113–14).

wrong with his hands and feet; altogether, "he appeared brighter and more active than did all those who use diversified diet and baths and a variety of clothing."[26]

Antony's regimen consisted of one meal of bread and salt per day, sometimes only every second or even fourth day, and water to drink. Neither he nor the other ascetics partook of meat or wine. He engaged in nocturnal vigils, not infrequently passing the whole night without sleep. The bare ground or a rush mat served as his bed, and he disdained to anoint his skin and did not even wash his feet.[27] Antony's mode of life broke all the rules of Hippocratic hygiene. He and his fellow ascetics not only deviated from Hippocratic medicine but also believed that their deprivations returned man to his pristine condition before the Fall: "body and soul together, to an original, natural and uncorrupted state."[28] The ascetics' healthy appearance was an almost necessary postulate of hagiography.

Whether or not one may think of Antony's life as conducive to health and longevity, the self-inflicted injuries of the pillar saints clearly belonged in the realm of the pathological.[29] Yet Simeon was said to have been about seventy-three years old at the time of his death, and his pupil, Daniel the Stylite, was over eighty-four years old when he died (in A.D. 493) after having spent thirty-three years and three months on his pillar.[30]

Ascetics were likely to look upon their self-inflicted hardships and injuries as sufferings that had to be borne. But not all hardship and injury was self-inflicted. Like other people, ascetics and saints were prone to diseases and accidents. What, then, was their attitude to secular help when they were sick, and what were their ideas about appealing for medical help?[31]

Their attitudes varied widely. In Nitria, in lower Egypt, where monks lived in a community (*cenobium*), physicians and even pastry-

---

26. Athanasius (55), *Life* 93; p. 97 (Meyer's translation).

27. Ibid. 7; p. 25 (which refers to his early ascetic life), and idem 93; p. 97.

28. Brown (115), p. 223. See idem, all of pp. 222–24; also idem, p. 294; and above, chap. 11, n. 41.

29. Apart from the harm to the circulation of the blood and to the joints caused by standing still for years, the filth and vermin covering and surrounding the saints ought to have caused all kinds of infections. But immunity from what was harmful to ordinary people was expected as a mark of the saint. Cf. above, text to n. 28.

30. Dawes and Baynes (162), p. 6. On the long life of holy men, Browning (121), p. 123, who gives more examples, remarks, "the holy man enjoys longevity, in spite of his exhausting life style."

31. For the distinction between the saint as patient and as healer, cf. Harvey (290), p. 89.

cooks were allegedly found.[32] The strict monastic rules of Pachomius made provisions for the sick brethren. They had their own quarters, which healthy persons were not allowed to enter,[33] and they enjoyed greater freedom regarding the quantity and quality of food, being also allowed wine and fish sauce.[34] Saint Benedict's rule made the care of the sick brethren a prime obligation "before and above" all others. The abbot had to see to it that they were not neglected, while they, on their side, had to keep in mind that they were servants of God and were obligated not to sadden the brethren serving them by making excessive demands.[35] No mention was made of physicians; but if inference from Cassiodorus is permissible, monks with some medical knowledge would have been chosen to look after the sick.[36]

Visitors reported that a certain Stephanus, who "had attained the highest degree of asceticism" and had cured "any kind of affliction," was suffering from cancer, and that they had found him in the care of a physician. "While his members were being cut away like locks of hair, he showed no sign whatsoever of pain, thanks to the superiority of his spiritual preparation." Stephanus explained to his visitors that "it may well be that my members deserve punishment and it would be better to pay the penalty here than after I have left the arena."[37] When Palladius, the biographer of the Egyptian monks, of whom he himself was one, became ill with dropsy, members of his cenobitic community sent him to Alexandria, and the Alexandrian doctors sent him on to Palestine because of its better climate.[38]

Of course, Heaven might take care of a saint. Saint Martin, Bishop of Tours, suffered a bad fall, causing many wounds that made him lie in his cell half-dead and tortured by pain. But in the night he saw an apparition, an angel who washed his wounds and anointed his bruise with a wholesome salve. The next day, he was completely cured.[39] This was a healing miracle in the manner of Asclepius.

Simeon the Stylite also was cured miraculously. His disease—like Job's—was caused by Satan, to whom God had given the power, and

32. For the monks or for guests? See Chitty (140), p. 31; also Volk (707), p. 35.

33. Pachomius (518), *Regulae* 23, 24, and 27; pp. 20–22 (Jerome's latin translation).

34. Ibid. 2, 25, and 26; pp. 12 and 21–22.

35. Benedict (89), *Regula* 36; p. 48. For Benedict's rules for the sick, cf. Amundsen and Ferngren (26), p. 16.

36. For the monks of Cassiodorus's Vivarium, see below, text to nn. 74 and 75.

37. Palladius (524), *Lausiac History* 2.24; pp. 83–84 (Meyer's translation).

38. Ibid. 35.11–12; p. 102. On the life and work of Palladius, see Coleman-Norton's introduction to Palladius (523).

39. Sulpicius Severus (660), *Vie* 19.4; p. 294.

his cure was the result of putting the Devil to shame and trusting in Jesus to the point of refusing all worldly help.[40] He had felt a sharp pain in his foot and was then covered with boils full of pus and worms. The stench was so bad that the disciples who had to climb up to him had to hold incense and perfumed oil before their noses. The saint could not be persuaded to climb down or to have the pillar lowered so that the physician might more easily administer plasters. Simeon told the bishops whom the emperor had sent to pray for him that Jesus "does not make me need physicians, roots, and medicines." [41]

The ascetics' diverse attitudes toward their own diseases corresponded to the ambiguous attitudes within Judaism and Christianity to disease and its secular treatments. In the final analysis, God was the healer. Without categorically rejecting secular medicine, Philo had allowed it no more than an insignificant place. Ecclesiasticus had offered a compromise: as God's creations, physicians and medicines could be decisive in the outcome of a disease. Thus the question of whether secular help should be sought or shunned remained open.[42]

Origen, though a partisan of secular medicine, nevertheless distinguished between the many who needed it and those who could turn to God directly: "A man ought to use medical means to heal his body if he aims to live in the simple and ordinary way. If he wishes to live in a way superior to that of the multitude, he should do this by devotion to the supreme God and by praying to Him." [43] For monks who aspired to the superior life, the question was of more than peripheral importance. An answer came from the homilies to monks written by a man who hid behind the name of Macarius the Egyptian.[44] With a slight textual deviation from Luke 16:10, Macarius quoted Jesus: "He that is faithful in that which is little is faithful also in much: and he that is without faith on that which is little is without faith also in much." [45] The little things were temporal matters such as food, clothing, and health, which the Lord had promised to give to believers and about which they were

40. Lietzmann (423), *Leben* 86—87 and 90; pp. 131–32 and 133.

41. Ibid. 87; p. 132 (quoted from Hilgenfeld's German translation). Harvey (290), pp. 89–90, thinks that "to declare one's commitment to the divine by divorcing oneself from the temporal realm . . . was a virtual requirement on the part of the ascetic, even as the healing of the lay populace was itself a requirement."

42. For Philo and Ecclesiasticus, see above, chap. 8.

43. Origen (510), *Contra Celsum* 8.60; p. 498 (Chadwick's translation). For this and the following, see also Amundsen (16), pp. 338, 341, and 347–48.

44. According to Dörries (433), pp. ix–xi, these homilies go back to the work of a heretic, Symeon, of the late third century. Edited around A.D. 1000, they were widely circulated in the medieval church.

45. Macarius (433), *Homilien* 48.1; p. 312, ll. 1–3.

not to worry. "That which is much" meant the gifts of the world of eternity, promised to the faithful, which they should ceaselessly aspire to and pray for. Everybody's faith in God was tested by the concern they showed for temporal things. And so Macarius addressed the monks:

> You say you believe that you are worthy of the kingdom of Heaven and are born again a son of God, to become a joint heir of Christ and to reign together with him for all times and, like God, to live in ineffable light for infinite and boundless ages? Undoubtedly you will say "Yes. Indeed it is for this reason that I have withdrawn from the world and have given myself to God." Then prove thyself.[46]

The proof consisted in acting in accordance with Jesus' words: "Take no thought for what you eat or drink or wear, for all these things do the gentiles seek," and "As the body is more precious than the raiment, so also is the soul more precious than the body."[47] Jesus came down to earth "that he might heal the souls of the believers of their incurable afflictions and purge [them] of the filth of the leprosy of evil, [he] the only true physician and healer."[48]

Macarius knew that his hearer would agree with these statements. But then he must also accept their conclusion and accept Christ as his physician in bodily ills:

> Know then, having searched yourself, [that] you must never bring the fleshly afflictions before mundane physicians, as if Christ, in whom you believe, were unable to cure you. See how you cheat yourself, because you think to have faith without yet believing, as you should, in accordance with truth. For if you believed that the eternal and incurable wounds and afflictions of evil of the immortal soul are healed by Christ, you would believe him capable of healing the transitory afflictions and diseases of the body as well, and would take refuge with him alone, disdaining medical practices and cures. For he who created the soul, he also made the body,[49] and he who heals what is immortal can also cure the body of its transitory afflictions and diseases.[50]

Macarius was addressing a monk who had given himself to God and believed himself worthy of the kingdom of God. Macarius's lengthy

46. Ibid. 48.2–3; p. 313, ll. 26–31.
47. Ibid 48.3; p. 313, ll. 39–40, and p. 314, ll. 44–45. Macarius quoted freely from Matt. 6:25–34.
48. Ibid; p. 314, ll. 48–50.
49. For Christ as creator, see Dörries (433), p. 314, apparatus.
50. Macarius (433), *Homilien* 48.4; p. 314, ll. 52–62.

argument made accepting Jesus as the perfect healer of soul and body a proof of faith, and entrusting oneself to doctors proof of a lack of it.[51] But Macarius's demand that doctors, whose ability to cure he did not deny, be rejected was not intended for ordinary Christians, or even for all monks. He conceded that his intransigence was inconsistent with the belief that God had created medicines and had provided for the existence of doctors.[52] To solve the contradiction, Macarius wanted it realized that God "in [His] great and limitless love for man and goodness"[53] had made these provisions for a fallen mankind, which had come under the power of darkness and had become faithless and subject to disease. Medicines and doctors were God's arrangements for the weak and for those without faith, because He had not wished to destroy utterly the sinful race of man. He also conceded the use of doctors and medicines to those "as yet unable to entrust themselves to God completely,"[54] monks included. The solitary hermit, however, to whom Macarius returned at the end of the sermon, who had become a stranger in the world, was "obliged to have a faith that is more novel and strange and, in contrast to all human beings of the world, a [different] purpose and citizenship."[55]

It was not unusual to make a distinction between those as yet weak in faith and those who were perfect. Thus Pachomius relates that an angel had given him a short set of monastic rules which, Pachomius complained, did not contain enough prayers. Thereupon the angel informed him that those rules were made "for the little ones . . . those who have not the true knowledge, so that they may fulfill the duties of their station in life like house-servants and so enjoy a life of complete liberty."[56] Those who were perfect needed no rules. Similarly, Benedict thought of his rules as necessary for beginners,[57] for the class of monks who lived in the monastery. Anchorites, capable of single-handedly fighting the devil and the vices of the flesh and of their thoughts, who with the monastery's approval had left its shelter, formed a different class.[58]

51. It is significant that Macarius relied on logical proof rather than on the Biblical evidence of Jesus' cures of bodily diseases. The latter could have been deemed unique historical events. On Macarius see also Frings (239), pp. 15–16; also Amundsen (16), pp. 338, 341, and 347–48.

52. Macarius (433), Homilien 48.5; p. 314. This is a conscious or unconscious acceptance of Ecclesiasticus.

53. Ibid. 48.5; p. 315, ll. 68–69.

54. Ibid. 48.6; p. 315, l. 81.

55. Ibid. 48.6; p. 315, ll. 85–87.

56. Palladius (524), Lausiac History 32.7; p. 94 (Meyer's translation).

57. Benedict (89), Regula 73; p. 74.

58. Ibid. 1; p. 19.

What Macarius thought of as God's concession to human weakness and imperfection appeared as the rule of ordinary life to Diadochus, a fifth-century bishop of Photica. "There is nothing to forbid the summoning of doctors at the time of disease," he declared. "Indeed, since the [medical] art was bound eventually to come into existence through human experience, medicines, therefore, came into existence earlier." [59] To this he added the caveat "Except that one must not put one's hope for healing in [the doctor] but in Jesus Christ, our true savior and physician." [60] Diadochus was speaking not just of laymen but also of ascetics, especially those living in monasteries or in cities, whom force of circumstances prevented from practicing their faith consistently. Employing medicines and doctors would also prevent ascetics from succumbing to vainglory and the temptation of the Devil, whereby some of them were made to proclaim publicly that they had no need of doctors. [61]

The matter was different for anchorites who lived in lonely places with two or three like-minded brethren. "In whatever affliction may befall him, he should submit himself in faith to the Lord, who heals every disease and every weakness of ours." [62] Besides, solitude mitigated diseases effectively; in solitude, nothing detracted from one's faith and there was no opportunity to make a display of one's virtue and endurance. [63]

Diadochus held the existence of disease to be necessary and desirable. Paul himself (2 Cor. 12:7) had believed that his infirmity was given him lest he be exalted beyond measure by the superabundance of his revelations. In former days, Diadochus thought, the persecutions had kept the saints above sinful passions. Now, however, since the church lived in peace, the bodies of the champions of piety needed disorders and their souls needed evil thoughts so that they might prove themselves. If we gratefully submit to the will of the Lord, "continuing disease and the battle against devilish thoughts will be accounted to us as a second martyrdom." [64] Too great a detestation of bodily disorders proved that the soul was still enslaved by the body's desires. The soul wanted material well-being, was reluctant to give up the good things of life, and thought it very burdensome not to be able to enjoy them. But if the soul accepted the distress caused by disease gracefully, it ap-

---

59. Diadochus (170), *Hundred Gnostic Chapters* 53; p. 115, ll. 2–3. On Diadochus, see Nutton (489), pp. 5–6.
60. Diadochus (170), *Hundred Gnostic Chapters* 53; p. 115, ll. 5–7.
61. Ibid. 53; p. 115, ll. 7–13.
62. Ibid. 53; p. 115, ll. 15–17.
63. Ibid. 53; p. 115, ll. 17–21.
64. Ibid. 94; p. 156, ll. 21–23.

proached insensibility to suffering[65] and looked forward with joy to death as a preface to a truer life.[66]

Such an outlook on life and disease conflicted with Hippocratic medicine, which counted on the patient's willing cooperation in the quest for health.[67] So far as ascetic doctrine can be summarized briefly, it can be said to have viewed complete reliance on God and Jesus in all disease, to the exclusion of all medical help, as ideal. The fulfillment of this ideal could be expected of those who had reached perfection in their faith. For all others, laymen as well as monks, God had provided doctors and medicines as help in their weakness.

The emphasis on the weakness of faith was an unavowed admission of trust in the help provided by secular medicine, a trust that even ascetics, when ill, might harbor. But when monks, holy men, and saints are seen not in their concern for their own souls but in their charity toward others, the matter looks somewhat different.

C. Monks, Saints, and Holy Men as Healers

Philanthropy or agape[68] (Latinized as *caritas*), be it translated by charity, love, or benevolence, became a virtue that Paul (1 Cor. 13) made a cornerstone of Christian ethics, placing it above faith and hope. Like the philanthropy of the Stoics, the Hebrew love of one's neighbor, and the modern respect for life, charity could be commanded; it could be a general attitude to be assumed toward all and toward no one in particular; and it might or it might not be imbued with a feeling of love and of compassion toward those who suffered, particularly the poor, the hungry, and the sick.[69]

During an epidemic in the third century, Christians set a shining example of "a discipline and a test," as reported by Dionysius, the bishop of Alexandria.

> In their exceeding love [*agapē*] and affection for the brotherhood, [most Christians] were unsparing of themselves and cleaved to one another, visiting the sick without a thought as to the danger, assiduously ministering to them, treating [θεραπεύοντες] them in Christ. So they most

65. Ibid. 54; p. 116, l. 9: ἀπαθείας. On the meaning of the word ἀπάθεια, see idem, pp. 14–15. Cf. idem. 84.3; idem 17; p. 94; l. 7; and idem 72; p. 131, l. 13.
66. Ibid. 54; p. 116.
67. See Hippocrates (302), *Epidemics* 1.11; 1:164.
68. The words "agape" and "philanthropy" came to be used synonymously in Christian literature; see Amundsen and Ferngren (26), pp. 12–13.
69. See the Epilogue.

gladly perished along with them; being infected[70] with the disease from others, drawing upon themselves the sickness from their neighbors, and willingly taking over their pains. And many, when they had tended to others' disease and restored their strength, died themselves, thus transferring their death to themselves.[71]

During the Athenian plague, some people, though aware of the danger, had visited their sick friends, just as the Alexandrian Christians had visited their fellow Christians. However, the motives attributed to them differed: "People," Thucydides wrote, "either from fear, did not visit one another . . . or, if they did, were lost, especially those with a claim to virtue; for out of a sense of shame they visited [their] friends, unsparing of themselves."[72] The pagans wanted to remain (or to appear) loyal to their image of a virtuous person, whereas the Christians—equal to the martyrs, as the bishop thought—died in consequence of "much piety and strong faith," and were followed by those who lovingly took care of the bodies of these "saints."[73]

The rules of Pachomius and of Benedict made provision for the care of sick monks, and Cassiodorus coupled the monks' charitable duty to the sick with the requirement that they obtain some rudimentary instruction in Hippocratic medicine, thus initiating the period of "monks' medicine." Cassiodorus addressed his

> illustrious brethren, who deal with the welfare of the human body with diligent inquisitiveness and devote the services of holy piety to those who take refuge in the abodes of the saints, who are saddened by others' sufferings, who grieve over those in danger, are pierced by the pain of those you take into your care, and [are] always stunned by grief over the misfortunes of others.[74]

This Christianized paraphrase of the Hippocratic saying concerning the physician's toil serves as a preamble to Cassiodorus's exhortation to the monks to serve the sick as the knowledge of the medical art directs, but

70. Ἀναπιμπλάμενοι, literally "being filled up." The image is quite different from the Latin *inficere*, "to stain."

71. Eusebius (211), *Ecclesiastical History* 7.22.6–9; 2:184–87 (Oulton's translation, modified). See also Neuburger (480), 2:41; Amundsen and Ferngren (26), pp. 14–15; and idem (22), p. 47, regarding John 3:16: "Hereby receive we the love of God, because he laid down his life for us: and we ought to lay down our lives for the brethren."

72. Thucydides (685), 2.51.5; 1:122.

73. Eusebius (211), *Ecclesiastical History* 7.22.8; 2:186.

74. Cassiodorus (133), *Institutiones* 31.1; pp. 78–79. See also Temkin (672), p. 14 and p. 24, n. 51; and MacKinney (434), pp. 50–52.

not to put their "hope in the herbs" nor their "trust in human counsel
... Medicine is ordained by the Lord [he continued], yet it is without
doubt He who makes [man] healthy and who grants life." [75]

It should not be left unremarked that Bishop Dionysius and Cassiodorus interpreted the behavior of the Alexandrian Christians and of the
monks, respectively, in the light of Christian love and duty. These are
examples of the substitution of a religious creed for individual motives
of which nothing is known. [76]

The origin of the hospital as an outgrowth of monastic zeal belongs
to the East. [77] Rightly or wrongly, the credit for having founded the first
hospital is given to Basil, whose Basilias (named after him), [78] located
near Caesarea, certainly became famous above all other early hospitals.
In the funeral oration for his friend, Gregory of Nazianzus spoke of "a
new city" in which "disease is studied, [79] misfortune is called a blessing,
and compassion is put to the test." [80] He focused attention on the admission of lepers, "human beings, dead before death, most limbs of
their body withered away, expelled from cities, houses, public places,
waters, [81] and those dearest to them, recognized by [their] names rather
than [their] bodies, not represented in assemblies and gatherings of societies and fellowships, nor commiserated with on account of [their]
illness, but despised—masters of pitiful songs, if even a voice is left to
any of them." [82] Gregory singled out the welcome given to lepers as a
mark of Basil's concern for "the sick and for the healing of injuries and
for the imitation of Christ, who cleansed leprosy not by talk but by
deeds." [83]

Basil himself, who had to defend his action to the governor, described the place as a complex consisting of "a sumptuously furnished
house of prayer to our God" surrounded by an arrangement of quar-

75. Cassiodorus (133), *Institutiones* 31.1; pp. 78–79.
76. The practice of substituting religiously prescribed thoughts and feelings for
the conscious or unconscious thoughts and feelings of the individuals concerned also
extends to philosophical tenets and socially accepted beliefs.
77. On the subject, see Miller (463), and the review by Nutton (495).
78. Sozomen (639), *Kirchengeschichte* 6.34.9; p. 291, ll. 19–22.
79. Νόσος φιλοσοφεῖται.
80. Gregory of Nazianzus (273), *Oratio XLIII*, art. 63; col. 577C.
81. Ὑδάτων, which here probably means public baths, fountains, and springs.
82. Gregory of Nazianzus (273), *Oratio XLIII*, art. 63; col. 580A–B. Although
Aretaeus already had mentioned the social consequences of the disease for the leper
(see Grmek [278], p. 171), Gregory's seems to be one of the earliest detailed descriptions.
83. Gregory of Nazianzus (273), *Oratio XLIII;* art. 63; col. 580C. The text is
ambiguous; the cleansing of leprosy can be referred to Basil as well as to Christ.

ters: one for the head of the institution; others, more lowly ones, for the servants of God, the use of which was free for the governors and their retinues. Then Basil continued:

Whom do we harm by building lodgings for strangers: for those visiting us while passing through, as well as for those in need of some attendance because of [their] infirmity, also providing the necessary comfort for them: men who nurse, those who give medical care, beasts of burden, and escorts? Crafts too must be associated with them, those needed for living and such as have been invented for living decently, also [there must be] other houses to serve as work places. All of this [is] an ornament to the place and a cause for pride to our governor, since the praise redounds to him.[84]

The Basilias certainly included a leprosarium and quarters for travelers, with provisions for those who had fallen ill. The existence of a general hospital is not equally well attested.[85] It has to be remembered that in the early days those who benefited from hospitalization were people who could not obtain proper care at home, that is, travelers, lepers, and the indigent. Others were likely to be taken care of by their families and their servants, and by doctors.

Basil did not say whether his hospice was open to pagans, nor did he speak of physicians (ἰατροί). The expression he used, "those who give medical care [ἰατρεύοντας]," rather suggests monks who possessed medical knowledge such as he himself had acquired as a student in Athens. According to Gregory, "the ill-health of [his] body as well as the care of the sick" had made Basil direct his attention to medicine.[86] Together, Basil and Gregory had studied the basis of the care of the sick (νοσοκομίαι) and of medical treatment.[87] Basil penetrated more deeply into the philosophical principles of medicine than his friend, though, as Gregory's unclear expression suggests, this did not include clinical instruction.[88] At any rate, Basil was well prepared for his hospital and was qualified to judge what good there was in Hippocratic medicine for devout Christians.[89]

84. Basil (81), Letters 94; 2:150–152. Cf. Miller (463), pp. 86 and 125.

85. Amundsen and Ferngren (26), p. 15, characterize the Basilias as including "rooms for lepers and lodgings for travellers." For the terminology of charitable institutions, see Patlagean (531), p. 193; and Miller (463), pp. 23–29.

86. Gregory of Nazianzus (273), Oratio XLIII, art. 23; col. 528B.

87. Ibid. 61; col. 576C.

88. According to ibid. 23; col. 528B, Basil's study went as far as the structure (ἕξιν) of the art, "not as far as it relates to what is visible and that which lies underneath, but as far as it is based on principle [δογματικόν] and is philosophical."

89. See below, chap. 13.

While patriarch of Constantinople (A.D. 398–404), John Chrysostom founded "several hospitals and also appointed two pious presbyters as well as physicians [ἰατροὺς], cooks, and efficient workmen, who were single, to serve them, so that visiting strangers and [people] seized by disease [especially the one called sacred][90] might find care."[91] This description resembles that of the Basilias. What kind of physicians John installed remains uncertain.

Eventually, professional doctors infiltrated the hospitals and replaced the monks, but this process does not seem to have gained momentum before the middle of the fifth century. Whatever the early hospital may have contributed to Hippocratic medicine, as a training ground or otherwise, has not left an imprint on the extant Hippocratic medical literature of late Antiquity.

Apart from the organized medical charity of monastic institutions, there were holy men who had the power to heal. This power emanated from them as their sanctity increased; it was not imparted at a particular moment or by a particular act.[92] Through Antony, so his biographer wrote, "the Lord cured many of those present who were afflicted with bodily ills, and freed others from impure spirits."[93] Antony rebuked demons, and he healed by praying to the Lord. He impressed upon his fellow monks that it was not given to them to perform signs, as Jesus had done, and he quoted the words of Jesus to the seventy disciples, warning them not to rejoice that the spirits were subject to them, but to rejoice that their names were written in heaven (Luke 10:20).

However, holy men did not restrict themselves to prayer and to rebuking demons. The association between demons and disease was close, and the variety of ills healed was great, ranging from leprosy to gout and dislocated joints.[94] Such miracles as were performed by holy men also took place at the graves of martyrs and saints, and this became the predominant mode of religious healing in the West.[95] In the East, the aspiring holy man assumed a special social function, of which

90. Which here probably meant leprosy rather than epilepsy (see Temkin [666], p. 19). The editors excluded these words as belonging to a gloss.

91. Palladius (523), *Dialogus* 5; p. 32, ll. 13–15.

92. Healing power was "perhaps the commonest manifestation of Holiness" (Browning [121], p. 131).

93. Athanasius (55), *Life* 14; p. 32 (Meyer's translation).

94. See Dawes and Baynes (162), pp. 153, 175, and 144 (from Saint Theodore of Sykeon). See Patlagean (531), pp. 101–2, on the prevalent diseases with which the saints had to deal.

95. See Brown (116).

healing became a prominent part, once his holiness was recognized.[96]

It is not possible to generalize regarding the attitudes of holy men toward secular physicians; they varied just as the attitudes of ascetics varied toward their own diseases. Even those who could be expected to refuse medical aid for themselves might take a liberal attitude toward it for others. For instance, a man attacked by bandits who wounded him severely and "cut the sinews of his knees" was brought to nearby Ancyra, whose bishop ordered him "to be conveyed to the hospital and cared for there." His wounds healed but he could not walk, and upon his request, the bishop (at his personal expense) had him transported to the enclosure of Daniel the Stylite (near Constantinople). Though the man's legs "hung down as if they did not belong to him," he was miraculously cured after having been anointed "with the oil of the saints" and brought to the saint's enclosure at prayer time. The hospital had done its part, and the holy man did his. There was no friction between the two; Daniel even "sent thanks to the bishop for the kindness he had shown the man."[97]

Whereas Basil had acquired medical knowledge by study, Theodore of Sykeon had acquired it during the course of his religious activities, which abounded in healing, freeing people from demons, and all kinds of miracles. He combined miraculous power with medical experience and cooperation with physicians.

> If any required medical treatment for certain illnesses or surgery or a purging draught or hot springs, this God-inspired man would prescribe the best thing for each, for even in technical matters he had become an experienced doctor. He might recommend one to have recourse to surgery and he would always state clearly which doctor he should employ.[98]

Basil, on the other hand, though a learned man, was also a saint, believed to be endowed with healing powers. When his son fell severely ill, the Arian emperor Valens sent for Basil, though on the night before he had condemned him to banishment. "Immediately on the arrival of

96. See Brown (118), who focuses on the holy men of Syria (later also Asia Minor and Palestine) in the fourth and fifth centuries and emphasizes that their relationship to society differed from that of the monks of the Egyptian desert (see especially idem, p. 82). I am using the term "holy man" comprehensively, disregarding regional differences.

97. Dawes and Baynes (162), "St. Daniel the Stylite" 87; pp. 60–61 (Dawes and Baynes's translation).

98. Ibid., "St. Theodore of Sykeon" 146; p. 182 (Dawes and Baynes's translation).

Basil, the prince began to rally; so that many maintain that his recovery would have been complete, had not some heretics been summoned to pray with Basil for his restoration."[99] Everybody, the emperor included, believed that the prince's death was due to the wrath of God over the intrigues against Basil.[100]

The ways in which miraculous cures were achieved varied considerably. On one end of the spectrum, there was prayer and the laying on of hands, in accordance with the resurrected Jesus' statement to the apostles that those who believed their preaching "shall lay hands on the sick, and they shall recover" (Mark 16:18). This practice must have been used frequently. Simeon the Stylite told a man who sought his help: "I am a sinful man and lower than all human beings. My hand is not like that of all other bishops and monks who have laid [their] hands on you."[101] It seems that Simeon did nothing to the sick man; but at the end of his customary prayer he kicked his footstool so hard that everybody was frightened and arose, the sick man too, healed and praising God.[102]

On the other end of the spectrum, there was surgery, of which the most famous case was the replacement of a diseased lower leg with that of a corpse. The sufferer had "a pointed foreign body [σκόλοπα] in his right lower leg, and the doctors had lavishly spent all his belongings and had not brought him any help."[103] Rather, the evil was getting worse. Having heard of the miracles performed by the famous *anargyroi* Cosmas and Damian, he went to their house and begged them to cure his leg. The saints had to cover their noses, for he already stank, because his bone too was festering. The saints told him that they could not treat the wound, and they referred him to the healing grace of Jesus Christ. But upon his insistence, they ordered him to go inside the house, to rest and pray to God, while they too would pray to the Lord, who would show them what they might do for him. In the night the angel Raphael appeared and directed them to a church where they would find a dead man whose right lower leg they should give the wounded man. "On the day of resurrection each may take his own member, because [the man] went to you with great faith in God. For the Lord also wishes

99. Sozomen (638), *Ecclesiastical History* 16; pp. 267–68 (Walford's translation).

100. Ibid.; p. 266.

101. Lietzmann (423), *Leben* 64; p. 112, ll. 23–25 (from Hilgenfeld's German translation).

102. Ibid.; pp. 112–13.

103. Deubner (169), miracle 48; p. 207, ll. 10–13.

to extol the holy anargyroi." [104] The saints cut off the right lower leg of the corpse at the knee, and likewise that of the wounded man, and exchanged the two. The patient had witnessed the operation in his sleep: "In a dream I saw that men came, cut off my leg, and I was endowed with the leg of another man." [105] The whole story resembles an incubation miracle, with the saints taking the place of Asclepius.

Having been taught the holy books by their mother, Cosmas and Damian

> were taught the medical science [ἐπιστήμην] by the Holy Ghost: to heal in accord with the Gospel "all manner of disease" [Matt. 4:23], not only in human beings, but in cattle as well, that the prophetic oracle might be fulfilled: "O Lord, thou preservest man and beast" [Ps. 36:6].[106] The afflictions that the holy Cosmas and Damian cured were these: to the blind they gave sight, in the name of Jesus Christ, [they] made the lame walk, [they] made cripples sound, [and] by the grace given them they cured all badness within human bodies. Although they cured, they never accepted anything whatsoever from anybody, neither rich nor poor, fulfilling the saying "Freely ye have received, freely give" [Matt. 10:8].[107]

The biography of Cosmas and Damian shows the strong link between the activity of the anargyroi and the precedents set by Jesus. The lists of the diseases they cured are reminiscent of the one Jesus sent to John the Baptist,[108] and the very first case reported in their biography has a precedent in the story of the woman with the bloody flux as told by Luke (8:43–48). A bedridden woman had spent all she had on the doctors without being helped by them. Seeing her faith, the saints readily and quickly effected a cure.[109]

The biography also explained the appellation of "anargyroi" (literally, "without money"). The anargyroi were physician-saints who cured without any remuneration. The legendary life of Saint Cyrus, another anargyros, explains the nature of their activity:

> In his wordly calling, the saint was a physician. This regards the outside, not, however, the mind. In his cures, he healed not only the bodies

---

104. Ibid.; pp. 207 (l. 31)–98 (l. 1). The miracle, as an enhancement of the saints' prestige, puts them into a competitive position.

105. Ibid.; p. 208, ll. 52–53.

106. In the Septuagint, this is Ps. 35:7.

107. Deubner (169), *Leben* 1.9–19; p. 88. Cf. idem, miracle 48; p. 207, ll. 6–9.

108. See above, chap. 9, text following n. 18.

109. Deubner (169), *Leben* 2.2–3; p. 88.

of the sick but also [their] precious souls from whatever diseases had befallen them. And in his visits he led [them] away from that which is alien to the faith, not by addressing the sick [by words out of] Galen and Hippocrates and authors similar to them, but by leading them on to the true strength and life by prophetic, apostolic, and evangelic counsel.[110]

Cyrus was not a combination of physician and priest; he was a doctor of the body and of the soul such as Hippocratic doctors were not.

Holy men could perform miracles, that is, they could do what doctors could not. Theodore of Sykeon, who was not averse to cooperating with physicians, proved able to cure the son of the emperor Maurice after the physicians had got nowhere.[111] This feature was and is common to religious healing from Asclepius on. Besides, saints and holy men either exacted no remuneration—like Jesus and the apostles before them—or, like Asclepius, required a very small contribution that even poor people might be able to afford.

The saints' charity contrasted with the avarice of which physicians were liable to be accused.[112] The legends often tell of sick people's wasting money on drugs and various kinds of healers. The Life of Saint Simeon the Stylite contains several examples: a boy suffering from stone of the bladder;[113] a man with a bent neck, who had also consulted sorcerers and magicians, and whom Simeon told that no man could heal another without God's will;[114] a man with severe head pain;[115] a paralyzed Persian boy whose father had spent a fortune on magicians and sorcerers;[116] and a scoundrel of high rank with a swollen belly.[117] Before coming to Simeon, they all had sought help vainly. After the holy man's death, the mourners asked where they would find a doctor equal to him.[118]

The ineffectiveness of doctors was forcefully brought home when Hippocratic doctors were involved. The emperor had turned over a sick monk to the care of physicians who were at the very top of their profession and among his own intimates. "Employing many of the things out of Galen and Hippocrates as well as [things] reputed to act di-

---

110. Sophronius (635), Vita et conversatio 6; col. 3680D–3681A.
111. Dawes and Baynes (162), "St. Theodore of Sykeon" 97; p. 153.
112. For examples, see Magoulias (438), pp. 131–32.
113. Lietzmann (423), Leben 37; p. 99.
114. Ibid. 64; p. 112.
115. Ibid. 66; p. 114.
116. Ibid. 67; p. 115.
117. Ibid. 92; p. 135.
118. Ibid. 128; p. 73; similarly, idem 129; p. 174.

rectly,[119] [and] toiling vainly day by day, they were put to shame and could not find a remedy advantageous to [the monk] or ward off evil." [120]

Holy men's claims of superiority over doctors could take the form of hostile gloating over their foolish pretensions, as when Saint Artemius asked, "Where now are the loudmouthed Hippocrateses and Galen and [the] other tens of thousands who pretend to be physicians?" [121] Another example, from the wonders of Cyrus and John, involved the physician Gesius,[122] who is said to have declared that the miracles of the saints had been derived from the works of Hippocrates, Galen, and Democritus. However, when ill himself, he could not find relief in the medical art but was cured after obeying the saints' command: he was to have himself pulled around the church with a horse's bit in his mouth, an ass's packsaddle over his shoulders, and a large bell around his neck, all the while shouting, "I am a fool." Having proved their power, the saints asked him: "Tell us where Hippocrates set down the medication for your infirmity? Where does Democritus prescribe anything?" [123]

Behind the disparagement of physicians and the reproach of those so foolish as to spend money on them, there was a covert reprimand of those who did not entrust themselves to Jesus and to God. This reproach took an overt form in a story that Jerome told of Saint Hilarion, to whom a monk brought a woman blind for ten years. She had spent all she had on doctors. "If you had given to the poor what you have lost on the physicians," the saint told her, "the true physician Jesus would have cured you." With those words the matter seems to have been closed for the holy man. When the woman cried and asked for compassion Hilarion "spat in her eyes . . . and the example of the Savior [Mark 8:22–26] was followed forthwith by the same [healing] effect." [124]

The above are samples of the attitudes of holy men toward medicine, and particularly Hippocratic medicine and physicians, as reflected

119. Ἁπλῶς, which means specific drugs.

120. Deubner (169), miracle 47.31–36; p. 206.

121. Papadopoulos-Kerameus (528), miracle 24; p. 34, ll. 18–20: Ποῦ τοίνυν οἱ κομπορρήμονες Ἱπποκράται καὶ Γαληνὸς καὶ ἄλλοι μυρίοι τὸ δοκεῖν ἰατροί?

122. Probably the Alexandrian commentator and editor of Galenic works; see Duffy (192), p. 23.

123. Quoted from Magoulias (438), pp. 130–31. According to Baldwin (72), p. 18 and n. 40, Gesius was converted to Christianity; however, see Nutton (489), p. 6.

124. Jerome (342), Vita Hilarionis 15; col. 36A.

in the hagiographies. Hagiographic literature, even if presented as funeral oration or biography, has a legendary character. Usually written a shorter or longer time after the saint's death, it does not represent the saint as he acted and felt in historical reality.[125] There is not sufficient material to allow a general evaluation of the relationship between these religious healers and the physicians, and the extent to which they cooperated with, competed with, or were isolated from one another. Conditions varied regionally, and whether the services of Hippocratic doctors were readily available in rural areas is doubtful anyhow.[126] In the cities of the East, physicians were not swept aside by the saintly healers and the miracles wrought by them. Relatively little was heard of secular doctors during the early Middle Ages of the Latin West,[127], but this may have been due to social changes, such as the desolation of the cities and the parceling of the land into feudal estates, rather than to a conflict between secular and religious healing. The existence of such a conflict cannot be denied,[128] but the fact that ancient medical writings were copied in monasteries and that monks were known to have written short medical treatises for practical use argues against a widespread suppression of secular medicine, even if medicine was not practiced by many learned secular healers.

The hagiographic literature suggests the inadequacy of any simple characterization of the relationship between holy men and physicians. This much, however, can be said: Such Christian antagonism as existed against Hippocratic medicine in Late Antiquity found a more deeply *felt* expression among some of the holy men (as they were seen by their biographers and eulogists) than in the literature of the theologians, be they monks or secular Christian authors. Strong as the influence of the ascetic movement was, it did not dictate the official attitude of the church.

125. Fox (230), pp. 18–20, cites the legendary life and activity of Hilarion as an illustration of the aims of hagiography.

126. Hippocratic doctors were more likely to be summoned to rural places than to settle there; cf. below, chap. 17.A, Paul of Aegina's explanation of the need for a manual.

127. According to Müller (473), p. 204, both Ambrose and Augustine remarked that there were few who practiced medicine as a profession.

128. See Sudhoff (657).

13

HIPPOCRATIC MEDICINE
AND SPIRITUAL MEDICINE

The welcome extended to men of the church who could care for both the soul and the body, as well as the acceptance of secular medical care as a common practice for ordinary Christians, go to show that secular medicine, Hippocratic medicine in particular, played its part in the Christian civilization of the East. Nor was it lacking in the Latin civilization of the West as long as Roman culture and Mediterranean economic life prevailed. East and West, however, are broad terms that conceal the regional differences within each of the two territories.

Yet though Hippocratic medicine was welcomed, or at least accepted on sufferance, there was no consensus as to its place in Christian theology, nor was there anything that might be called "the Christian attitude" toward Hippocratic medicine and physicians. Outspoken hostility also existed and cannot be disregarded, even though it was harbored by an extreme wing. In the circumstances, one can do no more than present a view that integrated many of the existing tendencies, avoided one-sidedness, and represented the opinion of an influential churchman in touch with medicine. The combination of these qualifications gives importance to the position of Basil the Great.

As part of the general thesis "that God is not the author of evils,"[1] Basil argued that

---

1. Basil (82), *Quod Deus non est auctor malorum.*

disease is neither unbegotten nor [is it] God's work. Living beings were created with a structure fitting for them in accordance with nature, and they were brought into life with limbs complete. Yet they became ill when diverted from [their] natural state. For they are deprived of health either because of a bad regimen or because of a morbific cause, whatever it may be. Thus God created the body, not disease. Also, God made the soul, not sin. Yet the soul became vitiated when diverted from [its] natural state.[2]

By declaring body and soul to be healthy in their natural, God-created state and ill when diverted from it, and by stressing bad diet as a morbific cause where the body was concerned, Basil gave a theological foundation to the question "Whether it is in accordance with piety to use what comes from medicine?" Both the question and its answer appear in a text entitled *More Extensively Treated Rules,* which belongs to Basil's ascetic writings.[3] The rules are not a monastic code; they are "spiritual counsels and commentaries on Scripture"[4] addressed to monks and devout and dedicated Christians. And the question concerns possible benefits for the body as well as for the soul, as becomes very clear at the very beginning of the answer.

God granted to mankind such arts as agriculture, weaving, architecture, and medicine, which were needed after the expulsion from paradise. But at the same time, medicine, apart from serving man's material needs, was intended for a higher purpose:

> Our body, prone to affliction, is subject to sundry harm, some befalling from outside and other engendered within, from food. It suffers from surfeits and depletions. Therefore the medical art, which counsels the removal of what is superfluous and the addition of what is wanting, has been conceded to us by God, who orders all our life, as a model for the therapy of the soul.[5]

The definition of medicine given here is Hippocratic.[6] The theme of Hippocratic medicine as a model for the healing of the soul is elabo-

---

2. Ibid. 6; col. 344A. For man's natural, God-created state, cf. above, chap. 12, n. 28, and the text to that note.

3. Basil (84), *Regulae fusius tractatae,* interrogatio 55; cols. 1043–52: Εἰ τοῖς ἐκ τῆς ἰατρικῆς κεχρῆσθαι κατὰ σκοπὸν ἐστι τῆς εὐσεβείας. Although this question has been covered by Frings (239), pp. 12–14; and by Amundsen (16), pp. 338–39, I have, in spite of considerable overlap, retained my interpretation for the sake of a coherent argument.

4. Knowles (366), p. 22.

5. Basil (84), interrogatio 55, art. l; col. 1044C.

6. Hippocrates (306), *On Breaths* 1; p. 92, ll. 8–9.

rated throughout, and is here presented in a version in which the paradigmatic use of somatic medicine is one of God's aims, if not the major aim, in His bestowing medicine on mankind.

Basil's attitude to somatic medicine was positive. He established a basic identity between materia medica and what we eat and drink. This again is a basic principle of Hippocratic-Galenic medicine. It allowed Basil to warn against the luxury of the table as well as against the over-elaboration of hygienic and therapeutic prescriptions: "Christians must abstain from what is contrived and elaborate, what diverts strongly from other things, and turns our whole life, as it were, over to the care of the flesh." [7] The admonition not to make the body life's main concern was directed to all Christians.

Medicine, Basil thought, was given to mankind to provide "a certain measure" [8] of help to the sick. [9] This may seem to be a more realistic evaluation of medicine, especially as it then was, than the self-assured therapeutic optimism of Galen. But realism as a possible factor is made less likely by Basil's adding: "and we must take heed to use the [medical] art, if ever needed, so as not to invest it with the entire cause of [our] being healthy or sick. Rather, we must receive the use of what belongs to medicine with a view to the glory of God and as an example of the care of the soul." [10]

If medical help is not available, we must not give up hope. Scripture offers several examples of divine cure, and we must bear in mind that God will not try us beyond our endurance. God acts in many ways; thus a lengthy dietetic treatment may be suitable not only for the body but for the soul as well. "It is fitting to rid oneself of what is foreign and to get hold of what is according to nature, because God made man upright[11] and for good works that he might walk in them." [12] Probity and uprightness, to Basil, belong to the natural state of the soul.[13]

We must not reject all of medicine's benefits because some people misuse it. We make use of cooking and weaving, though they too are misused. It is unreasonable to slander God's gift. To place the hope for one's health in the physician's hands, "as we see some wretches do who are not averse to calling them saviors," [14] is acting like sheep. On the

7. Basil (84), interrogatio 55, art. 2; col. 1045B.
8. Κατὰ τὸ ποσόν.
9. Basil (84), interrogatio 55, art. 1; col. 1045A.
10. Ibid. 2; col. 1045B.
11. Εὐθῇ; cf. Septuaginta (617); and Eccles. 7:29.
12. Basil (84), interrogatio 55, art. 2; col. 1045C–D.
13. See above, n. 2.
14. Basil (84), interrogatio 55, art. 3; col. 1048B.

other hand, it is obstinate to flee from medicine entirely. We should act as King Hezekiah did, to whom Isaiah gave "a lump of figs" to put on his boil (2 Kings 20:7). The king did not consider the lump of figs an ultimate cause of health nor the cause of his recovery. Rather, he gratefully glorified God for the creation of figs. We ought to ask God His reason for inflicting His blows on us, then ask for the removal of the pain, and finally, ask Him to grant us endurance.

Basil accepted Hippocratic medicine, but not as existing independently of God. All healing had to be accepted gratefully, regardless of whether God's help worked invisibly—this probably referred to spontaneous healing—or through bodily means. The latter could even be more conducive to making us aware of God's favor. Often, when disease befalls us to teach us a lesson, we are condemned, as part of our education, to submit to very painful therapy. Sound reasoning tells us "not to refuse cutting or burning, nor the pain caused by sharp and toilsome drugs, nor a rigorously measured diet, nor abstinence from noxious things." [15] And all the time, we have to keep in mind that what is done somatically was intended to serve as a model for the care of the soul.

This is the religious framework within which Basil accepts Hippocratic medicine, but its validity is limited. He believed that not all diseases belong to the realm of nature and befall us because of a faulty diet or some other somatic cause—that is, not all diseases are of the kind against which medicine is sometimes useful. To think that all afflictions require medical help is vain and dangerous. Diseases can also be scourges for our sins and can lead to our conversion. Once we realize that we are being judged and chastised by God [16] and recognize our sins, we must discard medical help and bear what we have brought upon ourselves in accordance with the saying "I will bear the indignation of the Lord, because I have sinned against him" (Mic. 7:9). Diseases may also arise at the prompting of the Evil One, as was the case with Job; or as with Lazarus (Luke 16:20), they may be inflicted to provide an example for those who are not capable of bearing suffering until death. Another cause of disease is found among the saints, as in the case of the apostle Paul, who for his entire life carried a disease, lest he be thought to surpass the limits of human nature and his natural constitution be thought to be out of the ordinary. [17] How could such people

---

15. Ibid. 4; cols. 1048D–94A.
16. Ibid. 4; col. 1049A–B; Basil quotes Prov. 3:12 and 1 Cor. 11:30 and 32.
17. As happened in Lycaonia (Acts 14:11–13); Basil (84), interrogatio 55, art. 4; col. 1049A–D.

benefit from medicine? Would there not be danger of their swaying from the right word (of God) to the care of the body?[18]

Basil's dichotomization of diseases into those that have a natural origin (while remaining under God's authority) and those that have a supernatural[19] cause and purpose seems clear enough. The first class is amenable to medical treatment, the second is not. But the dichotomy involves a practical difficulty that Basil does not address explicitly: What symptoms and diagnostic signs assigned a person's disease to the first or the second category? The absence of somatic causes and the failure of medical therapy, as well as the awareness of personal guilt, could be indicative but were neither comprehensive nor reliable. An incorrect medical diagnosis and poor treatment might be responsible for the failure of medical treatment, while a ready admission of guilt could result from the imaginings of a person convinced of his own sinfulness and worthlessness. But this diagnostic difficulty has been inherent in all attempts—be they pagan, Christian, or secular—to dichotomize diseases into those of the body and those transcending it and can still be found in modern attempts to distinguish between somatic and psychogenic factors in disease.

Toward the end of his discussion, Basil summarized the acceptable view of medicine:

> This art must neither be shunned altogether, nor must all hope be set on it. Rather, as we use agriculture and yet ask God for the fruits and [as we] entrust the rudder to the helmsman but pray God that we may safely return from the sea, so in summoning a physician when this is reasonable[20] we do not renounce the hope that should be put in God.[21]

Moderate ascetics came into their own in his final eulogy of the spiritual value of medicine. Because of its dietetic strictures, "the art also contributes not a little to self-discipline" and "calls want[22] [the] mother of health."[23] Thus, what dietetic medicine demanded for the welfare of the body was also demanded by asceticism for the welfare of the soul. Above all else, Christians who loved God should accept from medicine its guidance toward a saintly life. And so Basil concluded with

18. Basil (84), interrogatio 55, art. 5; col. 1052A.
19. Basil does not use this word.
20. Basil (84), interrogatio 55, art. 5; col. 1052B: ὅτε λόγος συγχωρεῖ. This may also mean summoning the doctor when it does not conflict with God's word.
21. Ibid.; col. 1052A–B.
22. As contrasted with surfeit and satiety.
23. Basil (84), interrogatio 55, art. 5; col. 1052B.

the words of Paul (1 Cor. 10:31): " 'Whether therefore ye eat, or drink, or whatever ye do, do all to the glory of God.' "[24]

Christian theology, the biblical symbolism of disease, and biblical examples of diseases of the soul transformed the pagan medicine of the soul into a spiritual medicine. Hippocratic medicine retained its function of providing the necessary mundane analogues. But this function was now seen as one of God's purposes—actually His chief purpose—in granting medicine to mankind. It was the main benefit that piety could and should derive from medicine.

Spiritual medicine had its beginnings long before Christianity and before Basil. It had been adumbrated by the Psalms and by the Prophets, and it had been in the thoughts of Origen.[25] The Apostolic Constitutions, with its detailed comparison between the treatment of sinners and the medical treatment of wounds,[26] had provided an example of its practical application. In centuries to come, spiritual medicine was a major guide for the activities of preachers and confessors.[27]

Basil chose Hippocratic medicine as the mundane analogue for spiritual medicine for both personal and theoretical reasons. In Athens he had studied the philosophical basis of medicine, and in a passage of his homiletic work on the origin of man,[28] he appears as an admirer of the Hippocratic tradition as represented by Galen:

> If you go to medicine, you will find out how many things have been described regarding the use of what is ours, how many hidden paths it has discovered in the course of anatomical administrations:[29] invisible junctions, a complete cooperation [of the parts] of the body,[30] ducts for [the] breath, conveyances of the blood, [the] pull of inhaling, [the] domiciling of the hearth of heat in the heart, [the] continuous movement of the pneuma around the heart.[31]

---

24. Ibid.; col. 1052C. For the spiritual meaning of health and disease among ascetics, see Harvey (290), pp. 87–93.

25. See above, chap. 11, especially the text to nn. 73 and 74.

26. See above, chap. 11, text to nn. 64–66. Miller (463), p. 60, gives another example of the wound metaphor.

27. The theme of the *medicina celestis* and its relationship to mundane medicine has been given elaborate treatment by Agrimi and Crisciani (4).

28. Basil's authorship of homilies 10 and 11 on the Hexameron has been convincingly argued by Smets and Van Esbroeck in their introduction to Basil (85).

29. Ἐν ταῖς ἀνατομικαῖς ἐγχειρήσεσιν. The title of Galen's main anatomical work was Περὶ ἀνατομικῶν ἐγχειρήσεων (*On Anatomical Administrations*).

30. Μίαν σύμπνοιαν ἀπὸ τοῦ σώματος, which Smets and Van Esbroeck (85), p. 169, translate as "la concertation du corps pour respirer." Σύμπνοια may have been used with reference to the Hippocratic σύμπνοια μία, πάντα συμπαθέα (Hippocrates [306], *On Nutriment* 23; p. 81, ll. 5–6).

31. Basil (85), homily 1.2; p. 168, ll. 2–9. Instead of περικαρδίου I read περὶ

Somewhat later Basil adds, "and having understood the art [vested] in me, with what wisdom the body of mine has been constructed, I have from this small structure perceived the great Maker [δημιουργόν]."[32] This was Galen's natural theology, with nature, Galen's demiurge, replaced by God.[33]

By making available a wide variety of medical analogues, Hippocratic medicine became a vital part of Christian theological exegesis and pastoral practice. The relationship was not reciprocal, for medicine obtained relatively little in return, unless its adoption by the church is considered ample compensation. At the head of spiritual medicine stood Christ, the physician of the soul.[34] As a physician, Christ added luster to the medical profession,[35] without however entering into the substance of the science and the art of Hippocratic medicine. A doctor might invoke "Jesus, our real physician for ever and ever,"[36] but this was a testimonial to the physician's piety rather than an essential part of his medical reasoning. Fundamentally, "Christ the physician" was a religious theme.[37]

[τὴν] καρδίαν. On this passage, cf. the excerpt by Gregory of Nyssa, quoted above, chap. 11, text to n. 41.

32. Ibid., p. 170, ll. 19–22.

33. See below, chap. 14, text to nn. 78–84. The Christian recognition of the material world as the beautiful, orderly, and beneficent creation of God goes at least as far back as Origen's fight with the Gnostic heretics; see Chadwick (138), p. 104.

34. For the close relationship between spiritual medicine and the theme of "Christ the physician," see Agrimi and Crisciani (4), chap. 3 ("Medici e sacerdoti"); also Miller (463), pp. 58–61.

35. See above, chap. 11, text to nn. 95–99.

36. Theophilus (680), *On Excrements;* 1:408. Theophilus probably belongs to the seventh century.

37. See Arbesmann (38) for the religious role of the *Christus medicus* motif in the work of Augustine. The predominantly religious (rather than medical) significance of the motif also is evidenced by the examples cited by other authors; see Fichtner (223), Honecker (314), Schadewaldt (609), and Schipperges (610).

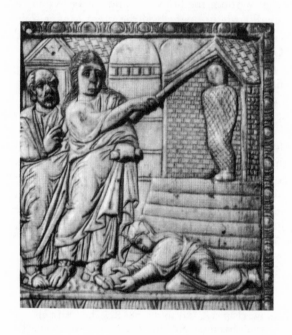

Christ as miracle healer. Detail of an Italian diptych, ca. 450–
460. From Peter Brown, *The World of Late Antiquity: Marcus
Aurelius to Muhammad.* London: Thames and Hudson, 1971,
p. 55.

VI

Hippocratism Encounters Christianity

The attitudes of Christians and of their church toward Hippocratic medicine defined the conditions under which this medicine and its doctors were acceptable to Christianity. That left open the question of how Hippocratic doctors looked at the new religion, and of the conditions under which they might exercise their art.

Tertullian had said that Christians were made, not born. It probably was true that during the first two and a half centuries, pagan physicians who converted did so for religious reasons. But with the ascent of the church to power, the reasons for conversion often were other than religious. Gradually, moreover, Tertullian's dictum ceased to be true, and physicians too were born Christian and lived in Christian surroundings.

Whether converted or born into the faith, there was the question of whether a doctor could be a true believer and at the same time practice Hippocratic medicine, that child of pagan culture. Were there no pagan elements intrinsic to this medicine that would stand in conflict with Christian beliefs and dogmas and that the church could not, or would not, tolerate? What compromises, if any, were needed on the part of physicians and of the church in order to establish a *modus vivendi?* The cult of any pagan god intimately associated with the practice of medicine, and the immanence of the belief in any divine power other than God in the theory of medicine, would obviously be obstacles to the conversion of Hippocratic doctors. To put it more concretely: Was there a Hippocratic religion binding Hippocratic doctors professionally to the cult of Asclepius? Was Hippocratic theory founded on the belief in nature as an autonomous divine power?

14

WAS THERE A

HIPPOCRATIC RELIGION?

A. The Cult of Asclepius

The cult of Asclepius suggests itself as the most important of the cults for several reasons. The Homeric Asclepius, before becoming a god of healing, may have been the patron saint of the doctors. The Asclepiads traced their genealogy to him, and "sons of Asclepius" became a popular term for physicians.[1] The Hippocratic oath invoked the healing god, his legendary father Apollo,[2] and two goddesses of his family. The history of the oath during the early Christian centuries thus is of some importance regarding the relationship of physicians for Asclepius. At least from the first century on, the oath attributed to Hippocrates was held in high regard; it was alluded to in the poem of Sarapion, and it entered into the early medieval and Arabic texts that have been loosely grouped together as the Testament of Hippocrates. "Be mindful of the Hippocratic Oath, and abstain from all guilt and especially from immorality and acts of seduction,"[3] says one text, and another says, "He who wishes to begin the art of medicine and the science of nature ought to take the oath and not shrink in any way whatsoever

---

1. See above, chap. 7.
2. However, the oath called him "Apollo the physician" without any reference to his fatherhood.
3. Quoted from MacKinney (435), text 4; p. 12.

from the consequences."[4] Since swearing the Hippocratic oath seems to have been common in Alexandria in the fourth century,[5] "the oath" here probably meant the Hippocratic oath. At any rate, the Hippocratic oath in its pagan form was certainly a major document of medical ethics until at least about the end of the fourth century.

The ethics of the oath harmonize so well with Judaeo-Christian morality that an early influence of the oath has been conjectured in the so-called *Didache,* or *Teaching of the Twelve Apostles.* It commanded, "You shall not murder an infant by means of an abortifacient nor kill [it] after [its] birth."[6] But this prohibition was too much in line with Judaeo-Christian thinking to prove that the *Didache* had borrowed from the pagan medical text. All expectation to the contrary, the oath did not feature prominently in Christian writings of the early centuries. Jerome knew the oath, and wrote to a young priest that

> before he will teach [them], Hippocrates entreats his pupils seriously and compels them to swear obedience to him. He exacts silence from them by an oath; he lays down for them their language, approach, dress, and manners. How much greater an obligation is laid on us who have been entrusted with healing the souls, [and] with loving the houses of all Christians as if they were our own.[7]

In addition to the scanty Christian references, a passage in the funeral oration of Gregory of Nazianzus for his brother Caesarius hints at a Christian's refusal to swear the oath. Caesarius's studies in Alexandria had included medicine, which he then practiced in Byzantium to great acclaim. "Because he was beloved by all for his moderation, he was entrusted by them with what is most precious. He had no need of Hippocrates to administer the oath to him."[8]

---

4. Quoted from ibid., text 11; p. 15. On the Testament of Hippocrates, see above, chap. 11, n. 84.

5. See below, text to n. 8.

6. See *Didache* (172), 2.2; 1:310–12. *Epistle of Barnabas* (75), 19.5; p. 402, has the same interdict of abortion and infanticide. The interdict is thus part of the earliest Christian tradition. Pines (550) has drawn attention to parallels between the Hippocratic oath, the pertinent part of the *Didache* (i.e., "The Doctrine of the Two Ways," which he [p. 227] considers to be probably "a Jewish pre-Christian text"), and the Hebrew oath in the *Sefer ha-Refuot* of Asaph the Jew.

7. Jerome (339), *Epistulae* 52.15; pp. 438–39; and Wright (341), p. 224. My translation deviates from that of Wright (followed by MacKinney [435], p. 3), which suggests that Jerome confused the oath and other deontological texts.

8. Gregory of Nazianzus (272), *Oratio VII,* art. 10; col. 767A. Quoted from McCauley's ([270] p. 12) translation. Keenan (360), p. 11, seems to believe that Caesarius was not required to take the oath in Byzantium, where he was practicing medicine.

By about A.D. 500, parts of the Hippocratic oath were incorporated into the Hebrew oath.[9] At some uncertain time, a Christian paraphrase appeared: "From the Oath according to Hippocrates in so far [sic] as a Christian may swear it. Blessed be God the Father of our Lord Jesus Christ, who is blessed for ever and ever; I lie not. I will bring no stain upon the learning of the medical art. Neither will I give poison to anybody though asked to do so, nor will I suggest such a plan," and so on.[10]

Too little is known about the circumstances of swearing the Hippocratic oath to tell how serious an obstacle the swearing was to the conversion to Christianity. At any rate, it would be unwarranted to infer from its existence and its moral weight that a specifically medical cult of Asclepius had existed, which made physicians servants of the god. The belief of many, if not most, doctors in Asclepius's power to cure is indisputable. Around A.D. 200, a physician from Smyrna donated a statue of "king Asclepius" as "a visible offering" for having many times avoided sickness by following the god's counsel. The physician called himself a "servant [θεράπων]" of Asclepius.[11] Another doctor, Nicias, offered frankincense daily to a statue of Asclepius.[12] Rufus of Ephesus, one of the greatest clinicians around A.D. 100, related that an epileptic had been cured of his epilepsy by Asclepius, who first changed it to quartan fever, a form of malaria, with which the doctors knew how to cope. This moved Rufus to comment that a doctor able to provoke fever deserved to be considered a god.[13] In a lengthy poem on theriac, Asclepius was invoked to cure the emperor Marcus Aurelius:

Be gracious, blessed healer [Παιών], you who fashioned this remedy, whether the Triccaean ridges hold you, O divine being [δαῖμον], or Rhodes, or Cos and Epidaurus on the sea; be gracious, send your always gracious daughter, Panacea, to the emperor, who will propitiate you with pure sacrifices for the everlasting freedom from pain which you can grant.[14]

9. See Pines (550), pp. 230, 241–44, 246, 255, and 257; for the Hebrew oath, see above, n. 6.

10. Quoted from Jones (350), p. 23.

11. Edelstein and Edelstein (197), T 600 (the Edelsteins' translation). In a similar inscription (T 599), the same doctor calls Asclepius "saviour" instead of king.

12. See Festugière (221), p. 144, n. 15.

13. Oribasius (505), *Collectiones* 45.30; 3:192. Pace Kudlien (386), pp. 122–25. In my opinion Rufus did not believe man to be capable of causing quartan fever.

14. T 595 (the Edelsteins' translation; modified); from Galen (241), *De antidotis* 1.6; 14:42.

Galen also knew of cases of miraculous cures by Asclepius[15] and acknowledged that he himself had been saved by the god. When the emperor Marcus Aurelius wished to take Galen along to the wars, he was persuaded to withdraw his request, "having heard," as Galen said, that "the ancestral[16] god Asclepius of whom I declared myself a servant [θεραπευτὴν], since he saved me when I was in a deadly condition from an abscess, had commanded otherwise."[17] Galen probably meant no more than that he had become a devout worshipper of Asclepius. But the fact that this happened only after the god had given him life-saving advice argues against the assumption that mere membership in the profession bound doctors to the cult.

A clearer picture of how doctors behaved toward Asclepius and what they thought of his power emerges from the *Sacred Tales* of Aelius Aristides. A famous orator and, like his contemporary Galen, a man of independent means, Aristides was plagued throughout much of his life by illnesses in which the somatic and the mental components were indissolubly combined. After having sought help from Serapis and Isis,[18] he turned to Asclepius and spent two years (A.D. 145–47) in Pergamum. He observed his symptoms lovingly and, in his *Sacred Tales*, described them minutely,[19] together with the treatment Asclepius prescribed to him in his dreams. Many of Asclepius's prescriptions were bizarre and, as Aristides himself said, likely to make physicians "shudder whenever they hear many of these practices."[20] Yet Aristides claimed to be alive because at various times, thanks to the god, he had escaped "from things which no physician knew what to call, to say nothing of cure, nor had seen befall the nature of man."[21]

Aristides did not reject medical science and had physicians in his

15. See T 459 and T 436.

16. Πάτριον, which probably referred to the sanctuary in Galen's native Pergamum.

17. Galen (242), *De libris propriis* 2; 2:99, ll. 8–11. My translation differs somewhat from the Edelsteins' T 458 (cf. also T 358 and T 413). On this whole episode, see Nutton (250), p. 212. Wilamowitz-Moellendorff (721), 2:506, n. 1, referred to Galen's "*Ausrede*."

18. For Isis and Serapis as healing gods, see Kee (358), pp. 67–68. Healings by Isis as described by Diodorus of Sicily (181), 1.25.2–7; 1:80–83, resemble healings by Asclepius to a degree that suggests adaptation to the Greek god.

19. For analyses of his illnesses, see Behr (87), chap. 7 ("Disease and Medicine"); and Gourevitch (267), pp. 38–70. I confess skepticism regarding the possibility of understanding most of Aristides' illnesses in modern diagnostic terms.

20. Aristides (42), *To Plato* 70–71; p. 323 (Behr's translation). On Aristides' bizarre prescriptions, see Behr (87), p. 36.

21. Ibid. 67; p. 321 (Behr's translation).

entourage who visited him and dispensed medical advice. During one of his illnesses, he was receiving instructions from Asclepius when his physician arrived, ready "to help, as much as he knew how. But when he heard of the dream, being a sensible man, he also yielded [ὑπεχώρει] to the god. And we recognized the true physician, fitting for us, and we did what he prescribed." [22] This is how Aristides formulated his relationship to doctors and to Asclepius in serious illness:

> Even when we were stricken in body, we did not come to ignoble supplication of the doctors. But although, to speak by the grace of the gods, we possessed the friendship of the best doctors,[23] we took refuge in the [temple] of Asclepius, in the belief that if it was fated for us to be saved, it was better to be saved through his agency, and that if it was not possible, it was time to die.[24]

To this the translator remarks that "it was only after unsuccessful experiences with human doctors that Aristides turned to Asclepius." [25]

It was just the paradoxical in Asclepius's cures that attracted Aristides, and by which he felt honored.[26] For instance, once, during the winter, when the north wind was blowing and the cold so great that pebbles were frozen to one another, Asclepius commanded him to bathe in the river. Obeying the dream, Aristides went down to the river escorted by "friends and various doctors, some of them acquaintances, and others who came either out of concern or even for the purpose of investigation." [27] A physician, a companion of Aristides, later confessed that he was convinced that at best Aristides would suffer from trouble in his spine or something similar. Arriving at the river, Aristides, "still full of warmth from the vision of the god," went in where it was deepest, swam about, and came out, all his skin rosy and his body comfortable. The assembled crowd shouted, "Great is Asclepius." [28]

22. Aristides (44), *Orationes* 47.57; pp. 389(l. 30)–90(l. 3). I have utilized the translations by the Edelsteins, T 418, and by Behr (87), p. 287.

23. For the physician as a friend, see Celsus (137), *De medicina*, prooemium, art. 73; 1:40; also Seneca (see below, chap. 16, text to nn. 38 and 39). Apparently Aristides considered turning to physicians ignoble. As he saw it, he happened to have physicians among his friends who offered him their advice.

24. Aristides (44), *Orationes* 28.132; p. 183, ll. 11–15. Quoted from Behr's ([43], p. 134) translation.

25. Behr (43), p. 387, n. 188.

26. T 317.8. Cf. Aristides (43), pp. 248–49.

27. Aristides (44), *Orationes* 48.20; p. 399, ll. 8–15 Quoted from Behr's ([43], p. 295) translation.

28. Aristides (44), *Orationes* 48.21; p. 399. Quoted from Behr's ([43], pp. 295–96) translation. This exclamation was a "typical expression of the act of faith" (Festugière [221], p. 100).

For Aristides, Asclepius was a physician superior to all secular doctors and to be followed when the latter failed or when their opinion conflicted with the god's. Moreover, Asclepius was not only the great physician but also the god who had made Aristides' illnesses "worthwhile [λυσιτελῇ]."[29] The manifestations of the god—in dreams that were halfway between sleeping and waking[30]—gave him an indescribable feeling of closeness to the divinity. "If any man has been initiated he knows and understands."[31] In view of the temple of Zeus Asclepius in Pergamum, Aristides accepted Asclepius as the ruler of the universe and the savior of mankind. By saving mankind from extinction, Asclepius had made the race immortal. In contrast to Christianity, this doctrine did not give eternal life to the individual. As physician and as savior, Asclepius aided men in all troubles, somatic and mental, that befell them in this world.[32]

The physicians around Aristides did not view Asclepius with equal fervor. Only if they were persuaded by their patient did they yield to the god when his command ran counter to their own, and they praised him if convinced by the outcome. Their reluctance to give up their opinion, and their subsequent change of mind can be discerned in the episode of the tumor in Aristides' thigh. Insignificant at first, it progressed to a monstrous size, the groin was engulfed, everything was swollen, terrible pain followed, and there was some fever. "The doctors cried out all sorts of things, some said surgery, some said cauterization by drugs, or that putrefaction would develop and I must surely die."[33] But Asclepius would have none of this: Aristides must endure! It was clear to him that he must follow the god rather than the physicians. When the tumor enlarged still more, some of his friends admired his endurance, while others censured him for relying too much on dreams or accused him of lacking courage because he allowed neither surgery nor cauterization by drugs. But Asclepius remained adamant and, amazingly, during the four months that all this lasted, Aristides' head and upper abdomen felt quite comfortable, and he even delivered speeches from his bed.

While the inflammation was at its height and had almost reached the navel, the god ordered Aristides to do various strange and arduous things. Then Asclepius prescribed a drug, and upon its application,

29. T 402.16 (from *Oratio* 23), see also T 317.6.
30. See Aristides (44), *Orationes* 48.18 and 32.
31. Ibid. 48.33; p. 402, ll. 3–4. Quoted from Behr's ([43], p. 298) translation.
32. See Aristides (44), 48.4–7. On Zeus-Asclepius, see Benedum (90).
33. Aristides (44), *Orationes* 47.62; p. 391, ll. 4–6. Quoted from Behr's ([43], p. 288) translation.

"most of the tumor quickly flowed away."[34] From this point on, "the doctors stopped their criticisms, expressed extraordinary admiration for the providence of the god in each particular, and said that it was some other greater [μεῖζον] disease, which he secretly cured."[35] Still, they thought that surgery was indicated to remove the loose skin, now that "what concerned the god had been wholly accomplished."[36] But again Asclepius objected, and achieved a perfect cure.

Generally speaking, doctors of the second century not only believed in Asclepius but conceded that he was a greater healer than they. They may even have welcomed his cult because it offered them the possibility of referring hopeless or difficult cases to him.[37] Nevertheless, their naturalistic training made them hesitate to accept paradoxical treatments. Thus, Aristides' doctors assumed that Asclepius had diagnosed and treated a "greater" disease behind the tumor—a disease that had escaped them.[38] There were also doctors who were skeptical of Asclepius's cures. A patient told his doctor that Asclepius had advised him to anoint his eyes with boar's fat dissolved in vinegar. The physician "sarcastically [εἴρων]" explained that "one part of the [prescription] contracted the swelling by its acidity and the other anointed the eyes and nourished them gently."[39]

In later centuries, eminent Hippocratic physicians resisted the advance of Christianity. Loyalty to the cult of Asclepius does not seem to have been the reason for their resistance. Eventually the devotional and liturgical cult of God and Christ replaced the cult of Asclepius, which even the works On the Sacred Disease and On Airs, Waters, Localities had not rejected.[40]

The Hippocratic On Regimen took a very positive attitude toward the gods who "ordered [the] nature of all [things]."[41] The fourth book,

34. Aristides (44), Orationes 47.66; 2:392, ll. 2–3. Cf. Behr (43), p. 428, n. 89.
35. Aristides (44), Orationes 47.67; 2:392, ll. 4–6. Quoted from Behr's ([43], p. 289) translation.
36. Aristides (44), Orationes 47.67; 2:392, ll. 9–10. Quoted from Behr's ([43], p. 289) translation.
37. See Edelstein (198), pp. 245–46.
38. I see no reason to assume that this means a disease of a divine order.
39. T 405 (the Edelsteins' translation, modified). Kudlien (386), pp. 124–25, mentions this, as well as another instance of medical skepticism. However, regarding Galen's "implicit criticism of an Asclepius cure" (Kudlien (386), p. 124, with reference to T 401), I think that Galen merely stressed what some people's belief will do, without himself approving or disapproving of the god's orders.
40. They did not, however, mention it.
41. Hippocrates (302), On Regimen 1.11; 4:248, l. 13. On this work, cf. Diller (178), pp. 70–88.

devoted to dreams, in certain cases even ordered prayers to specific deities.[42] The author was concerned with dreams in which the soul, awake while the body slept, indicated somatic changes and hence the proper prophylactic treatment. Prayer was particularly indicated in dreams that involved the heavenly bodies or the earth.[43] But with all his respect for prayer, the author did not consider it a substitute for medical action. "Prayer indeed is good, but while calling on the gods a man should himself lend a hand."[44]

The later *Decorum* claimed that "knowledge about the gods" was "woven into the mind of medicine." In most cases of disease, "medicine is found to be held in honor by the gods. And the physicians have yielded [παρακεχωρήκασιν] to the gods. For in medicine the ruling power is not unessential. In fact, though the physicians take many things in hand, many [diseases] are also overcome for them spontaneously."[45] Spontaneous healing was thus ascribed to the gods, and in those cases the doctors yielded to them, who were the ruling power. Thus the author of *Decorum* could say that "knowledge about the gods" was "woven into the mind of medicine."[46] Aristides' doctor also had yielded to the god when confronted with Asclepius's orders.[47] Here it was the superiority of an individual god. But when *Decorum* speaks of the gods as the ruling power, it may well be asked whether it refers to the gods of the cult or to divine power in general. The divine is repeatedly mentioned in the Hippocratic writings and is often identified with phenomena that we call natural. Was spontaneous healing the deliberate act of a god, or was it a natural process considered to be divine because nature itself was divine?[48] No clear-cut answer is forthcoming, nor is it justified to expect of the ancient physicians a radical distinction rooted in the Judaeo-Christian notion of the natural as subordinated to the divine, the truly "supernatural."

The concept of nature and its close relationship to thoughts about

42. Hippocrates (302), *On Regimen* 4.89 and 90; 4:436 and 440. On dreams in this work, see Diller (178), pp. 70–83.

43. Hippocrates (302), *On Regimen* 4.89 and 90. This hints at a link between the original gods and their secularization as climatic and cosmic factors of disease.

44. Ibid. 4.87; 4:423 (Jones's translation).

45. Hippocrates (306), *Decorum* 6; p. 27, ll. 13–18. Quotation modified from Jones's ([302], 2:289) translation.

46. Cf. Edelstein (198), pp. 216–217, on the connection between the divine and spontaneous healing. I think, however, that this connection does not exist in all cases, especially in *Prognostic* 1, cited below in text to n. 61.

47. See above, text to n. 22.

48. See above, n. 46.

the divine were so deeply grounded in Hippocratic medical thinking as to force the question of whether Hippocratic medicine was inseparably bound to a religion of nature.

B. Nature

The cult of the gods, including Asclepius, belonged to the realm of supplicant piety.[49] The gods were expected to respond to prayer and sacrifice. But ever since Xenophanes of Colophon, toward the late sixth century B.C., had criticized as anthropomorphic the gods of myth and of the poets, philosophers had begun to develop notions of the divine that tried to avoid anthropomorphism. They demythologized the gods and identified the divine with nature as a power ruling the universe with immanent necessity[50] (i.e., without regard to human wishes). As a rule of law, nature was both order and norm. What was natural was normal, that is, it was as it should be, and it was just.[51] For the enlightened Greeks, it has been said that nature was "the real and truly divine . . . before which [man] must prostrate himself in veneration." Theirs has been called "a physiological piety [a piety with nature, *phusis*, as its object], more or less harmoniously united with the cult of the traditional gods and accepted by the authors of the Hippocratic collection."[52]

The influence of pre-Socratic philosophy on the authors of the Hippocratic Collection is well established, and some of their writings carry the stamp of the Sophistic enlightenment of the fifth century. But instead

49. I use the term "supplicant piety" as more serviceable than Festugière's (221) "popular piety," which he opposes to the "reflective piety" of the philosophers. The two forms of piety, supplicant and reflective, were not as isolated from each other as I make it appear for the sake of clarity, and their interconnection was rather intricate and by no means entirely logical.

50. For details of the development of natural theology, see Jaeger (337), especially pp. 1–4. For necessity (ἀνάγκη) as immanent in nature, see below, text to nn. 58 and 74.

51. On law and justice (δίκη) with reference to the Hippocratic writings, see Lloyd-Jones (428), p. 80. On φύσις in general, see Diller (177), pp. 144–61; Grant (268), chap. 1 ("Nature") and chap. 2 ("Laws of Nature"); Lloyd (426), pp. 49–58; and Vlastos (705), pp. 13–22 (discussing nature as the principle of a rational universe).

52. Laín Entralgo (408), p. 57. Though the Greeks had a word for "piety," they lacked a word for "religion" (Wilamowitz-Moellendorff [721], 1:15). The absence in classical Greek of a term for religion "as we use it" (Nock [483], p. 10) suggests caution in speaking of Greek "religion" and "religiosity."

of studying influences and relying on inferences from philosophy, it will be more to the point to see whether a "religion of nature" was intrinsic to the Hippocratic art and science, so as to make them incompatible with Christianity.

According to Hippocratic science, everything, including diseases, had its nature, and natural events were neither due to the caprice of gods nor subject to human will. The natural order was also the norm: the human body had its nature, that is, its constitution, and as long as the body and its parts were healthy (i.e., in the state in which they ought to be), they were "according to nature [κατὰ φύσιν]" or, as we would say, normal. Any illness or other deviation from nature was "against nature [παρὰ φύσιν]," or abnormal. In addition to these two major categories, a third one, "not by nature [οὐ φύσει]" assumed importance in post-Galenic medicine.[53] "Not by nature," in medicine, designated those things (res non naturales in medieval Latin terminology) which, though necessary for life, were not part of man's natural endowment.[54] Galen listed them as follows: contact with the air, motion and rest, sleep and wakefulness, food, excretion and retention, and passions.[55] They were the factors that determined whether the body was healthy or diseased, and their regulation formed the science of hygiene and of dietetic treatment.

The notion of nature as a principle of order, regularity, and normalcy, open to observation and rational calculation, was fundamental for Hippocratic medicine; it pervaded most writings of the Collection and of later Hippocratic physicians. Its elimination meant changing the theoretical basis on which scientific Hippocratic medicine rested and denying to its practitioner the intellectual tools with which he approached disease, hygiene, and therapy. It was left to the Empiricists to believe that nature was incomprehensible, and to the Methodists, inclining toward a mechanistic philosophy, to distrust any teleological connotation.[56]

Hippocratic naturalism was accepted by the Christian church, provided that nature and natural phenomena were acknowledged as God's work and were not given a divine character of their own. According to Eusebius, the whole realm of nature was God's creation, and natural laws could not be transcended except by Him, who was above nature,

53. On the origin of the term, see Diller (178), pp. 24–25.
54. See Bylebyl (129).
55. Galen (241), Ars medica 23; 1:367, ll. 13–18. Cf. Rather (579).
56. For the Empiricists, see Celsus (137), De medicina, prooemium, art. 27; 1:16. The denial of teleology was one of Galen's main accusations against the atomistic philosophers and indirectly the Methodists; see below, text following n. 78.

and by those delegated by Him.[57] Greek pagans, however, tended to look upon as divine all powers that were outside of human control. This included not only the gods but also cosmic phenomena, fate, and even necessity.[58] Philosophers and Hippocratic physicians might strip these of their original identification with gods, yet with the possible exception of Epicurus, they did not thereby take away their religious aura.

The author of *On the Sacred Disease* proved in great detail that the disease was neither sacred nor a defilement by any god. It had its nature, its natural etiology, and its natural pathogenesis. It was both human and divine—divine because of its dependence on the sun, the moon, the stars, and the winds. But these divine entities exerted their influence by heating, cooling, drying, and moistening—that is, by the same forces that were active in other, mundane processes. In this manner, astrophysical factors could be—and were—distinguished from divine wrath and demoniac possession.[59]

While it was possible to avoid the overt association of Hippocratic naturalism with gods and other divine beings, the notion of the divine was not thereby eliminated. The concept was sufficiently vague to cause difficulty for any commentators. One of the books of the Hippocratic Collection began a discussion of "the nature of woman and her diseases" with the statement that "the divine is the main cause among human beings . . . He who works skillfully must first begin with the things divine." [60] Equally puzzling, and more important because of the great practical significance of the work, was a passage in *Prognostic*. The author insisted on the necessity of knowing the nature and the force of acute diseases that might be fatal before medical help could be rendered, and also "whether there is something divine in the diseases." He urged that the prognosis of "these [τούτων]" also be studied thoroughly.[61] However, the Hippocratic text that Galen used read differently,[62] so that Hippocrates could be understood as having insisted on studying the prognosis of that which was divine. This led Galen to a

57. Eusebius (212), *Treatise* 6; p. 496. See also Saler (600), on the development of the concept of the supernatural. Vlastos (705), p. 18, rightly remarks on the anachronism in the use of the term for the pre-Socratics.

58. Hippocrates (302), *On Regimen* 1.5.13; 4:236: πάντα γίνεται δι' ἀνάγκην θείην. Cf. below, chap. 15, text to n. 60.

59. See Temkin (666), pp. 91–96.

60. Hippocrates (309), *De natura muliebri* 1; 7:312. In Jaeger's ([337], p. 203, n. 44) opinion, the divine here has the same meaning as in *On the Sacred Disease*.

61. Hippocrates (8), *Prognostic* 1; p. 194, ll. 3–5.

62. Galen (247), *In Hippocratis Prognosticum* 1.4; p. 199, l. 1 up: τουτέου instead of τούτων; also idem; pp. 205–6.

discussion of earlier interpretations that had identified the divine with divine wrath, epilepsy, love, and those days on which the illness was likely to undergo a crisis. Obviously, the ancient commentators not long after Hippocrates already did not know what "the divine" meant here. Galen dismissed "divine wrath" with the remark that "not in one of his writings does Hippocrates seem to have referred the cause of a disease to the gods." [63] Dismissing the other explanations as well, Galen offered as his own opinion the contention that Hippocrates meant the air surrounding us, and had used the word "divine" as an abbreviation for what he had taught in *Aphorisms* and *Epidemics*.[64]

Stephanus, a late Alexandrian, followed Galen and made no protest against this identification of the air with the divine. Stephanus gave an original twist to Hippocrates' claim that a physician who knew prognosis might be "justly admired and be a good physician." Hippocrates, so Stephanus commented, believed that the doctor who also prognosticated whether there was anything divine in the diseases was certain of success. "Such a person fully and justly deserves our admiration because the doctor, by using prognosis, is assimilated to God as far as [this is] possible for human beings." [65] Prognosticating was close to prophesying, and the concept of assimilation to God was shared by Platonic and Neoplatonic philosophers as well as by Christians.[66]

The overt acknowledgment of celestial bodies as divine was not essential for Hippocratic naturalism, and the Christian church was not rigorous in eradicating occasional literary slips, nor were the latter significant by comparison with pagan practices such as magic and the use

63. Ibid.; p. 206, ll. 9–10.

64. Ibid.; pp. 206(l. 15)–9(l. 6). Nestle (479), p. 3; Laín Entralgo (409), pp. 315–19; and Kudlien (388) may be right in agreeing with Galen's interpretation. In case of an epidemic, the physician could base his prognosis on the course of other cases.

A scholium of uncertain date lists and criticizes various interpretations of "the divine." The word has been used in reference to a god-sent disease, to national dietary "superstitions" such as those of the Jews and the Egyptians, to enthusiasm (τὸ ἐνθουσιαστικὸν πάθος), to pestilence, to the critical days, and to love. The scholium is preserved in a text of *On the Sacred Disease* (Hippocrates [309], 6:22–23) but has its logical place in *Prognostic;* see Galen (247), p. 206, apparatus.

65. Stephanus (647), *Commentary on the Prognosticon of Hippocrates* 1.18; p. 64 (Duffy's translation, modified).

66. For Plato, "becoming like the divine as far as we can" meant "to become righteous with the help of wisdom" in order to flee the evil unavoidable in the human world (Plato [555], *Theaetetus* 176A–B; p. 87 [Cornford's translation]. On the Platonic and Christian ὁμοίωσις, see Ladner (405), pp. 63–66, and Festugière (221), p. 2. According to Nilsson (482), p. 44, in late Antiquity the aim of the mysteries was to elevate man to the realm of the divine and to confer immortality upon him.

of superstitious formulas and symbols, which even Hippocratic doctors occasionally employed.[67] Such remnants of pagan religiosity as were retained in meteorological medicine, and probably helped to give to air, climate, and the constellations of stars medical eminence beyond their empirical value, [68] were no longer overt in works such as *Epidemics*. But was this also true of the concept of nature itself? Was nature a mere rational principle of order, or was the power that governed the life of plants, animals, and human beings and set the norm for what they ought to be and to do,[69] not itself the real divine "before which [man] must prostrate himself in veneration"?[70]

A note of admiration, if not veneration, is unmistakable in many Hippocratic utterances. "Nature is sufficient in all for all," [71] and "in everything nature [acts] without having been taught." [72] Here the famous Hippocratic dictum about the healing power of nature has its place. "In people, [their] constitutions [are the] physicians of their diseases. Nature itself, and for itself, finds the ways [and] not as a result of reasoning . . . Being educated [73] without having been taught, [nature] does what is necessary." [74] People, it was thought, did not realize that their arts but imitated nature. Thus, healing and banishing pain by the removal of the cause of disease were the tasks of the medical art, yet "nature of herself knows [how to do] these things." [75] These apophthegms belong to different works of the Collection, a fact that goes to show that admiration of nature beyond its recognition as a super-

67. See above, chap. 10.C, and below, chap. 17.A (Alexander of Tralles).

68. Cf. Nestle (479), p. 23.

69. Jaeger (335), p. 18: "Greek paideia, which had always derived its norms of human and social behavior from the divine norms of the universe, which were called 'nature' (φύσις)."

70. See above, text to n. 52.

71. Hippocrates (306), *On Nutriment* 15; p. 80, l. 11. Quoted from Jones's ([302], 1:347) translation. On the difficult dating of this work, see Diller (178), pp. 17–29.

72. Hippocrates (306), *On Nutriment* 39; p. 82, l. 28; also see idem (302), p. 356.

73. The reading of εὐπαίδευτος instead of ἀπαίδευτος has been argued in detail by Manetti (440), pp. 177–79 and 200–206.

74. Hippocrates (309), *Epidemics* 6.5.1; 5:314. This famous passage establishes the principle of the healing power of nature, which is not to be confused with the self-termination of disease. The passage refers to the fact that all healing processes are natural processes, which medicine can support but not replace. Belief in the healing power of nature can well go together with active therapy.

75. Hippocrates (302), *On Regimen* 1.15; 4:252 (Jones's translation, modified). On the character and date of this writing and its comparison of therapy and natural healing, see Diller (178), pp. 71–88.

human intelligence was common to many, if not to all, Hippocratic authors. But admiration and veneration were not essential to Hippocratic science and art and could be replaced. Christian theologians could not do without the concept of nature as norm any more than the pagans did. Basil spoke of the natural condition of the soul as its healthy condition.[76] Yet he did not look upon nature as divine. In admiring nature, Christian theologians admired God's work,[77] and physicians could do the same without infringing on their science. It was a matter of personal choice whether they did so or whether they retained the pagan sentiments that their great authority Galen had built into a true religion of nature.

Following in the footsteps of Aristotle, Galen demonstrated the perfect adaptation of every part of the body to its functions. In his *On the Use of Parts,* he described the structure of each part and then showed that a better and more useful structure was not even thinkable. Such knowledge was needed in medicine, for the physician had to know the goal of his treatment: the natural state he was attempting to restore. But the book went beyond medicine. Nature had built the human body from the material available to it; an absolute creation as postulated for the God of Moses was an absurdity. With this limitation, nature was the builder of man's body, the power that fashioned it in conception and growth and enabled man to maintain himself and his kind. Nature was powerful; it did nothing in vain; it was provident, wise, good, and just.[78]

Galen spoke of nature, the demiurge, as if it needed defense against the atomists, the shameless accusers and detractors who believed in the working of chance. From the knowledge of nature that his work provided, Galen inferred the existence of an intelligence (νοῦς) that hailed from the heavenly bodies,[79] the substance of which was much superior to that of the earth, superior even to the minds of such men as Plato, Aristotle, Hipparchus, and Archimedes.[80] The air too, since it was able to partake of the light of the sun, must be full of its power. And thus, Galen thought, his book

> will be reckoned truly to be the source of a perfect theology, which is a thing far greater and far nobler than all of medicine. Hence such a work

76. See above, chap. 13, text to n. 2.
77. See below, text to n. 84.
78. For details and references, see Temkin (667), p. 25.
79. Galen (244), *De usu partium* 17.1; 2:446. This was Stoic philosophy as confirmed by pseudo-Galen (241), *De historia philosophica* 427: 19:252–53.
80. Galen (244), *De usu partium* 17.1; 2:447, ll. 2–3.

is serviceable not only for the physician, but much more so for the philosopher who is eager to gain an understanding of the whole of Nature. And I think that all human beings of whatever nation or rank who honor the gods should be initiated into this work, which is by no means like the mysteries of Eleusis and Samothrace. For feeble are the proofs that these give of what they strive to teach, whereas the proofs of Nature are plain to be seen in all animals.[81]

Galen completed his glorification of nature by comparing it to an epode, the third part of a lyric poem, sung in praise of the gods.[82] Here indeed was naturalism fashioned into a religion after the Stoic pattern.[83] There was much that conflicted with Christianity: nature, the demiurge, was not the God who "in the beginning" (Gen. 1:1) had created heaven and earth; nature and cosmic intelligence were immanent in the cosmos and were not separate from it as God was; and the cosmic intelligence emanated from the stars, which to Jews and Christians were bodies created by God, and not even on the first day of the Creation.

Galen's paganism was undeniable, like that of Plato and Aristotle. And also like them, he could be made useful for Christians, to whom his On the Use of Parts offered a perfect work on the wisdom and the providence of God in his creation of man. All that was needed was to look at nature as a manifestation of God's intelligence and power. Thus reinterpreted, natural theology presented one of the major arguments for God's existence. Speaking of the human body, Augustine exclaimed, "What goodness of God, what providence of the great Creator is apparent!" [84]

As to Galen himself, his excursus from nature to the cosmic intelligence was not an essential part of his medical philosophy. He thought himself to be at one with Hippocrates, who "extols and admires [nature's] power," but "does not go as far as to declare what the substance

81. Ibid; 2:447(l. 16)–48(l. 9). Quoted from May's ([251], 2: 731) translation, modified. On mysteries, cf. above, n. 66.

82. Galen (241), De usu partium 17.3; 2:451. See May's ([251], 2:733) translation.

83. Grant (268), p. 14: "[Galen's] demiurge, like the Stoic god, is nature, not standing outside nature"; to which cf. Seneca (616), On Benefits 4.7.1; 3:216: "Quid enim aliud est natura quam deus et divina ratio toti mundo partibusque eius inserta?" See Grant (268), pp. 10 and 14–18, for Galen's view of nature as compared with the Christian view. Moraux (470), pp. 101–2, notes a deviation from Stoicism insofar as Galen follows Aristotle in limiting nature's providence to man as a species, excluding the individual.

84. Augustine (58), City of God 22.24; 2:526 (Dods's translation).

is of the nature that forms and governs us." [85] Galen's agnosticism and his disinclination to engage in contemplative philosophy also made him assert that "we must wonder at the craftsman who fashioned our body," yet add, "whichever god he is." [86] He himself had stated that his theology went beyond medicine; therefore there was no need for Hippocratic physicians to follow his example.

Yet his picture of a rational cosmos of providential nature within which gods and humans had their place was not without grandeur. To some physicians, it may well have seemed more attractive and more in harmony with Hippocratic principles than the ascetics' sin-laden world of the crucified Christ, whose worshippers promised eternal bliss after death at the price of the suppression of the flesh, the degradation of earthly life, and contempt for sensual beauty.[87] To such doctors, the sacrifice of their pagan universe may have appeared more repulsive than the mere replacement of Asclepius by Christ.

Where such sentiments existed, they probably restrained those who harbored them from conversion. However that may be, the majority of physicians can be assumed to have professed Christianity by the end of the fifth century and to have disavowed an outright religion of nature. A more insidious threat to their orthodoxy offered itself in some inferences from Hippocratic naturalism, whereby limits were put to God's will and to man's dependence on Him.

85. Galen (248), *De placitis Hippocratis et Platonis* 9.8.27; 2:596, ll. 26–29 (De Lacy's translation). Elsewhere, in a discussion of the meaning of the term "nature," Galen merely referred to the essence of things and what followed from it. This limitation was adequate for his commentary on the Hippocratic *On the Nature of Man*. See Galen (245), *In Hippocratis De natura hominis* 1.1; pp. 3–7.

86. Galen (248), *De Placitis Hippocratis et Platonis* 9.8.22; p. 596, ll. 5–7. Cf. Moraux (470), p. 100.

87. More will be said on this in the Epilogue.

15

NATURALISM

The naturalism of pre-Socratic philosophers and of Hippocratic physicians had originated in a pagan society that demanded respect for the gods but left much freedom for speculation about the divine. This society, moreover, was secular; concern for life in the hereafter did not weigh heavily on human affairs.[1] Virtue was good in itself and in its contribution to human happiness. With the change from respect for the gods to submission to the Christian God[2] and acceptance of His kingdom, Hippocratic naturalism did not automatically lose the traces of its birth. Potential conflict existed between the natural explanation of disease and the concept of disease as imposed by God; between the corporality of the soul and its immortality and subjection to God's judgment; and between the physician's role as an autonomous healer and his function as a mere agent of God, the true healer. In the East, the works of the Hippocratic Collection were there to read, and who could tell whether a Christian doctor went along with their authors or had attained a truly Christian frame of mind?

1. That is to say, if compared with Christian otherworldliness. The undeniable fear of death and of the uncertainties of the hereafter did not dominate life.
2. I.e., the God of the Trinity.

A. Supernatural Disease and Possession

Basil had drawn a sharp demarcation line between disease from natural causes, in which dietetic medicine had a place, and diseases inflicted by God for purposes of His own.[3] However, if applied to medical practice, this posed a difficulty similar to that seen with "something divine" of the Hippocratic *Prognostic*.[4] How was the doctor to recognize whether the disease came from God? A guilt-laden soul might call out with the prophet Micah, "I will bear the indignation of the Lord, because I have sinned against him" (Micah 7:9), or others might point out sins that the patient had committed. Basil himself had mentioned the failure of medical treatment as a distinguishing sign. But this diagnosis *ex non iuvantibus*[5] inflicted a period of unrelieved suffering on the patient; it also left undecided the length of the period after which the doctor was to acknowledge defeat.

The medical literature of the last centuries of Antiquity paid little attention to the existence of divine diseases; the physician's domain was the medicine of the body, while supernatural diseases were left to others, presumably to the priests. This was important for rendering Hippocratic medicine religiously neutral. There are signs that the neutralization of medicine was a process that may have gone as far back as the retreat from the Greek "enlightenment." Galen, who thought that Hippocrates had nowhere referred the cause of a disease to the gods, added; "In *On the Sacred Disease* more has been written in censure of those who believed diseases to originate from the gods."[6] But there existed a note reporting that Galen had ascribed the book to a clever man but asserted that it was not on the level of Hippocrates' style and way of thinking.[7] No commentary on the book is known, nor did it appear on the syllabus of twelve Hippocratic works that Arabic historians ascribed to late Alexandria.[8]

On Airs, Waters, Localities, however, was considered important

---

3. See above, chap. 13.
4. See above, chap. 14, text to n. 61.
5. "From what is not helpful."
6. Galen (247), *In Hippocratis Prognosticum* 1.4; p. 206, ll. 13–15.
7. See Grensemann (277), p. 48. Stephanus (647), p. 54, ll. 23–29, paraphrased Galen but wrote ἔχει instead of γέγραπται, thus saving the authority of Hippocrates.
8. For this syllabus and the syllabus of Galenic works, see Duffy (192), p. 22, n. 5; Iskandar (334); Lieber (422); Temkin (668), pp. 74–77; Ullmann (697); and Westerink (717).

enough to receive a commentary by Galen and to be listed in the Hippocratic syllabus. In the twenty-second chapter of this Hippocratic work, the Scythians' belief that the disease prevalent among them was imposed by the gods was led *ad absurdum,* and in its place a natural explanation was given. Galen's commentary on this chapter did not enter into the religious argument. It confined itself to an interpretation of the term *kedmata* used by Hippocrates, and a discussion of Hippocrates' views on the blood vessels behind the ears and the impotence caused by bleeding from them.[9]

Although the religious neutralization of medicine was not initiated by the encounter with Christianity, Christians were aware of the gulf between their own views and those embodied in the two Hippocratic writings. A Byzantine scholium commented:

> Even if among the pagans disease did not arise on account of the wrath of gods, yet among us diseases are sent because of the wrath of God and to try [us], or even because of [our] haughty bearing. "For in a slight affliction," says the Psalmist [Isa. 26:16][10] "your chastisement is [upon] us," and the most divine Paul [says], "There was given to me a thorn in the flesh, the messenger of Satan to buffet me, lest I should be exalted above measure" [2 Cor. 12:7], and in Job [2:7] the sores [were said to arise] in the same manner, and other things in other [people]. Here then is the divine [inherent in our] trials. As to wrath, the plagues in Egypt may have been a lesson to you as also the leprosy of Gehazi [2 Kings 5:27] and, according to us, [you will find] many more instances if you care to search for such things.[11]

Essentially, the scholiast repeated what Basil had said, though his denial of divine wrath among the pagans is ambiguous. It could mean that among the heathen, divine wrath was not acknowledged as a cause of disease. Stephanus, writing in the sixth century, denied the wrath of God as a cause of epilepsy. "Neither," so he wrote in his commentary on the *Prognostic,* "does the condition of epileptics have divine wrath as a cause of its generation; rather, epilepsy develops according to a

---

9. I am greatly indebted to Gotthard Strohmeier of the Akademie der Wissenschaften (Berlin) for having made available to me his preliminary translation from the Arabic of Galen's commentary on that chapter.

10. I have translated these few words as quoted by the scholiast, who deviates from the text of the Septuagint.

11. Translated from Galen (247), p. 205, apparatus, where the editor has also cited the Biblical references. The Greek scholium is found in a manuscript containing Galen's commentary on the Hippocratic *Prognostic.*

particular phase of the moon, by which I do not mean that the wrath of God sends the disease to men through the movement of the heavenly bodies." [12]

Epilepsy, once the sacred disease, was particularly apt to cause a confrontation between the Hippocratic physician and Christian theologians. Defending the demoniac origin of the fits of a lunatic boy, Origen noted that physicians upheld the purely somatic nature of the affliction against the existence of an unclean spirit, and that "as natural philosophers they have to maintain that the contents of the head are set in motion according to [their] sympathy with the lunar light, which is of a moist nature. We, however, also believe the Gospel . . ." [13]

Disease caused by demons and manifest possession by a demon were among the principal forms of supernatural affliction. Their existence was attested by the Gospels, though theologians might argue about whether demons were capable of causing organic disease.[14] Pagans shared such beliefs; Apollonius of Tyana exposed a demon as the cause of an epidemic, and Tertullian reminded his pagan readers of the fame Christians enjoyed as exorcists.[15] As time went by, the fear of demons became well-nigh ubiquitous, philosophers also incorporating them into their systems.[16]

If Plotinus is to be believed, philosophers and "reasonable people" in the time of Origen still adhered to the naturalistic explanation of disease. According to Plotinus, the Gnostics, instead of purging themselves of disease "by temperance and an orderly regimen" claimed that diseases were demons whom they could remove with their words. These Gnostics might impress the crowd, who admired the powers of magicians, "but they were not likely to persuade reasonable people that diseases were not caused by toil or surfeit or deficiency or putrefaction and, all together, by changes that originate outside or inside [the body]." [17] Diseases were eliminated by copious bowel movements, medicines, bleeding, or restriction of food—and where, Plotinus asked, were the demons during this process? He ridiculed the idea (actually

12. Stephanus (647), p. 56 (Duffy's translation). On Stephanus see below, chap. 17.A.

13. Origen (508), *Commentarium in Matthaeum* 13.6; col. 1105. Cf. Temkin (666), p. 92.

14. See above, chap. 10.C.

15. See above, chap. 6, text to nn. 160 and 162; and chap. 10, text to n. 39.

16. See Geffken (256); and Brown (120), pp. 53–56.

17. Plotinus (560), *Against the Gnostics* 14 (Ennead 2.9); 2:279 (Armstrong's translation, modified).

held by Tatian) that, together with the natural cause of the disease, the demons were also at hand, as if standing by.[18]

In the late fourth century, Posidonius, a physician much interested in diseases of the brain, contradicted the popular opinion that nightmare was caused by Ephialtes, a demon with whom it shared its name: "Ephialtes is not a demon but a premonition and preface to epilepsy, mania, or apoplexy."[19] This report by the medical encyclopedist Aetius is supplemented by a heretic historian of the church, according to whom Posidonius had a poor opinion of demons' capabilities. Human beings "did not become frenzied [ἐκβακχεύεσθαι] through the onslaught of demons; rather, the bad composition of certain fluids caused the disease. For altogether there was no power in demons to harm human nature."[20] The historian did not fail to call this opinion "incorrect." But why did he go out of his way to record it at all? Was it because Posidonius represented the medical opinion of his time, or because such opinion had become "a rare exception"[21] by the end of the fourth century?

The medical literature of late Antiquity gives no answer to this question. But it kept alive the naturalistic tradition regarding a closely related matter, possession by a god—"enthusiasm" in the literal sense of the word, that is, the god-inspired state of bacchants, prophets, and priests of orgiastic cults. A Hippocratic physician of the fourth century B.C. explained that the affliction of divine possession (ἐνθεαστικὸν πάθος) "had its seat in the region of the heart and the aorta."[22] Later, Aretaeus, whose dates have not been ascertained (unfortunately so, because he ventured upon the religious territory),[23] classified the condition as "another form of mania." This form was to be found among people who "cut their limbs in pious fantasy, as if thereby propitiating peculiar divinities. This is a madness of the apprehension [ὑπολήψιος] solely; for in other respects they are sane. They are roused by the flute and frolicking, or by drink, or by the urging of those around them." Are-

18. Ibid., pp. 278–80. For Tatian see above, chap. 10.C.

19. Aetius (2), *Libri medicinales* 6.12; 2:152, ll. 13–14.

20. Philostorgius (542), *Kirchengeschichte* 8.10; p. 111, ll. 11–15.

21. See Neuburger (480), 2:53. Kudlien (396), p. 424, has suggested a possible identity of this Posidonius with the Stoic philosopher of the first century B.C. I still believe that Aetius had in mind the physician mentioned by Philostorgius.

22. Steckerl (644), frag. 71; p. 81; see Temkin (666), p. 87. For the whole complicated matter of enthusiasm among the Greeks, see Rhode (589); Dodds (187), pp. 64–101; and Smith (631).

23. Kudlien has assigned Aretaeus to the first century; cf. above, chap. 3, n. 104.

taeus acknowledged the religious nature of the condition: "This madness is of divine character [ἔνθεος] and when they recover from the madness they are cheerful and free of care as if initiated to the god."[24] As "a madness of the apprehension solely," Aretaeus placed it outside the realm of the medicine of the body, into an intellectual sphere. He emphasized the religious experience by comparing it to an initiation mystery. But he returned to the somatic (i.e., medical) aspect by adding that because of their wounds, the enthusiasts remained pale and thin, and were weak for a long time.[25]

Aretaeus was a pagan. To Jews and Christians, such divine frenzy as he described would suit priests of Baal and of Cybele, lunatics, and demoniacs. Since the pagan gods had become mere demons, the divine possession of the Greeks was now demoniac possession. But the Jews also had their prophets upon whom the Spirit of God had come (1 Sam. 10:5–6 and 10); Jesus' disciples were "filled with the Holy Ghost, and began to speak with other tongues" (Acts 2:4); and Paul had declared prophesying and speaking in tongues to be gifts of the Spirit (1 Cor. 13:10).

The medical texts of late Antiquity took little notice of the profound difference between demoniac possession as the work of the Devil, and divine possession by the spirit of God. Possession appeared as madness in the Latin work of Theodorus Priscianus of the fourth century,[26] and at the very end of Antiquity, Paul of Aegina also included *enthousiasmos* in his chapter on madness.[27] The terminology remained traditional and thus also noncommittal.

Regarding the whole field of possession and demoniac disease, the classical medical literature of late Antiquity retained its naturalistic tradition. It also increasingly gives the impression of a facade behind which individual doctors could follow their personal inclinations. Augustine knew of a physician in Carthage, a sufferer from gout, who on the day preceding his baptism dreamed of "curly-haired black boys, whom he recognized as demons, who forbade him to be baptized this year."[28] He resisted them and did not defer "being washed in the laver of regeneration," though the demons trod on his feet and caused him

---

24. Aretaeus (39), 3.6, pp. 43 (l. 29)–44 (l. 3). Quotation modified from Adams's ([40], p. 304) translation. Aretaeus obviously describes episodes of religious ecstasy.

25. Aretaeus (39), 3.6; p. 44, ll. 3–4.

26. Theodorus Priscianus (678), *Euporiston* 2.17; p. 152, l. 6.

27. Paul of Aegina (532), 3.14; vol. 9.2, p. 156, ll. 20–22.

28. Augustine (59), *City of God* 22.8; 7:224. The man may of course not have been a Hippocratic doctor.

greater pain than he had ever experienced. With baptism, the pain as well as the disease disappeared.[29] On the other hand, the nonmedical literature also mentioned Christian physicians who did not hide their skepticism even in such a dogmatically important matter as the resurrection, at least the resurrection of the body.

B. The Soul

From the beginning of Christianity, the resurrection of the body had been hard to accept for pagans as well as for many followers of the new faith. Medical naturalism would make acceptance of the resurrection particularly difficult, and it is not surprising to find a Christian physician given the role of disputing its possibility and using a Hippocratic work[30] to prove the truth of "earth thou art and shalt become earth" (Gen. 3:19).[31]

Somewhat later, around the beginning of the fifth century, Augustine knew of a doctor (whether pagan or Christian he does not say) whose attitude toward the resurrection of Lazarus was flippant if not cynical. This man was consulted by a devout Christian woman of high rank for cancer of the breast. According to the doctors, Augustine informed his readers, such cancers were incurable by any drugs. Either the breast had to be amputated or, "according to Hippocrates,[32] it is said, all treatment had to be omitted" so that the patient might live a little longer.[33] This having been conveyed to the patient by the doctor, she turned in prayer to God and was cured miraculously. Having convinced himself that the patient was healed, the physician, an experienced man and an intimate of her family, was eager to learn the remedy "by which the maxim of Hippocrates could be confounded."[34] Easter was then approaching, and in a dream the woman had been ordered to have the sign of the cross made over her breast by the first woman who emerged baptized from the baptistry. Upon hearing this, the doctor, to the horror of the newly cured patient, said "with scrupulous urbanity" but contemptuously in voice and expression: "'I thought you were going to tell me something momentous . . .What [is] great in Christ's

---

29. Augustine (58), *City of God* 22.8; 2:490 (Dods's translation).

30. Hippocrates (302), *Humors* 11; 4:82.

31. Methodius (455), *De resurrectione* 1.9.14; p. 233 (from Bonwetsch's German translation of the Syriac text). The work was written in about A.D. 300.

32. Hippocrates (302), *Aphorisms* 6.38; 4:188.

33. Augustine (59), *City of God* 22.8; 7:220.

34. Ibid.; p. 222.

curing a cancer, seeing that he resuscitated a person who had been dead four days.' "[35]

Although stories of this kind were balanced by others of doctors not lacking in faith, they could support doubt concerning the depth of the physicians' faith. Most scandalous to the religious minds of late Antiquity, however, Christian and pagan alike, was the fact that Galen had pushed his naturalism so far as to doubt the immortality of the soul, which Plato himself had acknowledged. Galen admired Plato almost as much as he admired the venerated Hippocrates, but he was not prepared to follow him on this point. In a little book with the revealing title *That the Faculties of the Soul Follow the Temperament of the Body*, Galen the natural philosopher and physician expounded his views. Melancholia, phrenitis, and mania made it obvious that the blemishes of the body dominated the soul.[36] Food and particularly wine, as Plato himself had taught, influenced the soul.[37] Galen insisted that Plato and Aristotle had endorsed his thesis and that Hippocrates in *On Airs, Waters, Localities* had shown the part that climate played in shaping the behavior of nations.[38]

Galen did not exclude man's moral character from dependence on the body, and faced the consequence arising therefrom. If it was true that

> neither are all human beings born enemies of righteousness nor [are] all its friends but become such because of the temperament of their bodies, how then, it may be asked, can anybody rightly be praised and blamed, hated and loved, since he has become evil or good not by himself but on account of the temperament that he seems to have acquired from other causes?

Galen made short shrift of this inference. "Because [he said] it is in all of us to welcome the good, to approve [of it], and to love [it], yet to turn our backs upon the bad to hate and to flee it without first considering whether it has a genesis or not." [39] Galen's recourse to an inborn moral instinct[40] was not very far from the assertion of free will as a subjective experience independent of the inquiry into its determining psychological or somatic causes.

However, Galen did not find it equally easy to deal with another

35. Ibid.
36. Galen (242), *Quod animi mores* 5; 2:49, ll. 1–3.
37. Ibid. 10.
38. Ibid. 9.
39. Ibid. 11; 2:73 (l. 10)–74 (l. 1).
40. See Moraux (469), 2:794 and 803, n. 468.

consequence of his naturalistic stance. Like Plato before him, Galen believed that the soul was tripartite—comprising the concupiscent soul, the passionate soul, and the rational soul—and that each of these three parts had its organic center. There was no difficulty in identifying the concupiscent soul with the temperament of the liver and the passionate with that of the heart. That meant that the qualitative dispositions of these two organs expressed themselves in appetites and passions. The same then also ought to be the case with regard to the rational soul: our thoughts, feelings, and voluntary actions ought to depend on the temperament of the brain. Hence the soul was neither incorporeal nor immortal. Although Galen's inclination toward this conclusion was rather obvious, he confined himself to declaring his inability to share Plato's assurance, and to pleading an agnostic attitude.[41]

Christian theologians, such as Tertullian, could accept the notion of the soul as a fine substance of a unique kind. From a Christian point of view, this kind of naturalism only needed to be supplemented by trust in the survival of this material soul. The main issue was not the immateriality of the soul, which was hard to imagine anyhow, but the relegation of the soul to the status of a mere temperament of a perishable organ.

The bishop Nemesius recognized that Galen's approval of the notion of the soul as temperament was implied rather than openly maintained, and he tried to disprove the possibility.[42] Around the same time, Isidore of Pelusium, in a letter to a physician, attacked Galen, who, he said, was skilled in treating the body but ought not to have meddled in areas where he was not competent. If the soul were a mere cerebral condition, it was mortal, and we could not look forward to reward and punishment after death. All praise and blame would become meaningless.[43] The Neoplatonic philosopher Proclus, of the fifth century, held Galen no less in disfavor than did the Christian theologian. Galen had erred in deviating from Plato and making the body the soul's substratum. On the contrary, the body was an impediment to the soul.[44]

41. Galen (242), *Quod animi mores* 3; p. 36, ll. 12–16; also idem 5. See Temkin (667), pp. 44–45 and 83–84; and Moraux (469), 2:784–85.

42. Nemesius (477), *De natura hominis* 2; pp. 86–87. Cf. Temkin (667), pp. 81–82 and 87.

43. Isidore of Pelusium (331), *Epistolae* 4.125; cols. 1197–1204A. The letter was addressed "to Proeschius Scholasticus, physician." In blaming Galen for meddling with matters outside his medical competence, Isidore anticipated Maimonides; cf. Temkin (667), pp. 77–79.

44. Proclus (572), *In Platonis Timaeum* [44B]; 3:349–50. For a French translation, see idem (571), p. 231.

In the case of the nature of the soul and its immortality, as in the case of Galen's theology, Hippocratic physicians were under no constraint to follow the great master in his metaphysical speculations. But the pagan naturalism in which Hippocratic medicine was embedded made the idea of the soul as a function of the brain a persuasive logical consequence.[45] Moreover, naturalism carried the risk of bringing the doctor into conflict with the Christian demand that he humbly acknowledge God rather than the physician as the true healer of all illness.[46]

C. The Doctor and His Art

"Three things make the [medical] art: the illness, the patient, and the physician. The physician is a servant of the art; the patient must oppose the illness together with the physician."[47] This famous passage from the Hippocratic *Epidemics* is as remarkable for what it does not say as for what it says. No divinity is mentioned as a factor in the art of healing. Hippocratic doctors were not atheists; some authors gave the gods a place, and the possibility of something divine in disease was not overlooked. At least one late voice even called the doctor an agent of a god.[48] Many doctors probably believed that their healing endeavors would be in vain if carried out without the help of the gods, or against their resistance, and may have offered a libation to them before beginning their work.

However far the pagan Hippocratic doctors' piety may have gone— and it probably differed much according to their philosophical orientation—it stopped short of seeking religious justification for their existence. In contrast to Ecclesiasticus, doctors were not to be honored because they were part of the divine creation. Rather, in making medicine a gift of the gods, the Greek myth implied that medicine was a valuable art. And the divine ancestry of Hippocrates did not save doctors from being attacked and ridiculed. "If doctors did not exist, there would be nothing more stupid than the grammarians," somebody remarked at a

45. It has remained so to the present day.
46. Ambrose (11), *Cain and Abel* 1.7.25; p. 384, held forth against people who "tend to refer the results to their own particular virtues and to consider that they, and not the Author of the favors, are responsible for their success" (Savage's translation).
47. Hippocrates (302), *Epidemics* 1.11; 1:164, ll. 12–15.
48. See above, chap. 7, text to n. 35.

symposium.[49] The gods punished hubris, but Greek polytheism did not demand that doctors justify their existence in the face of the divine healers and that they humble themselves before their gods. Christianity, however, demanded that doctors feel humility and pay tribute to God as the true and only healer, and it warned the faithful not to put their final trust in physicians and medicines.[50]

Side by side with the myths of medicine as a gift of the gods, there existed a Hippocratic work, *On Ancient Medicine*, that attributed the origin of dietetic medicine to human ingenuity driven by necessity. The author opposed the reliance on unstable hypotheses about "hot, cold, moist, or dry, or whatever else they may wish," [51] the truth of which could not be tested.[52] Instead, he traced the way in which the only true method of medicine had been invented. In times past, the suffering inflicted by eating raw food led to the discovering of cooking, which rendered food fit for consumption by healthy people. But ordinary food did not satisfy the needs of the sick. Step by step, by trial and error, diets suitable for the constitutions of sick people were discovered, and medicine came into existence. "Necessity itself has made human beings seek and find medicine." [53] Full of admiration for the manner in which the ancient investigators had made their discoveries, the author believed that they themselves had "deemed the art worthy to be ascribed to a god as is actually believed." [54] To be worthy of a god is not the same as being due to a god. The passage was a tribute to the glory of the discovery.

On Ancient Medicine was on a track different from the one leading to the classical humoral theory with which Hippocrates is associated. It was not unique in identifying dietetic medicine with the medical art, as if surgery and pharmaceutics were not part of it. The discourse *On the Art* also concentrated on dietetic medicine, though not quite as exclusively. Here, too, the defense of medicine as a real and effective art was constructed without reference to the gods. The absence of any mention of the divine in the bulk of the technical Hippocratic writings made them appear religiously neutral from the beginning.[55]

---

49. Athenaeus (56), *Deipnosophists* 15.666a; 7:66–67.

50. See above, chap. 12, text to nn. 74 and 75; and chap. 13.

51. Hippocrates (306), *On Ancient Medicine* 1; p. 36, ll. 3–4.

52. Ibid.; p. 36, ll. 20–21.

53. Ibid. 3; p. 37, ll. 24–25. For necessity (ἀνάγκη), see below, text to n. 60.

54. Ibid. 14; p. 45, ll. 17–18. This was an allusion to Apollo and Asclepius as the legendary inventors and founders of medicine.

55. On this neutrality, however, see below, chap. 17.B.

The concept of medicine as an art worthy of a god appeared again in the second letter of the Pseudepigrapha, only this time Hippocrates was praised as its leader, a descendant of gods.[56] The ideal physician of the Sarapion poem was compared to a healing god.[57] The physician who embraced the correct philosophy was godlike.[58] All this was a far cry from Ambroise Paré's pious avowal "Je le pansay, Dieu le guarit." [59]

It might be objected that necessity, driving man to devise dietetic medicine, was itself divine.[60] It was divine as nature was divine, a force that could not be petitioned to dispense favors. It was not like the gods of the Hippocratic oath, who watched the doctor in order to see whether he lived up to what he had sworn. He had sworn to guard his life and his art "in purity and holiness," [61] serving his patients and abstaining from many specific actions. If he remained loyal to his oath, he hoped that enjoyment of "life and art," as well as eternal fame, would be his, and that the reverse would be true if he did not live up to his promise. Obviously, the oath was a religious document, with which the doctor put himself within the power of the gods. They would watch whether he lived righteously; his behavior would determine his fate. But he did not expect to be a mere instrument in their hands. The "ens Dei," to speak with Paracelsus, was not a constituent part of medicine itself.[62]

It was not easy to read a Hippocratic doctor's mind and find out whether he believed in supernatural diseases, possession, the resurrection of the body, and the immortality of the soul. It is well-nigh impossible to look into his heart and see whether he humbly felt himself to be a mere tool in God's hand. Complacency and false pride were—and have remained—sins from which even the pious might not be free.

56. See above, chap. 6, text to n. 130.
57. See above, chap. 6, text to n. 136.
58. Hippocrates (306), Decorum 5; p. 27, l. 3. See above, chap. 3, text to n. 51.
59. "I dressed him, God healed him." This dictum is inscribed on Paré's statue; see Garrison (255), p. 255. The cure of every individual is in God's hand; by contrast, the healing power of nature is a providential property of man's constitution.
60. See above, text to n. 53; and chap. 14, text to nn. 50, 58, and 74.
61. See above, chap. 3, n. 26.
62. On Paracelsus and the ens Dei, see below, chap. 17.B.

Christianized Hippocratic Oath in form of a cross. Codex Abrosianus B 113 sup. fol. 203ᵛ (Milan), fourteenth century. From W. H. S. Jones, *The Doctor's Oath*. Cambridge: University Press, 1924, p. 26.

VII

Hippocratic Medicine and Triumphant Christianity

The inter-relationship between Christian faith and Hippocratic principles did not, by itself, determine the situation of physicians, because religion was also intertwined with political and social developments. With the death of Julian the Apostate, paganism had lost its last battle to regain its former supremacy. But the polarization of pagans and Christians continued, and physicians were to be found on both sides. Another polarization, that of the *honestiores*, the rich, powerful, and educated, as against the *humiliores*, the poor and uninfluential, not only persisted but became accentuated by the championship of the poor by a church that took over religious and social institutions. Medical ethics were not to remain entirely uninfluenced by the changing zeitgeist.

Barbaric invasions, rebellions, assassinations, and intrigues among the secular leadership, as well as bitterly fought dogmatic struggles, among which the Arian and Monophysite schisms were politically the most destructive, made the time of the Christian reconstruction of society very turbulent. The social aspirations of doctors and the conditions of their practice were affected by the external events no less than by the religious struggles for their beliefs and their sympathies.

16

PUBLIC ASPECTS OF
HIPPOCRATIC MEDICINE

A. The Polarization of Christians and Pagans

In the absence of numerical data, the rate at which doctors converted to Christianity remains undetermined. Individual cases only show that around A.D. 300, the time of the great persecution of Diocletian, there were among the Christian physicians men of learning as well as individuals inclined toward a life of piety. Thus Bishop Theodotus of Laodicea "had reached the summit of the science [ἐπιστήμης] regarding the healing of bodies, and in [the art] of curing souls he was second to none among men, because of his philanthropy, sincerity, compassion, and zeal toward those that sought his help; also he was greatly practiced in the study of divinity."[1] If there is truth in the story allegedly told to Saint Antony, there was a man in Alexandria, "a physician by profession, who is like you, who gives his abundance to those in need, and who every day with the angels sings the Trisagion[2] to the harp."[3]

The Christianization of doctors during the three centuries following the edict of Milan may have proceeded at a rate proportional to that seen in the urban population, or it may have had its own development. It is certain that there was resistance extending into the end of the fifth

1. Eusebius (211), *Ecclesiastical History* 7.32.23; 2:241 (Oulton and Lawlord's translation, modified). In idem 8.13.4; 2:294, Eusebius names Zenobius, presbyter in Sidon, "the best of physicians," among the martyrs.
2. The "holy, holy, holy"; see Isa. 6:3.
3. *Apophthegmata patrum* (32), "De abbate Antonio" 24; col. 84B.

century. In Oribasius the fourth century had a physician who was a dedicated pagan and a follower of Hippocrates and Galen, with whom he shared Pergamum as his native city. He was physician and friend to Julian the Apostate, whom he accompanied on his Persian campaign and who died in his arms.[4] During the ensuing Christian reaction, Oribasius fell on bad times. His admiring biographer,[5] himself a convinced pagan, praised him as the model of a genuine philosopher. Though nothing is known about his philosophical views, he must have laid claim to the status of a philosopher, as is evidenced by a letter from Isidore of Pelusium "to Oribasius the physician":

> According to Democritus, medicine cures diseases of the body, whereas wisdom relieves the soul of passions.[6] Now since you lay claim to both, and use the one[7] to cure the affliction of the body in other people, heal yourself properly with the other[8] by acquiring also the health that you lack [and] without which you will be neither an outstanding [ἄριστος] physician nor a real sage.[9]

Only a Christian could be a perfect physician of body and soul, and since truth rested in the Christian faith, no pagan could in fact be a sage.

Oribasius was depicted as a leader among the Alexandrian physicians of the mid fourth century.[10] Galenic Hippocratism did not originate with him, but it was formally installed by him in the medical literature of late Antiquity.[11] Oribasius was the most comprehensive of the medical encyclopedists, and with him, the last stage of ancient medicine may be said to begin.

About a century after Oribasius, at the time of the Eastern emperors Leo I and Zeno, another group of pagan physicians was more or less

---

4. See Bowersock (110), p. 116. Philostorgius (542), *Kirchengeschichte* 7.15; p. 103, ll. 3–4, names "the excellent physician Oribasius, the Lydian . . . from Sardes" as having attended Julian. To this compare Baldwin (73), p. 87.

5. Eunapius (209), *Lives;* pp. 532–37.

6. Cf. above, chap. 2.

7. I.e., medicine.

8. I.e., wisdom.

9. Isidore of Pelusium (331), *Epistolae* 1.437; col. 424A–B. On the career of Oribasius, see Baldwin (73). Baldwin (72), p. 18, believes that the letter was too late to have been addressed to Oribasius, the friend of Julian. Could there possibly have been two physicians by the same name (see above, n. 4)? But even if the letter was not addressed to Oribasius of Pergamum, it expressed Christian unwillingness to recognize a pagan as a true physician of the soul.

10. Eunapius (209); *Lives,* pp. 532–37.

11. See above, chap. 3 text to n. 3.

closely associated with the Neoplatonism of the Academy of Athens.[12] The most outstanding of these was Jacob, son and pupil of the physician Hesychius and, in turn, the medical teacher of the philosopher, scientist, and physician Asclepiodotus. Jacob practiced medicine in Constantinople with such spectacular success that he was called "savior."[13] He carried the nickname *Psychristes,* (from the Greek verb "to cool"), allegedly because he favored a cooling diet, seeing that "most people were very busy and covetous of money."[14] Since he received a salary from the city,[15] he must have functioned as an archiater.

Among the iatrosophists (professors of medicine) in Alexandria, a certain Agapius (who later moved to Constantinople) was a pagan,[16] and so was Gesius until his alleged conversion at an uncertain time during his career.[17] Gesius was famous as a teacher and a practitioner. He amassed great riches and was given extraordinarily high honorary positions in the state. The Arabic historians of medicine listed him among the Alexandrians who had canonized sixteen Galenic books for teaching and study.[18] A Christian hagiographer cited him as a disbeliever in Christian miracles whom personal experience forced to a very humiliating recantation.[19]

The fame of these pagan physicians may partly be due to the zeal of the pagan historians, who were liable to extol their fellow religionists. It should be taken into consideration that the free-born Hippocratic physicians, like other professionals, belonged to families who were among the honestiores of the cities. Roman aristocrats and intellectuals were leaders of the resistance to Christianity. Intellectually, the new religion had little to offer to persons brought up on Greek literature, philosophy, and an appreciation of secular beauty, on which fanatical Christians placed little value. Healing miracles, a strong inducement to conversion, were not likely to overimpress Hippocratic physicians, who recognized Asclepius as a god but liked to think of him as a supernatural Hippocratic physician working within natural boundaries.[20] The

12. See Neuburger (480), 2:73–75.

13. Asmus (53), p. 73, l. 16. This book contains a reconstruction (in German) of the biography of the Neoplatonist Isidore by his pupil Damascius of Damascus.

14. Alexander of Tralles (7), 2:163. See also Nutton (489), p. 4. The rationale of a cooling therapy for greed is not clear to me.

15. Asmus (53), p. 74.

16. Ibid., p. 115.

17. Ibid., p. 116.

18. See above, chap. 15, n. 8.

19. See above, chap. 12, text to nn. 122 and 123. The hostile tone of that story makes one wonder what the circumstances of Gesius's conversion were.

20. See also chap. 14, text to n. 38; and Kudlien (386). Healing miracles were

traditions of their class and the education they received tended to bind Hippocratic physicians to the old religion, though it is not possible to gauge the number of pagans in their ranks. It was bound to dwindle with the strides made by Christianity, and by the time of Justinian, physicians can be presumed to have been Christians nominally at least. As early as the fifth century, the Roman archiaters whose names are known from inscriptions were Christians.[21]

B. The Polarization of Rich and Poor

The education of a Hippocratic physician was demanding. Among the deontological Byzantine, Arabic, and early medieval Latin writings grouped together as the Testament of Hippocrates,[22] one Latin text stated that the future physician must study grammar, astronomy, arithmetic, geometry, and music. Philosophy, it was said, "should be taught together with medicine."[23] In other words, he should study the liberal arts, with the exception of rhetoric, "lest he talk too much."[24] This explanation sounds naive and casts some doubt on the insistence on what would otherwise be a complete liberal education. But the physician's need for some philosophical training, which would at least presuppose grammar and natural philosophy, is documented in the use of the term *physicus* as a medieval equivalent of "doctor."[25]

A liberal education, complete or incomplete, would be expensive, and indicates that the Hippocratic doctors originated from families belonging to the honestiores. Philosophy had long been one way of ele-

---

frequently seen, and evoked differing responses. The Gospels tell of mass conversions that followed Jesus' miraculous cures, but they also tell of the miracles being attributed to magic. According to Harnack (288), p. 131, Origen, polemizing against Asclepius, asserted that "the power of healing diseases is no evidence of anything especially divine." Emperor Julian (353), *Against the Galilaeans* 191E; 3:376, claimed that Jesus did nothing worthwhile, "unless anyone thinks that to heal crooked and blind men and to exorcise those who were possessed by evil demons in the villages of Bethsaida and Bethany can be classed as a mighty achievement" (Wrights' translation). Healing power was "perhaps the commonest manifestation of holiness" (Browning [121], p. 131). For Jewish miracle workers at the time of the New Testament, see Vermes (702), pp. 62–78.

21. See Nutton (487), pp. 208 and 225. MacMullen (436), pp. 68–73, has shown that the conversion of intellectuals became frequent in the late fourth century.

22. See above, chap. 11, n. 84.

23. Laux (412), p. 420, ll. 10–11, with the corrections of Deichgräber (167), pp. 94–96.

24. Laux (412), p. 420, ll. 9–10.

25. See Kristeller (376), pp. 159–60.

vating the doctor's status above that of a banausic craftsman, to speak with Plato. But in the Roman empire, a liberal education did not suffice to assure the doctor the status of a gentleman. Medicine was a craft, a "productive" craft with health as its product, according to Galen, who classed medicine with that part of architecture that engaged in the repair of houses.[26] On the other hand, he also ranked medicine as the highest of the intellectual arts. Hippocrates belonged together with Socrates, Homer, Plato, and their followers, "whom we venerate equally with the gods."[27] This double aspect expressed the uneasy social position of the doctor. "In the Roman consciousness," so it has been summed up, "there did not exist a uniform evaluation of medicine, of the medical profession, and of the physician, but a constant coexistence, nay a confusion of low esteem and high esteem."[28] It was all very well to argue that what medicine gave was beyond any monetary value[29] the fact remained that in the Roman world the well-born doctor shared the practice of medicine with slaves and freedmen. The latter engaged in it as a trade, and as the legendary Hippocrates had made it very clear, working for a fee had to be shunned.[30]

However, not every doctor possessed an independent income, as did Galen, that allowed him to practice without demanding a fee. The gift the physician accepted as a sign of gratitude from the patient was formalized as an honorarium, and its nature, in late Antiquity, becomes clear in the edict that Emperor Valentinian I issued in A.D. 368 regulating the institution of archiaters in the city of Rome.[31] The archiaters,

26. Galen (241), *De constitutione artis medicae ad Patrophilum* 2; 1:230.

27. Galen (715), *Adhortatio ad artes addiscendas* 5; p. 246, ll. 27–28.

28. Kudlien (397), p. 154. Idem, pp. 190–98 and 198–209, discusses "low esteem" and "high esteem," respectively. Harig (284), p. 2, discusses the *Zwitterstellung* of medicine between science and trade. See also Scarborough (604), chap. 8 ("The Doctor and His Place in Roman Society"), pp. 109–31.

29. Seneca (616), *On Benefits* 6.15.1–2; 3:392.

30. Hippocrates (307), *Letters* 11; p. 6, ll. 10–16. Cf. above, chap. 6, text to nn. 91–102; also cf. below, Epilogue. The legendary Hippocrates' view does not necessarily represent public opinion in the early Roman empire. According to Visky (704), especially pp. 268—71, the Romans believed that an art was not free if practiced for payment, even if the work was mental rather than physical. Visky has been contradicted by Kudlien (397), pp. 164–65.

31. *Codex Theodosianus* (153), 13. 3.8; vol. 1, pt. 2, p. 742. For an English translation, see Temkin (672), p. 6. The Latin text of this law, as well as of the supplementary law, *Codex Theodosianus* 13.3.9, regulating the promotion of an archiater in case of a vacancy, can also be found in Jones (349), 2:1293. For a discussion of the law, see idem p. 1012; Amundsen (21), pp. 556–57; and Nutton (488), pp. 208–10.

assigned one to every district of the city,[32] held a privileged position, attractive to persons of high social status.[33] They received a salary from public funds but were permitted, according to Valentinian's edict, "to accept what the healthy present to them for their dedication, not what those in peril of death promise for being saved."[34]

The problem of the physician's social status and of his remuneration went back into pre-Christian times and was not greatly influenced by the Christian transformation. Valentinian's edict, however, also exhorted the archiaters that in view of their salary, "they had better choose to dedicate themselves honestly to the poor than shamefully to serve the rich." Rich and poor were here put in sharp opposition. The edict, furthermore, tried to safeguard the election of new archiaters against the "patronage of the very powerful" and "the favor of one examiner." Valentinian was a Christian, a peasant's son, and his ancient biographer tells that he "hated the well dressed, the learned, the rich, and the high-born."[35] The emperor's social policy, his personal "interest in the welfare of the humbler classes,"[36] and Christian teaching,[37] thus met in contrasting the rich and the poor. The edict did not direct the archiater to cease treating rich people and instead to dedicate himself exclusively to the poor, that is, people of rather limited means but not necessarily indigent. It contrasted *honest* treatment of the poor with *shameful* service of the rich.

Seen from the point of view of members of the upper stratum of Roman society, such as Cicero, Seneca, and Aristides, medical science might deserve respect. But the physician was respected as a dedicated friend rather than as a craftsman. If the example of Seneca may be generalized, the rich and powerful were demanding. Doctors put the patient under obligation "not because of their art, which they sell, but because of their kindly and friendly goodwill."[38] The potential selfishness of this attitude shines forth in Seneca's remark about his own doctor: "Though a host of others called for him [i.e., his physician], I was always his chief concern; that he took time for others only when my

32. Except for the *portus Xysti* and the district of the vestal virgins; for textual details, see Nutton (488), appendix 2; and Fischer (226), p. 167 and p. 173, n. 25.

33. See Temkin (672), p. 24, n. 50.

34. The English quotations from the law are from Temkin (672), p. 6.

35. Ammianus Marcellinus (12), 30.8.10; 3:366–67 (Rolfe's translation).

36. Jones (349), 1:139.

37. Although Valentinian's edict was in line with Christian charity, Nutton (488), pp. 209–10, suggests that reasons of state rather than charity may have prompted the emperor. Regarding the classification of rich and poor, see Patlagean (531), pp. 25–35.

38. Seneca (616), *On Benefits* 6.16.1; 3:397 (Basore's translation modified).

illness had permitted him."[39] In such circumstances, little time may have been left for honest dedication to the doctor's humble patients.

This will explain Galen's contempt for those doctors who kow-towed to the rich and mighty, among whose friends they wished to be counted.[40] For Hippocratic doctors—and Valentinian's archiaters could be expected to have been well-educated Hippocratic physicians—the temptation to concentrate on the rich and powerful would have been enhanced by the conviction that dietetic medicine demanded an intimate knowledge of the patient's way of life, and thus justified concentration on a few patients. If Valentinian's edict is read as an admonition not to neglect the poor in favor of the rich and as an appeal to treat rich and poor with equal dedication, it is not as remote from pre-Christian medical ethics as it might appear to be. The sharp antithesis of rich and poor is not to be denied, but it is largely due to a political and social regrouping rather than to mere religious change.[41]

Hellenistic inscriptions praised doctors, especially communal doctors, for treating the rich and the poor equally;[42] the ideal physician of the Sarapion poem was told "like a savior god" to "make himself the equal of slaves and of paupers, of the rich and of rulers of men, and to all let him minister like a brother."[43] In the city-state as a community of all its citizens, benefiting by its prosperity and suffering in its adversity, equal treatment of all citizens was a desirable goal. Conflict between the classes—between rich and poor, between aristocrats and plebeians—was held to be calamitous. The parable that Menenius Agrippa once told the seceding plebeians—comparing the city-state to a body that needed the cooperation of all its parts—expressed the sense of organic unity. Coherence, cooperation, and internal peace became the concern of the empire after the city lost its autonomy. The church supported this tendency by its representation of the interests of the poor and its concern for their welfare.[44]

39. Ibid. 6.16.5; p. 397 (Basore's translation). On Seneca's (and Cicero's) attitude to doctors, see Scarborough (604), pp. 113–14 and 137. On Cicero, see Phillips (539), pp. 272–73.

40. See above, chap. 3, text to n. 24; also Temkin (667), p. 36.

41. See above, n. 37.

42. See above, chap. 3, text to nn. 8 and 10.

43. See above, chap. 6.C, text to nn. 136 and 137.

44. On the demographic and economic developments, see Patlagean (531), pp. 156–81; Miller (463), pp. 68–74; Jones (349), 2:1038–53; and Finley (225), *passim*. See also Brown (119), p. 115, for the increasing prosperity and population of the Syrian countryside in the fourth and fifth centuries. I fully recognize the importance of the demographic and economic situation of the time but do not feel competent to form a judgment reliable enough to allow far-reaching inferences.

Consideration for the patients' economic situation, once a matter of the physician's personal discretion, now became a social obligation. It is not as if pagan doctors as a class had been indifferent to poor people. Galen commended Hippocrates for treating the poor in some small cities rather than joining the court of the Macedonian king.[45] The adjustment of financial demands according to the patient's means was described as customary among some physicians, at least by John Chrysostom, the great Christian preacher of the second half of the fourth century;

> As physicians, healing the same disease, take a hundred pieces of gold from some patients, half [of it] from others, less [still] from others, and from some nothing at all, so Christ accepted much and marvelous faith from the centurion, less from this one [i.e., the paralytic of Matt. 9:2–8] and from the other [i.e., the invalid of John 5:5–9] not even a modicum—and, nevertheless, healed them all.[46]

John Chrysostom does not say that all these physicians were Christians, nor is this to be assumed as self-evident for the time of Oribasius. The curious comparison of monetary payment with faith in Jesus would have been tenuous had there not been physicians who gave the same attention to all their patients, regardless of the remuneration they received. Apart from the amounts mentioned (ranging from one hundred pieces of gold to nothing at all), the custom at the time of John Chrysostom seems to be the same as the graded fees that *Precepts* advised for philanthropic reasons.[47]

Was it pure love of man, compassion for a suffering fellow creature, that guided the physician as it was supposed to guide the monks of Cassiodorus's Vivarium?[48] Or were other motives involved, such as concern for one's reputation or a sense of equity? The motives were not mutually exclusive: in *Precepts*, too, philanthropy was not meant to supplant all personal interests. Moreover, individual doctors probably varied as they vary now, from the man whose heart was full of compassion, as Scribonius Largus had it, to the man with the cold heart who merely conformed with what was expected. Nor must the doctor be forgotten whose motive was neither emotional nor opportunistic, but simple belief in his religious or social obligation.

45. Galen (242), *Quod optimus medicus* 3; 2:5, ll. 10–12. Galen referred to the patients of the Hippocratic *Epidemics*.

46. John Chrysostom (322), *Homilia in paralyticum* 4; cols. 55–56. See also Frings (239), p. 91.

47. See above, chap. 3.

48. See above, chap. 12, text to nn. 74 and 75.

In a rhetorical exercise, a fictitious speech by a prosecuting lawyer, the orator Libanius, an ardent partisan of the Emperor Julian, had medicine itself express what was expected from physicians:

You desired to be one of the healers [of sickness], you had the benefit of having [good] teachers. Now, practice your art faithfully. Be reliable; cultivate love of man; if you are called to your patient, hasten to go; when you enter the sickroom, apply all your mental ability to the case at hand; share in the pain of those who suffer; rejoice with those who have found relief; consider yourself a partner in the disease; muster all you know for the fight to be fought; consider yourself to be of your contemporaries the brother, of those who are your elders the son, of those who are younger the father.[49]

This "quintessence of pagan medical humanism"[50] sounds like an elaboration of Sarapion's poem, which has been said to be Christian in tone.[51] Indeed, Christian borrowings cannot be excluded even from the utterances of pagans of Libanius's time.[52]

In the prosecutor's speech cited above, medical ethics were idealized to bring out the baseness of a physician accused of poisoning. The forensic hyperbole is obvious, as it also is in the following paragraph, which praises physicians' response to the precepts of the medical art:

[These precepts] have been heeded, gentlemen,[53] to our advantage, by all those physicians who, rather than striving for money, strive for the fame [derived] from having conquered disease. Indeed, I know many physicians who, instead of receiving [money], have themselves spent [money] for poor people. Reasonably so! For the art also affords them respect in the cities. And we look upon the most outstanding of them as if they were gods, believing that in them, next to the gods, lies our hope for deliverance.[54]

Philanthropy, especially for the poor, regard for reputation, and a sense of equity[55] are all here in this pagan salute to the doctors and their art.

49. Libanius (420), Κατὰ ἰατροῦ φαρμακέως 7; 8:184–85. Quoted from Edelstein's ([198], p. 345) translation.

50. Edelstein (198), p. 345, n. 46. However, it is medical humanism as conceived by a layman.

51. See above, chap. 6, text to n. 137.

52. See above, chap. 7, text to n. 35.

53. The prosecutor is addressing the court.

54. Libanius (420), Κατὰ ἰατροῦ φαρμακέως 8; p. 185, ll. 8–17.

55. The doctors owe philanthropic behavior for the respect they receive or, vice versa, the doctors are respected as philanthropists. Even if this portrayal is exaggerated, there must be some truth in it, since otherwise the prosecutor could not count on approval.

To these pagans, outstanding doctors were the focus of men's hope for deliverance from the evils of this world. No wonder that pagans called them saviors, a name repugnant to Christians for mere instruments of God. The pagan Jacob Psychrestes was called "savior,"[56] apparently by pagans but not necessarily by them alone. Christian physicians too did not escape the lure of this glorification. Agnellus, one of the late commentators on Galen, told beginners in the study of medicine that they should long "to grasp the fruit of future sweetness; so that holding in our possession an end worthy of our exertion, we might with regard to the working of medicine, be justly called physicians and saviors because of the multitude of people healed by us with God's help."[57]

Of the several kinds of physicians, only the anargyroi dispensed their help gratis.[58] If physicians were supposed to give free treatment to those who could not pay at all, the income from the rich compensated them. *Precepts* taught physicians to consider the affluence and the means of their patients, which allowed taking much from the rich, and the one hundred pieces of gold mentioned by John Chrysostom was a tidy sum.

The idea that rich patients should support the indigent sick was familiar to the fifth century. Jacob Psychrestes, though a pagan, would have been a man after Emperor Valentinian's heart. He "prevailed upon the rich [whom] he treated to assist ailing poverty and himself treats gratis, being content with the mere public provision"[59] that he received as head (*comes*) of the archiaters in Constantinople. In pagan times a doctor's philanthropy was his personal affair. There were physicians who practiced medicine for worldly advantages, and there were those, such as the legendary Hippocrates and others, Galen among them, who treated men for the sake of philanthropy.[60] But Christianity imposed consideration for the poor on all as a religious obligation, and taking from the rich could become an approved policy. John the Almsgiver, patriarch of Alexandria,

> used to say that if with the object of giving to the poor anybody were able, without illwill, to strip the rich right down to their shirts, he would do no wrong, more especially if they were heartless skinflints. For thereby he gets a two-fold profit, firstly he saves their souls, and secondly he himself will gain no small reward therefrom.[61]

56. See above, text to n. 13.
57. Agnellus (3), p. 2 (quoted with modification from p. 3).
58. While well-to-do physicians, such as Galen, and salaried doctors could dispense with fees, it is not clear on what the anargyroi were supposed to have lived.
59. Photius (545), vol. 1, col. 344a, ll. 27–29.
60. Galen (248), *De placitis Hippocratis et Platonis* 9.5.6; 2:565 ll. 26–30.
61. Quoted from Dawes and Baynes (162), p. 231.

John the Almsgiver took his cue from the tale that Saint Epiphanius (fourth century) "would skillfully steal away the Patriarch John's[62] silver and give it to the poor." [63] It is thus not surprising that Christian doctors, and perhaps others too, followed the same path but in a less saintly spirit. What in practice existed long before is found openly advised in a medieval text of the early ninth century: "If the patient be wealthy, let this be a proper occasion for profit; if a pauper, any reward is sufficient for you." [64] Still later, in the very popular poem known as *Schola Salernitana-(The School of Salerno)* or *Regimen sanitatis (Regimen of Health)*, the saintly spirit had given way to a very down-to-earth attitude. The physician was told: "Ask for the reward while the pain harasses the patient, for when the disease is gone, the giving stops and quarreling remains. Medicine bought dearly is wont to help; if given gratis, it is of little benefit." [65] Such advice was the reverse of what *Precepts* had taught, and makes the pagan philanthropy of the latter stand out more clearly.

C. Surgery and Doctors of Lower Rank

Motives might be hard to gauge, but practice was on public display. Among the miracles described by Augustine, one is particularly instructive because the scene includes the patient, his various doctors, and Christian clergy, and because the event affords insight into surgical practice, a subject too often neglected in discussions of medicine and religion.[66]

Upon their return to Carthage in A.D. 388,[67] Augustine and his brother were made welcome in the house of a pious Christian, a former civil servant. Their host was under treatment for multiple rectal fistulas[68] and had already undergone an extremely painful operation, but one of the sinuses had escaped attention. "Another doctor, who belonged to his household" [69] and whom the others had not admitted

62. Patriarch of Jerusalem.

63. Quoted from Dawes and Baynes (162), p. 231, where the story is said to hail from the Life of St. Epiphanius, chs. 44–45, ed. Dindorf, pp. 49–52.

64. Sudhoff (657), p. 237. See also MacKinney (435), p. 6.

65. De Renzi (168), 5:103. See also Temkin (672), p. 17 and p. 25, n. 67.

66. It is for this reason that I retell this story in some detail. (See especially Nutton [487], p. 173; and Ferngren [218], p. 502.)

67. Brown (114), p. 132.

68. According to Dr. Walter Birnbaum (see Augustine [59], *City of God* 22.8; 7:212–13, n. 3), it was a case of rectal abscess with the formation of multiple fistulas.

69. Ibid.; 7:214, l. 5: *alius medicus domesticus eius.* For the *medicus domesticus* as a personal doctor belonging to the household, see Phillips (539), p. 272.

to watch their operation, predicted the need for a second one. His irate patron, terribly afraid of that possibility, had him thrown out and readmitted him only reluctantly. The patient asked his physicians whether they would cut him again, and whether the domestic doctor was to prove right. They ridiculed "the ignorant doctor," [70] assuaged the patient's fears, and promised a cure with medicaments. In this they were supported by a famous elderly consultant; whereupon the patient, reassured by this man's authority, took fresh hope.

But the days dragged on, and finally he was told that there was no cure except by the knife. Pale with fear, the patient told his physicians to go away and not to come back. Yielding to necessity, he called in "a certain Alexandrian who was then reputed to be a marvelous surgeon." [71] The newcomer was so impressed by the work of his predecessors that he persuaded the patient to let them do the operation. "It was thoroughly inconsistent with his nature [he said] to win the credit of the cure by doing the little that remained to be done, and rob of their award men whose consummate skill, care, and diligence he could not but admire when he saw the traces of their work." [72] The former doctors were readmitted, and the operation was scheduled for the next day in the presence of the Alexandrian.

The patient was terrified, and the whole household was wailing in sympathy with him. In the evening "holy men," [73] including a bishop, and deacons of the church of Carthage, visited him as was their custom. With tears in his eyes, he asked them "to honor him with their presence next morning at what was to be his funeral rather than his suffering . . . They consoled him and admonished him to trust in God and to bear His will like a man." [74] Then they all prayed, but he flung himself to the ground and prayed so passionately, groaning, his tears flowing, and his whole body shaking, that Augustine, diverted from praying, could only say in his heart, "O Lord, what prayers of Thy people dost Thou hear if Thou hearest not these?" [75]

The dreaded hour has come. The doctors have arrived, and so have the servants of God. Everything is ready, the instruments are produced, and while those near to him try to cheer up the patient, his body is suitably arranged on the couch, and the diseased part is bared:

70. Augustine (59), *City of God* 22.8; 7:214, ll. 10–11: *medicum imperitum*, which could also mean unskilled or inexperienced.

71. Ibid.; 7:216, ll. 3–4. Nutton (493), p. 35, relates the story as evidence for the renown of Alexandria.

72. Augustine (58), *City of God* 22.8; 2:487 (Dods's translation).

73. Augustine (59), *City of God* 22.8; 7:216, l. 23: *sancti viri*.

74. Ibid.; 7:218, ll. 8–13.

75. Augustine (58), *City of God* 22.8; 2:488 (Dods's translation).

The doctor examines it, and, with knife in hand, eagerly looks for the sinus that is to be cut. He searches for it with his eyes; he feels for it with his finger; he applies every kind of scrutiny; he finds a perfectly firm scar! No words of mine [Augustine concludes the story] can describe the joy, and praise, and thanksgiving to the merciful and almighty God which was poured from the lips of all, with tears of gladness. Let the scene be imagined rather than described![76]

Some two hundred years earlier, a healing miracle had been greeted by the cry "Great is Asclepius," in which the doctors had joined, though with some reservations about the miraculous nature of the cure.[77] If Augustine is to be taken literally, this time the doctors too joined in giving thanks to God. Whether they did or not, Augustine and, as it would seem, all the holy men present accepted the doctors' role as a matter of course; they did the praying, the doctors did the surgery.[78] Perhaps the surgical nature of the disease, the obvious indications for what had to be done, had something to do with the churchmen's ready acquiescence. Celsus had called surgery the oldest part of medicine; it had been cultivated by Hippocrates, and its achievements were obvious, as compared with those of speculative dietetics.[79] Augustine's host was not unique in dreading the knife in the treatment of fistula. "If any person, out of cowardice, were to flee surgery, one should use the Hippocratic operation by ligature," was the suggestion of Paul of Aegina.[80]

A hundred years after Augustine, Alexandria was still a famous center of surgery.[81] The exquisite courtesy of the Alexandrian surgeon toward his colleagues stands out against Galen's tales of professional jealousy in Rome.[82] It also contrasts with the disdain with which these

76. Ibid. (Dods's translation, modified); for the Latin text, see Augustine (59), *City of God* 7:220 ll. 6–13.

77. See above chap. 14, text to n. 28.

78. Augustine's approval of the operation stands in contrast to his sharp attack on doctors, "so-called anatomists," who in their very cruel zeal have "torn in pieces [*laniavit*] and even vivisected human bodies. We must admire the beauty and usefulness of the body and of its parts but must not go below the surface (Augustine [59], *City of God* 22.24; 7:332). Ferngren (218), pp. 502–3, has rightly pointed out that laymen feel differently about therapeutically necessary procedures than the quest for knowledge, even if the latter is potentially useful. However, Augustine's thinking differs from that of Basil and Gregory of Nyssa (cf. above, chap. 11, text to n. 41; and chap. 13, text to n. 31), and even that of Ambrose (cf. above, chap. 11, text to n. 43).

79. Celsus (137), *De medicina* 7, prooemium, art. 2–3; 3:294.

80. Paul of Aegina (532), 6.78; 2:122, ll. 12–13. Cf. Hippocrates (309), *De fistulis*; 6:450.

81. See above, chap. 2, text to n. 13.

82. See above, chap. 3, text to n. 21. The Alexandrian surgeon's courtesy may

colleagues had treated the patient's domestic doctor. The fact that his master had "thrown him out of the house and had been reluctant to take him back,"[83] argues for his being of a different class than the others, who had been told "to go away and no longer come near him."[84] To what extent the attitude of these freely practicing doctors was snobbishness against a social inferior and to what extent it was contempt for an alleged medical ignoramus, the story does not reveal. However, it has some resemblance to the contemporary complaint of Oribasius regarding the great scarcity of true physicians and "the large number of those who pretend to the [medical] art and merely possess the name of physician." In particular, Oribasius denounces

> those having only learned to bleed, to cup, to scarify [or lance] and the other matters of menial skill, and who arrogate to themselves all medical treatment without knowing the quality or the quantity of remedies, and who do not find out the proper time or the order for [administering] them, which is the distinctive mark of the true physicians. [These people] take on diseases that are difficult to cure, or incurable, and they even kill some [persons].[85]

The tasks for which these second-class doctors were qualified were similar to those of the medieval barber surgeon. To the Hippocratic physician they were not true doctors, though they acted as though they were. Basil had spoken of persons engaged in healing at his hospital. Were they true doctors, or were they monks with some medical education?[86] The Justinian Code mentioned *parabalani,* men connected with the care of the sick[87] and expected to have some therapeutic experience.[88] At any rate, there existed men who formed a lower class of healing personnel and, identical with them or not, there were doctors whom Hippocratic physicians did not consider their equals.[89] For instance, the iatrosophist

---

have been due to his reluctance to get involved with a troublesome patient (I am grateful to Miriam Kleiger for this suggestion).

83. Augustine (59), *City of God* 22.8; 7:214, ll. 7–8.

84. Ibid.; 7:216, l. 1.

85. Oribasius (507), *Ad Eunapium,* preface; p. 317. Cf. above, chap. 3, text to n. 22.

86. See above, chap. 12, text to nn. 84 and 86.

87. *Codex Theodosianus* (153), 16.2.43; and *Corpus iurus civilis* (156), *Codex Iustinianus* 1.3.18.

88. *Corpus iuris civilis* (156), *Codex Iustinianus,* 1.3.18. For more details, see Temkin (665), pp. 218–19.

89. See below, chap. 17.A. In his section "The Lower Stratum [*Unterschicht*] of Physicians," Kudlien (397), p. 181, rightly denies the stratification of the Roman medical profession into higher, middle, and lower levels according to specialization

Palladius claimed that the "common [ἀγελαῖοι]" doctors bandaged broken bones without first applying traction and countertraction as the "rational [λογικοί]" doctors did.[90] How the Hippocratic doctor of the last century of Antiquity viewed himself as distinct from these men is made clear by Stephanus the Philosopher, one of the last ancient commentators on Hippocrates and Galen.

(e.g., surgery). Nevertheless, in the East at least, there existed medical men whom Hippocratic doctors did not recognize as true τεχνῖται, in full possession of the art. Horden (317), p. 10, is probably right in doubting that local Byzantine doctors gained "their knowledge from professional teachers or from access to large well-written manuscripts." For the West, Baader (65), p. 315, thinks that the slave doctor and his successors from the lower professional strata, rather than "the highly esteemed technites of the Greek world," formed the image of the doctor taken over from Antiquity in modified form by the Western Middle Ages. The appearance of terms that are not found in the traditional medical literature (e.g., "cephalic vein" and "hepatic vein") in Greek and early medieval phlebotomy texts points in the same direction; cf. Temkin (665), pp. 198–201.

90. Palladius (526), *Kommentar zu Hippokrates "De Fracturis"*; pp. 24–26. Palladius does not fail to point out the bad consequences of treatment by the common doctors. Regardless of whether these doctors were really guilty of such malpractice, their existence is certain.

17

HIPPOCRATIC MEDICINE IN THE TWILIGHT OF ANTIQUITY

A. Three Representatives

The works of three representatives of Hippocratic medicine of the very end of Antiquity illuminate three important aspects of the art: the classroom lecture (Stephanus), the medical manual (Paul of Aegina), and the work of the experienced practitioner (Alexander of Tralles).

Stephanus the Philosopher was the author of commentaries that were actually lectures to medical students in Alexandria.[1] One of these commentaries, on the first book of Galen's *Therapeutics for Glaucon*, deals with one of the works that formed the basis of the Alexandrian syllabus for beginners.[2] The commentaries, which deal with authoritative texts, carry the hallmarks of scholastic teaching.[3] Stephanus explains the author's meaning and, at the same time, presumes, proves, and elaborates the substantive truth of the content, but he provides

1. He was one of the "Alexandrians" listed by Arabic historians as editors and commentators of Galen; see Ibn abī Uṣaibiʿah (320), p. 103. Stephanus the Philosopher is identical with Stephanus of Athens.

2. See above, chap. 15, n. 8. Stephanus's (648) commentary on the first book of Galen's *Therapeutics for Glaucon* was edited by Dietz. The commentaries on Hippocrates' *Aphorisms* (sections 1–2) and *Prognostic* are now available in editions by Westerink (646) and Duffy (647), respectively.

3. Teaching in late Alexandria was discussed by Westerink in an unpublished lecture, "Academic Practice about 500: Alexandria." I am grateful to Professor Westerink for having made this illuminating lecture available to me.

little criticism. Dialectical argument and the refutation of contrary opinions often take the place of an appeal to empirical fact. For instance, in commenting on the Hippocratic dictum "The cavities are naturally hottest in winter and spring," Stephanus has to meet the objection that the body is desiccated in summer, when thirst prevails and "a burning, scalding heat . . . settles in the region of the stomach and in the depth of the body." Stephanus replies that Hippocrates is speaking of the natural [κατὰ φύσιν] heat of the stomach and "not the abnormal [παρὰ φύσιν] heat of fever patients, nor the non-natural [οὐ φύσει], adventitious heat that occurs in summer."[4] The innate heat that was part of the human constitution (in contrast to the nonconstitutional heat of the summer) was a concept of Hippocratic-Galenic medicine. The example also illustrates the use of the notion of the "non-naturals," which was to become prominent in Arabic and medieval medicine.

The commentaries include clinical subjects; they teach diagnosis, prognosis, and therapy; and they refer to fictitious cases as well as to cases from alleged medical practice. For instance, a number of hypothetical conditions of the stomach in youth serve as a basis from which to deduce confidently the situation in old age.[5] Stephanus also writes,

> when I visit a patient and find he is taking barley-water or fine bread in small quantity and is yet unable to digest it, it occurs to me that the retentive faculty of his stomach is atonic and weak; I then apply an infusion of absinthe, wine, oil, apple-juice and grape-juice, to stimulate its strength; after which the man who until now could not digest barley-water, is strong enough to convert even less digestible food.[6]

The case is to illustrate the Hippocratic aphorism that the cure will make it clear when disease has been caused by an abnormal abundance of food.[7] Is this case a fictitious example, or is it taken from Stephanus's own practice? More generally, was Stephanus the professor also a practicing physician, or was his use of the first person merely a rhetorical device for teaching how a Hippocratic doctor is to think and to proceed in practice. Since Stephanus speaks like a practitioner, there would have to be reasons for thinking that he was not actually one. Too little is known of Stephanus to give this question a definite answer. However, the cognomen "the Philosopher" and the possibility that he actually

4. Stephanus (646), *Commentary on Hippocrates' Aphorisms* 1.27; p. 107 (Westerink's translation).
5. Ibid. 2.20; pp. 176–83.
6. Ibid. 2.17; p. 173 (Westerink's translation).
7. Hippocrates (302), *Aphorisms* 2.17; 4:112.

taught philosophy do not suffice to rule out his engaging in medical practice.

Although he deals largely with clinical subjects, the lectures do not refer to the actual presence of patients. They are merely didactic, with a heavy emphasis on theoretical explanations, and the theory is that of Galenic Hippocratism. The commentary on the Hippocratic *Aphorisms,* which reads like an introductory text to Hippocratic medicine, contains a precise, short sketch of such fundamentals as the subdivisions of medicine and the humoral theory.[8]

As Oribasius had commended Galen for following the Hippocratic principles and doctrines,[9] so now Stephanus defined medical craftsmen [τεχνίτας] as "armed with the Hippocratic methods against diseases."[10] His pedagogic aim was to educate true craftsmen, that is, Hippocratic physicians. The Hippocratic doctor was sharply distinguished from the amateurish or incompetent doctor in such contrapositions as "a doctor [who] happens to be an amateur [ἰδιώτης]" as against "the Hippocratic physician,"[11] or "Let us suppose that a patient is visited by two doctors, the one ignorant (ἰδιώτης), the other Hippocratic."[12] This reflects the Hippocratic physician's complacent attitude toward the ignorant, incompetent, or amateurish doctor, an attitude that might well have impelled the doctors who attended Augustine's host in Carthage to show contempt for his domestic medical attendant.[13]

In Stephanus's lectures, the medical student was taught the Hippocratic-Galenic skeleton of medicine. Paul of Aegina's work informed the doctor of the principles and practice of medicine as considered acceptable around A.D. 600. Paul of Aegina is usually listed together with the two other, earlier encyclopedists, Oribasius and Aetius. But his aim was not to present a storehouse of medical knowledge, and his work was not shorter than those of the others because of any decrease in the quantity of available medical knowledge at the end of Antiquity.[14]

8. Stephanus (646), *Commentary on Hippocrates' Aphorisms* 1.1; pp. 34–38.

9. See above, chap. 3, text to n. 3.

10. Stephanus (648), *Commentarii in priorem Galeni librum therapeuticum ad Glauconem;* 1:238.

11. Ὁ δὲ Ἱπποκράτειος ἰατρός. Stephanus (646), *Commentary on Hippocrates' Aphorisms* 2.26; p. 196, ll. 4–9 (Westerink's translation, p. 197). (This is numbered as 2.27 according to Littré [309] and Jones [302].) For *idiota* as "unlettered" in the Latin tradition, see Brown (116), p. 137, n. 65.

12. Stephanus (646), *Commentary on Hippocrates' Aphorisms* 2.26; p. 196, ll. 19–20 (Westerink's translation, p. 197). Palladius contrasted the common doctors and the rational doctors (see above, chap. 16, text to n. 90).

13. See above, chap. 16, text to nn. 83, 84, 89, and 90.

14. This is not to deny that by A.D. 600 medical knowledge may have dimin-

Rather, it was something like a modern vade mecum, to be on hand wherever the doctor finds himself:

> It appears strange that lawyers should be possessed of compendious and, as they call them, popular legal synopses, in which are contained the heads of all the laws, to serve for immediate use, whilst we neglect these things, although they have it generally in their power to put off the investigation of every point not only for little but even for a considerable time, whereas we can seldom or very rarely do so; for, in many cases, necessity requires that we act promptly, and hence Hippocrates has properly said "the season is brief." [15]

Furthermore, Paul added, lawyers usually practice in cities where books abound, whereas physicians have to act not only in cities, in the field, and in isolated places but also aboard ship, where diseases strike suddenly, in which case delay means death or extreme danger.[16] Hospitals are not mentioned.

The parallel Paul drew between his manual and compendiums of law can also be drawn between the older medical encyclopedias and the codifications of law by the emperors Theodosius and Justinian. Oribasius and Aetius named their sources, just as the *Digest* (the compilation of excerpts from former legal authors that forms part of the *Corpus iuris civilis*) did.[17] The jurisprudence of continental Europe still rests largely on Roman legal concepts, and Anglo-American law considers older precedents set by the law courts.

A manual is not the place for expanding on the compiler's personal experiences. Paul said of his work, "I have compiled this brief collection from the works of the ancients, and have set down little of my own, except a few things which I have seen and tried in the practice of the art." [18]

Personal experience, however, was the very essence of the work that Alexander of Tralles wrote late in life. "Dearest Cosmas," the dedication begins, "you asked me to make public the cures that I frequently accomplished in diverse diseases on the basis of experience." He accedes

---

ished. For the West, such a trend can be taken for granted. For the East, however, its extent would still have to be explored.

15. Paul of Aegina (532), prooemium; 1:3, ll. 8–16; and idem (533), p. xvii (Adams's translation). Cf. Bloch (102), p. 549. Paul refers to the first Hippocratic aphorism; see Hippocrates (302), 4:98–99.

16. Paul of Aegina (532), 1:3, ll. 16–22; idem (533), 1:xvii–xviii.

17. Neuburger (480), 2:375, n. 1, has drawn attention to the similarity between scholastic reasoning and legal argumentation.

18. Paul of Aegina (532), prooemium; 1:3 (l. 24)–4 (l. 2); and idem (533), 1:xviii (Adams's translation).

to this wish: "Being an old man no longer capable of toil, I have written this book, bringing together the experiences in human diseases gathered with much perseverance."[19]

Unlike Stephanus, Alexander was not addressing medical students, nor was he the author of a medical compendium, as was Paul of Aegina. His work was not encyclopedic at all; it omitted surgery, and presents Alexander as a physician[20] who in his retirement looked back on his practice and recorded those things he had found valuable or worth communicating. His outlook may have been more independent than that of others, but the others of whom we know did not make personal experience the basis of their writing.

Alexander stresses the importance of correct diagnosis for proper therapy, and offers a good deal of humoral pathology and semeiology, as well as clinical description. His clinical descriptions are by no means negligible. He does not mind taking issue even with "the most divine Galen,"[21] for it was truth that encouraged him to contradict so outstanding a man; to keep silence seemed to him sinful (ἀσεβής). A physician who holds back with his opinion sins (ἀσεβεῖ),[22] and commits a great wrong. "Plato," he quotes elsewhere, "is my friend, but so is truth, and when the two are at issue, the truth must be preferred."[23] To put truth above authority was speaking in a Galenic spirit, and Alexander's intellectual independence does honor to him. Yet the actual disagreement with Galen that made Alexander quote the proverb about truth over friendship lies within the framework of Galenic pathology. Where viscous and thick humors blocked the lungs, Galen had prescribed a heating therapy and thinning drugs, as in asthma, yet he had not saved his patients. Instead, Alexander advises a well-blended, humectant, and moderately cooling diet such as he prescribed for a man who recovered after expectorating a stone from his lung.[24]

Alexander presents a hierarchy of treatments, beginning with dietetic therapy chosen according to the humoral pathology. Yet there are people who cannot follow the dietetic prescriptions,[25] and others, especially barbarians, who often do not obey them.[26] Then drugs come

19. Alexander of Tralles (7), 1:289.
20. In the sense of an internist. This does not prove, however, that Alexander never practiced surgery.
21. Alexander of Tralles (7), "On Fevers" 7; 1:407 and passim.
22. Alexander of Tralles (7), 2:155.
23. Ibid.; 2:155. This saying, best known in its Latin version, *Amicus Plato sed magis amicus veritas,* was proverbial.
24. I.e., a broncholith. Ibid.; 2:153–55.
25. Ibid.; 2:195.
26. Ibid.; 2:27.

into their own, and "there are remedies that reason as well as experience have attested to." [27] For most diseases, Alexander lists a large number of remedies, often in the form of complicated prescriptions. Such a multiplicity of prescriptions from which the physician (or the patient?) can choose can be a sign of uncertainty as to which drugs were really effective,[28] and occasional remarks throw some light on the clientele on which Alexander counted. For instance, a plaster made of olive oil and lead oxide (minium) "helps against many things and should not be despised because of the cheapness of its ingredients." [29]

Rational dietetics and drugs recommended by reason and experience constitute therapy according to "the art." Yet

> there are persons incapable of adhering to a strict regimen or of tolerating drugs, and [they] therefore compel us to use occult remedies and amulets in gout. I have taken up this [matter] so that the truly good [ἄριστος] physician may be well prepared in every respect to help all the sick in manyfold ways. But there being many such [things] that have it in their nature to act upon us, we describe those tested by much experience.[30]

Although this was said with regard to gout, it can be taken as Alexander's general opinion about occult remedies, especially in colic, epilepsy, and singultus. The justification for their use varied. "This then," he concluded his account of the regular pharmacological treatment of epilepsy,

> has been said regarding the remedies for epilepsy which I know and which long experience has taught. But because some people favor the occult [remedies] and amulets, are eager to use them, and actually attain the objective set for them, I have deemed it proper to communicate something about them for the friends of learning, that the physician may be well prepared in every respect to be able to help the sick.[31]

Here it was not the sick but the physicians who favored the occult,[32] men like Bolos, whom the good physician must not overlook.

Alexander's defensiveness and his misgivings about listing remedies outside the art are puzzling, since he was quite aware that for centuries Hippocratic physicians, for instance Archigenes, one of his main

27. Ibid.; 2:195.
28. But it also allows the physician to choose the drug best suited for the individual patient he is attending.
29. Alexander of Tralles (7), 2:119. Galen (241), 13:636, had previously remarked on the contempt for cheap drugs.
30. Alexander of Tralles (7), 2:579.
31. Ibid., 1:557.
32. Ibid., 1:437, ll. 15–16: ὑπὸ πάντων δὲ τῶν φυσικῶν ἰατρῶν.

sources, had also used them. When nothing that "the art" has to offer in singultus gives any relief, "it is by no means out of place also to make use of natural amulets[33] for the sake of saving the patient; indeed, it is even sinful to omit this kind [of remedy] and to become an obstacle to what will bring salvation to the sick, seeing that the most divine Galen and those before him also made use of them."[34]

The repeated insistence on the sinfulness of discarding any possible helpful remedy, together with the reference to Galen, suggests that Alexander's unease had a reason. Alexander recommended not only specifics, and drugs that acted by their whole substance;[35] he also included incantations and downright magic. Thus, digging for "the sacred plant, which is hyoscyamus," had to be done before dawn, when the moon was in the sign of Aquarius or Pisces, with the thumb and the index finger of the left hand, and without touching the root. At the same time, a formula had to be said, part of which read:

> I conjure you by the great name Iaoth, Sabaoth, the god who fixed the earth and stopped the sea . . . who dried up the wife of Lot and turned her into salt. Take of the spirit of your mother, the earth, and her power and dry up the flux of the feet and of the hands of this man or this woman.

On the following morning, before dawn, the plant was dug out with the bone of a dead animal, as these words were recited: "I conjure you by the holy names Iaoth, Sabaoth, Adonai, Eloi," and so on.[36]

Conjuring, even by the name of the Biblical God, was magic, but Alexander justified this sin by contending that it avoided the sin of allowing a patient to die, and he defended himself by citing the alleged authority of Galen. A work falsely attributed to Galen[37] related its author's conversion to the belief in magic:

> Some people believe that incantations resemble old wives' tales, as I [did] for a long time. Yet in [the] course of time I have been convinced

33. Τοῖς φυσικοῖς περιάπτοις, i.e., amulets that work by an occult power of nature.

34. Alexander of Tralles (7), 2:319. Although Galen (241), *De simplicium medicamentorum temperamentis ac facultatibus* 6.3; 11:859, used an amulet of peony in epilepsy, he made sure that the drying effect of the plant or of the air was the active agent; cf. Temkin (666), p. 25.

35. On this Galenic concept, see Temkin (667), p. 89.

36. Alexander of Tralles (7), 2:585.

37. The pseudo-Galenic work Περὶ τῆς καθ᾽ Ὅμηρον ἰατρικῆς is known from fragments only, of which Alexander's citation is one. See Kudlien (402), pp. 296–99, for a cogent argument of the pseudonymous character of this writing.

by manifest phenomena that there is power in them. For I observed [their] being of help to people wounded by a scorpion, and no less so when bones had stuck in the throat which upon an incantation were quickly spit out. There are many [remedies] that are excellent in their kind, and incantations also fulfill their purpose.

Fortified by what he believed to be Galen's conversion, Alexander added, "If then the most divine Galen and many others of the ancients bear witness, what prevents us from also communicating to you what we learned from experience and from friends." [38]

Alexander's unease was accompanied by a desire to keep the knowledge of the occult remedies confined to "the friends of learning" and "virtuous persons," and not to have it bruited about. The description of an iron ring inscribed with a gnostic character and the words "Flee, flee wee bile, the lark has searched for you" was followed by this explanation:

I have had much experience with this and thought it absurd not to pass on a power so strongly antipathetic to the affliction.[39] Yet I ask you not to show such matters to just anybody, but to persons who are virtuous [φιλαρέτους] and who can guard them, whence also the most divine Hippocrates in his insight admonishes: "Things that are holy are shown to holy persons but [to show them] to the profane is not right." [40]

Secrecy is a frequent companion of magic, be it to protect the public or the sorcerer, be it in the belief that spreading the magic power among the public would weaken it, or be it to enhance the mystic aura of the magician. In the Latin West, Marcellus of Bordeaux blatantly incorporated pagan incantations in his collection of medical recipes. A man of the highest rank,[41] and a Christian, who "beseeched the divine compassion" that his sons and their families might have no need for his reme-

---

38. Alexander of Tralles (7), 2:475. Cf. Bloch (102), p. 511; and Kudlien (402).

39. Colic.

40. Alexander of Tralles (7), 2:377, with reference to Hippocrates (306), *Law* 5; p. 8, ll. 15–17.

41. According to Kind (362), col. 1499, the surnames "Empiricus" and "Burdigalensis" (of Bordeaux) were later additions. Kind is undecided whether Marcellus was a physician; Kudlien (389), p. 50 and p. 57, n. 148, affirms it; and Baldwin (72), p. 18, cites him as a doctor in high places. Nevertheless, I agree with Baader (66), p. 426, in denying that the Marcellus who was a minister of Emperor Theodosius was a doctor. He counted himself among the men of learning who contributed to medicine without belonging to the medical profession; see Marcellus (443), "To His Sons" 1; p. 2, ll. 4–8.

dies,[42] he took the precaution of quoting the incantations in Greek, with which few people were still acquainted.

Alexander seemed to be apprehensive that he would be criticized by his contemporaries. His discussion of amulets against epilepsy ended with the affirmation that the physician must use "natural [remedies], informed reasoning, and [the] method of the art." He asserted that, he, Alexander¡ liked to employ all available methods in the interest of the sick, "but because at the present time the crowd is ignorant and finds fault with those who employ the natural [remedies], I have avoided making constant use of [the remedies] that are capable of acting by [their] nature and have endeavored to overcome the diseases by the method of the art."[43]

Alexander's occult therapy was not just an obtrusion of Byzantine superstition[44] but an essential part of the experience his book was meant to communicate. It is also this part that offers a glimpse into practices that were outside Hippocratic theory and the traditional material gathered by the encyclopedists. It confirms the long-standing existence of therapeutic practices that were outside the art, and even outside the law, and yet were never quite refuted by late Hippocratic physicians.

B. Neutral Medicine

Stephanus, Paul of Aegina, and Alexander of Tralles can be assumed to have been Christians, though the positive indications are not overwhelming. Stephanus's commentary on *Prognostic* closes with the words "Here, with God, is completed the present treatise, the commentary on *Prognostic*. Glory to God. Amen."[45] Similarly, the title of his commentary on *Aphorisms* invokes God's help.[46] But such formulas may even be additions by Byzantine editors and scribes.[47] The admis-

---

42. Marcellus (443), "To His Sons" 3; p. 2, ll. 20–21.

43. Alexander of Tralles (7), 1:571–73. This does not seem to be a part of Alexander's excerpts from Archigenes (cf. idem, p. 567).

44. Cf. Neuburger (480), 2:111; also Garrison (255), p. 124.

45. Stephanus (647), *Commentary on the Prognosticon of Hippocrates* 3.32; p. 292 (Duffy's translation, modified). See also idem, p. 26, for the Greek title of the whole work.

46. Stephanus (646), p. 28. See also the end of the first section, idem, p. 136. The fragment of Archelaus (71), p. 73, also ends "and God is [our] help."

47. According to its editor, the commentary on the first two sections of the *Aphorisms* only exists in an abridged edition prepared sometime "between ca. 900 . . . and ca. 1300" (Westerink [646], p. 16).

sion that "to know everything belongs to God alone"[48] and the references to "the will of the Higher Power"[49] and "the assimilation to
God"[50] are more indicative of Christianity, though not beyond all dispute.[51] The weakness of these indications stands out if they are compared with statements by Agnellus, another commentator of the period,
which leave little doubt of his Christianity. Agnellus urged his students
eventually to deserve to be "called physicians and saviors because of
the multitude of people healed by us with God's help."[52] He also paraphrased Galen in a Christian manner. Where Galen had an Empiricist
attacking the Methodists exclaim, "Ye gods, is the same therapy required wherever inflammation may develop, whether in the leg, the ear,
the mouth, or the eyes?"[53] Agnellus commented, "Here the empiricists,
furious with the methodist, say: 'How great a wrong you are doing,
you sin towards God, because you believe you cure swelling in every
part of the body whatsoever by a single treatment.'"[54]

Positive evidence of Christianity is weakest in the case of Paul of
Aegina, but at a time when hagiography told of an archiater carrying
his sickly son to the church that housed a relic of Saint Artemius, after
his own efforts had failed,[55] a pagan author would have been an exception. Alexander of Tralles was the brother of Anthemius, the architect
of the Hagia Sophia. His Christianity is suggested by his fear of having
sinned. The nature of these and possibly some other similar indications
of the Christianity of Stephanus, Paul of Aegina, Alexander of Tralles
demonstrates how little bearing their religion had upon their works.
For all practical purposes, these works could have been written by pagans.[56]

The form of teaching had changed, medical knowledge had grown,

48. Stephanus (646), *Commentary on Hippocrates' Aphorisms* 1.33; p. 122, l.
7. See also idem (647), p. 30, ll. 25–28.

49. Stephanus (646), *Commentary on Hippocrates' Aphorisms* 2.41; p. 230, ll.
7–8 (Westerink's translation). This is probably a Christian element, since "the will
of the Higher Power" here supersedes the Hippocratic prohibition of undertaking
to cure a terminally ill patient.

50. See above, chap. 14, text to n. 65.

51. See above, chap. 14, text to n. 66.

52. See above, chap. 16, text to n. 57.

53. Galen (242), *De sectis ad introducendos* 8; 3:21, ll. 4–7.

54. Agnellus (3), p. 127, ll. 11–15 (editors' translation). See also idem, p. 127,
ll. 37–38.

55. See Papadopoulos-Kerameus (528), 1; p. 2, ll. 9–22.

56. The same can be said of the iatrosophist Palladius and of the elusive John of
Alexandria, both of whom probably were Christians. Thus Palladius (526), p. 20, l.
27, writes μάθωμεν δὲ σὺν θεῷ. For Alexander, see Temkin (668), p. 68.

the interest in researching nature had waned, and many other things had changed in the course of the one thousand years since Hippocrates—but the substance of Hippocratic medicine had not changed. And since both the old and the new, from the bulk of the Hippocratic works to the works of the sixth century, were acceptable to the church, the conclusion might seem to be unavoidable that Hippocratic medicine had been religiously neutral from its very beginning.

Such a conclusion, however, is not tenable. Hippocratic medicine was not neutral in the sense in which mathematics and logic could be said to be neutral. It had fitted well into the religious outlook of pagan Antiquity. Even when shorn of frank polytheism, its remaining naturalism was a foreign body in any radically Christian culture. In Hippocratism, nature was and remained the final power.[57] Whether or not nature was considered to be God's creation was a decision outside the purview of medicine. From a radically Christian point of view, leaving it to the physician to implement his medical concepts with as many correctives as the depth and sincerity of his faith demanded was not permissible. The church could demand that the Christian doctor accept its teachings, yet its demands were addressed to the doctor as a Christian, not to the science and art he professed.

It can rightly be said that in other fields, too, pagan teachings were adopted on similar terms. The religion of the Aristotelian commentators in Alexandria of the period was not reflected in their commentaries.[58] The historian Agathias of Myrina, probably a Christian, wrote history in a classical style.[59] Hippocratic medicine can thus be seen as part of the pagan tradition that the Church admitted as a price to be paid for the Hellenization of Christianity. This is true but it does not go far enough. Whereas the arts and sciences were mainly a matter for the educated, medicine was part of everyday life in all levels of society. Medicine's stubborn insistence on natural explanations countered the popular beliefs regarding demons and regarding supernatural causes of mental disease. It was this medical tradition that secured a basis for the

57. Even for the very late authors, nature was a superhuman power. For instance, Stephanus (648), 1:344, could say that "nature fighting [ἀπομαχομένη] to drive off the superfluous humor through the upper [intestinal paths] helps in the contest." And according to idem (646), p. 124, l. 20, the physician remains "a servant of nature." Any theological reinterpretation of nature was outside the scientific text.

58. Praechter (568), p. 635: "Die alexandrinische Schule wurde allmählich zu einer neutralen philosophischen Bildungsanstalt ohne ein scharf ausgeprägtes platonisch-heidnisches Bekenntnis." See also Marrou (445), p. 140.

59. The question of Agathias's Christianity has been discussed by Cameron (131), chap. 9 ("Christian History in the Classical Manner"), pp. 89–111; see especially idem, p. 93.

development of modern medicine in the face of popular prejudices and religious objections, where these existed.

Hippocratic medicine of the sixth century was not truly neutral. A thousand years later, when the tradition of the Catholic Church came under attack, Paracelsus recognized the essentially pagan character of a medicine that omitted God from its concept of disease.[60] Fundamentally, Paracelsus repeated what Basil and others had said about the Christian's relationship to disease and healing. However, Basil had asked what Christians could accept from medicine,[61] whereas Paracelsus elaborated on what medicine ought to accept from Christianity: the presence of God, the *ens Dei,* in all diseases, regardless of whether they had arisen naturally or were a scourge of God.[62] The medical art explained diseases in the light of nature, and cured them accordingly. But to believe that this was the final explanation and the only cure was pagan. A Christian doctor who saw no further was as much a pagan physician as the infidel. Pagans who trusted in nothing but their art also achieved cures, if their endeavor coincided with the time God had set for the end of the disease. Every disease was a purgatory, and it ended when the purgatory was extinguished. The art helped only if and when the doctor and the patient got together at the right time, as determined by God.

To rephrase Hippocrates,[63] Paracelsus wanted God woven into the very texture of medical thinking and feeling. Love as the foundation of medicine, the doctor's duty to search for cures that would conquer allegedly incurable diseases, were postulates that grew out of Paracelsus's religious convictions. He did not hold the medical art to be antagonistic to healing by faith and prayer. God liked to act through human beings; if the faith were strong, as in the time of Jesus, miraculous cures could be performed, but if it were weak or absent, the doctor's art was needed. Much as his own naturalism differed from that of Galen, Paracelsus yet criticized naturalism as pagan only if it remained self-sufficient and without recourse to God.

Paracelsus belonged to a time characterized by a new admiration

---

60. The following sketch of Paracelsus's ideas is chiefly based on one of his early works, the *Volumen Paramirum,* in the edition of Karl Sudhoff (529). An annotated edition of the *Volumen Paramirum* was published by Joh. Daniel Achelis, Jena, 1928.

61. See above, chap. 13.

62. The *Volumen Paramirum* counts five *entia,* of which the first four (*ens astrale, ens veneni, ens naturale,* and *ens spirituale*) are pagan. The reader will find a brief account of the five *entia* in Sigerist (625), pp. 93–94.

63. Cf. Hippocrates (306), *Decorum* 6; p. 27, l. 13. See above, chap. 3, text to n. 56.

for Antiquity, but also by a wish to go back to early Christianity, un-contaminated by compromises.[64] Reformers and Puritans of the six-teenth and seventeenth centuries had a sharp eye for discovering heathen elements in the Catholic Church. They found such elements because, from the third century on, the church had gone the way of Hellenization and had integrated pagan thoughts and customs where this seemed necessary to make the new, missionary faith viable.

If then it is true that medicine at the end of Antiquity was un-Christian (though not anti-Christian) rather than strictly neutral, it is equally true that it was not polytheistic, Jewish, or Mohammedan, either. In this sense, it does deserve to be called neutral.[65] Jews and Mohammedans could—and did—adopt it and add to it what their re-spective faiths demanded. Modern medicine, with all its revolutionary changes, has retained this character, and scientific medicine can be taught in many countries, regardless of their religious preference. But there also has remained the nagging doubt that neutral medicine was compatible with truly Christian, Jewish, or Mohammedan religiosity. Once nature was reinterpreted in a mechanistic sense, as happened in the scientific revolution, neutral medicine also could be made to fit into an atheistic world view.

64. For example, the humanist Erasmus was the author of *In Praise of Folly,* with its endorsement of primitive Christianity.

65. Toellner (689), p. 746, speaks of "the relative neutrality" of this medicine with regard to religion, which "facilitates its recognition by theology and the church and its continued existence in Christianity." To quote Amundsen (17), p. 321, with regard to naturalistic medicine, its "religious neutrality allowed for natural pro-cesses of proximate causality within God's created order," and was thus acceptable to late Hellenistic Judaism.

18

HIPPOCRATES IN THE
CHRISTIAN WORLD

Christian culture needed Hippocratic medicine, but it did not need Hippocrates as a culture hero, for it had its apostles, its saints and martyrs, and its great theologians. In the eyes of strict Christians, he was not even a real sage, as Isidore of Pelusium had made clear;[1] he was not even a perfect physician like the anargyros Cyrus, who was capable of healing both bodies and souls.

In the Greek East, Hippocrates' writings, his *Vita*, the Pseudepigrapha, and the eulogies that Galen and others had bestowed upon him could still be read. A cultural decline, beginning in the sixth century and followed by a chaotic period of invasions and iconoclastic struggles, gave way, by the ninth century, to a renaissance,[2] during which the learned patriarch Photius wrote his *Bibliotheca*,[3] to which we owe much of our information about the Neoplatonists and the physicians of the fifth to sixth centuries. In the following century, there was compiled the so-called Souda, a lexicographic work by an unknown author, formerly believed to be one Suidas. It contains a biography of Hippocrates[4] as conceived at the height of the humanistic studies in the

---

1. See above, chap. 16, text to n. 9.
2. See Lemerle (417), p. 109.
3. Photius (545).
4. Souda (653), cols. 662–63. Three biographies of Hippocrates (Souda [653], Tzetzes [695], and Schöne [611]) were discussed by Edelstein (200), cols. 1292–93, who grouped them together as *Gelehrtenviten*.

Byzantine Empire. There is no mention of Hippocrates' descent from Asclepius, nor are there Christian allusions. It is mentioned that Hippocrates' great fame reached the Persian king, and the king's letter asking that Hippocrates be invited to his court is quoted, but not Hippocrates' reply. The stories of the cure of Perdikkas, king of Macedonia, and of the Abderites' request that Hippocrates cure Democritus are omitted. On the whole, the account is rather sober and avoids gossip. Hippocrates is not celebrated as the great Greek patriot or the self-sufficient scorner of money. All the more remarkable, therefore, is the hyperbole with which the physician Hippocrates and his works are praised:

> The books written by Hippocrates are very well known to all practicing the medical science, and they honor them like utterances of a god and not as coming from a human mouth. [This] aside, we too should keep in mind those that are foremost: first, the book containing the oath; second, that presenting the prognoses, third, that of *Aphorisms,* which transcends human intelligence. Let the fourth place be held by the much-discussed and much-admired work, consisting of sixty books, that encompasses the whole medical science and wisdom.[5]

The "utterances of a god" echoes Galen,[6] and the praise of *Aphorisms* is reminiscent of the preface to this work, which may have been the work of a Christian.[7] The article in the Souda was written for readers seeking information about Hippocrates, but not for physicians. It shows, however, in what high esteem the physician Hippocrates continued to be held in Byzantium, even if the enthusiasm for Hippocrates as a classical author were taken into account. The Souda followed the biographical line of the legend, even though it differed in some details. There also existed another biography, probably of Greek origin but preserved only fragmentarily in a Latin version of not earlier than about A.D. 500,[8] when the memory of Hippocratic times had already become hazy in the West.

This Latin fragment includes detailed lists[9] of Hippocrates' works, preceded by some remarks on his authorship. It holds that Hippocrates began writing after his return from the Median king "Arfaxad"[10] in

---

5. Souda (653), col. 662.
6. See above, chap. 5, text to n. 16.
7. See above, chap. 4, text to nn. 45–51.
8. Schöne (611), p. 66. According to Schöne, this biography is contained in the Brussels ms. no. 1342–50, fols. 52ᵛ–53ᵛ (see Schöne [611], p. 56).
9. The manuscript carries these lists in two different places, fol. 59ᵛ and fol. 3ʳ. See Schöne (611), pp. 58–61.
10. Fol. 52ᵛ spells the name "Arfaxath."

Ecbatana. He lectured in Athens,[11] and at the same time he accepted from Polybius, the son of Apollonius, seven books that came from Memphis. "These he carried hence with him to Cos, and from these books he composed the canon of medicine exceedingly well." [12] The visit to the king of the Medes and the dependence of Hippocrates' work on Egyptian wisdom conflict with the legend of the great Greek patriot. King "Arfaxad" was "Arphaxad, which reigned over the Medes in Ekbatane" of the Book of Judith,[13] which points to a late Judaeo-Christian intrusion into this biography.

This intrusion, if that is what it was, did not go far. Hippocrates' genealogy was traced to Asclepius. "To Asclepius two descendants were born from Epione, Hercules' daughter: Podalirius and Machaon"; Machaon, in most people's opinion, did not survive the destruction of Troy, whereas Podalirius had two sons (and so on).[14] This is the Homeric Asclepius rather than the son of Apollo; intentionally or not, there is no reference to Asclepius as the divine healer.[15]

Confusion and ignorance regarding ancient history marked Isidore of Seville's account of the founders of medicine: "Among the Greeks, the discoverer and founder of the art of medicine is said to have been Apollo." [16] This put the onus of the heathen god on the pagans. Isidore also disclaimed responsibility by reporting that "after Asclepius's death from a lightning bolt, *it is said*[17] that the healing art was forbidden" and died with Asclepius "until the time of Artaxerxes, King of Persia." The following blunder, however, seems to have been his own: "At that time, Hippocrates, born on the island of Cos and whose father was Aesculapius, restored it to light." [18] Isidore's blunder is not surprising. Some two hundred years before him, Marcellus had cited two letters of Hippocrates, of which one was supposed to be addressed to King Antiochus,[19] one of the Seleucid kings who lived in the third and second

11. Schöne (611), p. 58, list from fol. 3ʳ. According to the list from fol. 59ᵛ, Hippocrates wrote his books in Athens.

12. Schöne (611), p. 58 (fol. 3ʳ).

13. Apocrypha (29), Judith 1; p. 82 (Authorized Version). Cf. Schöne (611), p. 58, apparatus. Edelstein (200), col. 1293, misread (or conjectured?) Artaxerxes for Arfaxath.

14. Schöne (611), pp. 56–57.

15. The same is true of Tzetzes' genealogy of Hippocrates; see Tzetzes (695), *Historiae* 7.155.936–50; pp. 292–93 (see also below, n. 51).

16. Isidore of Seville (332), *Etymologiarum* 4.3. Quoted from Sharpe's ([333], p. 15) translation.

17. The emphasis is mine.

18. Isidore of Seville (332), *Etymologiarum* 4.3. Quotation modified from Sharpe's [333], p. 15) translations.

19. In the Greek original, the letter was by Diocles of Carystus.

centuries B.C., and the other to Maecenas,[20] a Roman patron of literature who lived in the first century B.C.!

Mistakes of this kind were common in the early Middle Ages, and during the sixth century historical ignorance in one place could coexist with serious study in another. Thus, Ravenna was a center for the translation of Greek medical texts, and here Agnellus lectured on Galenic writings.[21] Generally speaking, statements about "the Latin West" and "the Greek East" may often need qualification in view of regional differences and even small differences in time. The picture of Hippocrates prevailing in cities such as Constantinople, Alexandria, and Antioch probably differed from that in Cos, where local legends grew around its great citizen.

Throughout late Antiquity, Hippocrates was well remembered as a great physician and scientist. Whatever strict Christians might think of him, to an Alexandrian philosopher he was still the perfect physician, because he was capable of making physicians of others.[22] Alexander of Aphrodisias,[23] Tertullian,[24] and Theodoretus[25] all cited him among the authors who contended that the soul was located in the brain, though Tertullian rejected this view. Again, Hippocrates had defined wind as "a flow and a stream of air."[26] Aristotle questioned this opinion.[27] Regardless of whether Aristotle had had Hippocrates in mind, late commentators, including John Philoponus,[28] quoted Hippocrates, and Olympiodorus upbraided him: "You do not speak well, Hippocrates, that wind is air in movement."[29]

At times, however, Hippocrates had to share his scientific renown with others, notably Galen. Olympiodorus pointed out that the four

---

20. Marcellus (443), pp. 18–25 and 26–33.

21. See above chap. 17, text to nn. 52–54.

22. Asclepius (52), *In Aristotelis Metaphysicorum* 1021b12; p. 339, ll. 3–5 and p. 341, ll. 21–23. Pseudo-Galen (241), *Definitiones medicae* 25; 19:355, provides a more sensible definition: "a physician is perfect who is fully accomplished in theory and practice." Nachmanson (475) and idem (476) cited most of the following Hippocratic dicta occurring in pagan and Christian authors. However, philological interest made him concentrate on textual questions rather than on historical interpretation.

23. Alexander of Aphrodisias (5), *In Aristotelis Metaphysica* 1035b14; p. 508, ll. 29–35.

24. Tertullian (674), *De anima* 15.5; p. 19.

25. Theodoretus (677), *Curatio* 5.22; p. 232, ll. 20–23.

26. Hippocrates (306), *On Breaths* 3; pp. 92 (l. 22)–93 (l. 1).

27. Aristotle (47), *Meteorologica* 349a18; p. 88. See also idem, p. 89, n. 1.

28. John Philoponus (323), *De opificio mundi* 2.2; p. 63, ll. 2–4. Cf. Nachmanson (475), pp. 190–92, for textual differences in the quotations.

29. Olympiodorus (501), *In Aristotelis Meteora*; pp. 168 (l. 36)–69 (l. 1).

elements had existed even before knowledge of them was obtained by "the medicine of Hippocrates"[30]—which might mean Hippocrates alone or might include those who shared his medical opinions. According to Simplicius, Hippocrates and his followers pushed their analysis as far back as the primary qualities of the primary elements. In an argument directed against the philosophers and physicians who derived man from one single element, Hippocrates had written, "If man were a unit, he would never feel pain, for being a unit he would have nothing from which to suffer pain."[31] Galen had made this proposition the mainstay of his elaborated humoral theory, and it was also taken up by the Neoplatonist Proclus and his pupil Ammonius, as well as by Bishop Nemesius and John Philoponus in their defense of a plurality of qualities and elements.[32] John Philoponus, moreover, credited "the physician Hippocrates," together with Timaeus and Empedocles, with having established the theory of the four elements.[33] In view of Galen's admiration for Plato, it is very likely that John Philoponus was relying on Galen, and it was probably Galen who had directed attention to the Hippocratic thesis of the plurality of elements in the human body.

All this confirms the close association of the names of Hippocrates and Galen, but it also shows Galen as a potential spokesman for Hippocrates in scientific matters.[34] The two names could be coupled and treated as a unit. Asking his listeners not to bewail the death of his brother Caesarius, Gregory of Nazianzus balanced the losses and the gains caused by his death: "He will not study the works of Hippocrates and Galen and their adversaries? No, but neither will he be distressed by diseases and experience personal grief at others' misfortunes."[35] Some enemies of secular medicine, on the other hand, coupled the two names as representatives of godless healing and sources of disbelief.[36]

The relationship between Hippocrates and Galen was seen as giving

30. Olympiodorus (502), *Prolegomena*; pp. 108 (l. 37)–9 (l. 2).

31. Hippocrates (302), *On the Nature of Man* 2; 4:6, ll. 13–15. Galen believed the first part of *On the Nature of Man* to be genuinely Hippocratic.

32. Galen (241), *De elementis ex Hippocrate* 1.2; 1:415 Proclus Diadochus (572), *In Platonis Timaeum*; 2:28; Ammonius (13), *In Porphyrii Isagogen*; pp. 111 (l. 27)–12 (l. 3); Nemesius (477), *De natura hominis* 5; pp. 167–68; John Philoponus (324), *In Aristotelis De generatione et corruptione*; pp. 4 (l. 33)–5 (l. 1).

33. John Philoponus (325), *In Aristotelis Physicorum libros tres priores*; p. 24, ll. 2–3.

34. "Hippocrates came to the Greeks, one may formulate it somewhat pointedly, on Galen's towrope [*Schlepptau*]" (Ullmann [697], p. 248, n. 16).

35. Gregory of Nazianzus (272), *Oratio VII*, art. 20; col. 780C. Quoted from MacCauley's ([270], p. 21) translation. On Caesarius, see above, chap. 14, n. 8.

36. See above, chap. 12, text to nn. 110, 119, and 121.

luster to each. Hippocrates had written: "Exercise of the organs, toil, food, drink, sleep, sexual acts, [all] in moderation."[37] To this a commentator remarked:

> We have thus learned the hygienic prescriptions, yet this seems to give us reason to commend Hippocrates while censoring Galen. For behold, Hippocrates in a minimum of words taught all that pertains to hygiene. Why then did Galen use so many lines on hygiene? For just as Hippocrates taught some six things, namely toil, bath, food, drink, sleep, sexual acts, so Galen published six books on hygiene. In defense of Galen we say, however, that Hippocrates sowed, Galen did the farming. For it is not enough to give ear to "all in moderation"; for there are differences in what is moderate.[38]

The commentator then briefly pointed out the necessary details by which Galen amplified the seminal, but all-too-short, Hippocratic passages that foreshadowed the notion of the six non-naturals.[39]

Galen thought of himself as having clarified and brought to completion what was either obscure or incomplete in Hippocrates.[40] This close connection carried the risk that Hippocrates would be drawn into the attack of Christian and pagan theologians upon Galen.[41] Indeed, Galen had cited Hippocrates as a witness for his thesis of the soul's dependence upon the body, and the Hippocratic writings contained enough suspicious material.[42] The danger did not materialize; at least there seems to have been no specific attack on Hippocrates. Galen, the spokesman in scientific matters, drew the ire upon himself. He, not Hippocrates, had openly doubted the immortality of the soul and had confessed to a philosophy of agnosticism no longer welcome in an age that demanded faith and condemned all aberrations from absolute truth.

Galen, more than Hippocrates, represented science. On the other hand, Hippocrates, rather than Galen, represented clinical medicine and medical ethics. There are problems about the swearing of the Hip-

---

37. Hippocrates (309), *Epidemics* 6.6; 5:322–24.
38. Palladius (525), *Commentarii in Hippocratis librum sextum De morbis popularibus*; 2:157.
39. See above, chap. 14, text to nn. 53–55.
40. See Temkin (667), p. 33.
41. See above, chap. 15.B. Nemesius (477), *De natura hominis* 2; p. 87, ll. 4–5, noted that Galen had based his argument on Hippocrates.
42. Galen (242), *Quod animi mores* 7–9; 2:57–64. Galen cited chiefly *On Airs, Waters, Localities,* but also *Epidemics* 2 and 6 (see pp. 62–63). To these could be added Hippocrates (302), *Regimen* 1.25 and 26; 4:280–92, as far as intelligence is concerned.

pocratic oath by early Christian doctors.[43] But in medical education, the oath and the deontological writings of the Hippocratic Collection retained their moral force throughout Antiquity and the Middle Ages in the Orient and the Occident. Even today, in many institutions, the oath, often in a modified form, is sworn by medical students upon receiving their medical degrees. It is the oath that keeps the name of Hippocrates alive among a broad public that may have never heard of humoral pathology.

Hippocrates educated physicians in humaneness,[44] and Tertullian acknowledged him as a humane doctor. Tertullian condemned the killing of the living human fetus, while admitting that it was necessary in certain cases. Hippocrates and other physicians, he conceded, had used a pointed instrument for perforating the skull of the fetus when delivery of an intact child was impossible because, convinced that the fetus was a living being, and moved by compassion (*miserti*), they chose to kill such unfortunates lest they be dismembered alive.[45]

Hippocrates had complained that the doctor's lot was to harvest sorrows of his own from others' miseries. Thus, Gregory of Nazianzus had found consolation for his brother's death in Caesarius's release "from experiencing personal grief at others' misfortunes." [46] Cassiodorus had alluded to the Hippocratic saying when he described his monks' activities.[47] The dictum had also been applied to other professions, and then to Jesus, thus establishing a common bond between the physician and the "Savior." [48] By no later than the fifth century, probably much earlier, the saying had undergone a semantic change. It was no longer a complaint; rather, it was a description of a good physician, who took the burden of the miseries of the sick upon himself,[49] and it then became a demand that the physician shoulder his burden: "He should make the misfortunes [*casus*] of others his own sorrow.[50]

43. See above, chap. 14.A.

44. See above, chap. 4, text to n. 24.

45. Tertullian (674), *De anima* 25.4; p. 36, ll. 6–12; and idem, comments on p. 326. Tertullian's is a testimonial of a Christian's trust in the existence of compassion among pagan doctors.

46. Gregory of Nazianzus (272), *Oratio VII*, art. 20, col. 780C. Quoted from MacCauley's ([270], p. 21) translation.

47. See above, chap. 12, text to n. 74.

48. See above, chap. 11.C.

49. See above, chap. 11, text to n. 98.

50. MacKinney's (435), p. 14, text H, translation, modified. The whole passage reads, "Fortis autem [sit] ut possit per diem labores sustinere, quando videt horrenda et tangit insuavia, alienos casus suas faciat tristitias" (Rose [590], 2:244, ll. 14–16).

In the twelfth century, Tzetzes, a Byzantine grammarian and the author of *Histories,* wrote a chapter entitled "On the Hippocratic Words 'Harvesting Trouble of His Own.'"[51] The chapter gives a short biography of Hippocrates, derived from the *Vita,* and it ends with the words "This Hippocrates, the physician of Cos, son of Heracleides, said: 'What distinguishes the role of doctors is to harvest from others' misfortunes troubles of their own.'"[52] Probably meant as an extended literary reference, these lines, taken as expressing the ethical obligation of the doctor's calling, present a tribute to Hippocrates that both pagans and Christians might gladly pay.

51. Tzetzes (695), *Historiae* 7.155; pp. 292–94. The Hippocratic genealogy (see above, text to n. 14) is contained in this chapter.

52. Ibid. 7.979–81; p. 294.

EPILOGUE

Throughout the six centuries that established the relationship of Greek scientific medicine to the great monotheistic religions, Hippocrates, suitably elevated to legendary fame, represented one man's authority. He was the ideal of the great and good physician, to whom medicine owed a set of accepted principles and a body of proven experience laid down in the books that were attributed to him. Also, he was the medical lawgiver whose oath owed much of its power to his name.

Hippocrates maintained his authority, yet his cultural significance diminished. Neither in the East nor in the West did Christians need a pagan culture hero. In the West, his name, though not forgotten, and supported by such of his books as were translated into Latin, was enshrouded in the haze of a failing historical memory. In the East, the culture hero of pagan times was reduced to a pagan sage and an illustrious physician and scientist; he retained his authority among doctors, and his name was well known among the educated public.

His acceptance by the church attested to the need for his wisdom, and the continuing power of secular medicine over most of Eastern mankind. In pagan times, just as in Christian times, religious healing and secular healing existed side by side, with the difference, however, that for pagans this coexistence did not involve a troubled conscience. For pagans as well as Christians, Hippocratic medicine was involved in the competition between secular and religious healing. But its naturalistic basis gave it a non-Christian character and thus created a difficulty for Christians that did not exist for pagans.

However, this authoritative pagan, Hippocrates, had many faces, and the personalities behind them did not all relate to Christianity in the same way. As the descendent of the Homeric prince Asclepius, Hippocrates was a human being and was so treated by the Byzantine scholars.[1] However, Hippocrates the descendant of the healing god Asclepius, the son of Apollo, was of divine lineage and endowed with a divine nature, which conflicted with Christian beliefs.

Less obvious yet more to the point were cases where Hippocrates appeared in his role as physician. In *Epidemics,* he declared the physician to be the servant of the art (techne).[2] In the most elementary sense, this suggests the conscientious craftsman who took pains to produce good work, at considerable inconvenience to himself, if necessary. Neither pagan nor Christian could object to honest work. In a more sophisticated sense, the techne was an art that included rules based on theoretical insights. For Hippocrates the Dogmatist, that meant insights into the workings of nature. That nature was the healer of disease was one of the fundamental insights,[3] and it made the physician the servant of nature.[4] Nature alone could (and can) mend a broken bone, and the doctor could (and can) help her by setting the fractured bone, and by splints and bandages (and open reduction, to bring the matter up to date). Whether this left the doctor in a humble position or not depended on whether nature or her helper was treated as the protagonist.[5]

There was little modesty in the way Hippocrates of the legend conceived of his role as assistant to nature. In his reply to the Abderites, he wrote as the defender of free medicine, which was not to be debased by the physician's accepting a fee. Indignant though he was over their offer of money, he explained his acceptance of their invitation as follows:

> Convinced that [the] arts are favors of the gods and human beings works of nature, it seems to me—be not angry, men of Abdera—that not you but nature herself calls me to restore a work of hers that is in danger of disintegrating under the disease. Thus I now obey nature and the gods rather than you in curing sick Democritus.[6]

1. See above, chap. 18.
2. Hippocrates (302), *Epidemics* 1.11; 1:164.
3. Cf. Sigerist (623), p. 31. See also above, chap. 14, text to n. 74.
4. Stephanus (646), p. 124, l. 20.
5. For nature's priority over human endeavor, see above, chap. 14, text to n. 75.
6. Hippocrates (307), Pseudepigrapha 11; p. 6, ll. 10–13. Cf. above, chap. 6.B.2.

These were the proud words of a pagan mindful of what his art owed to the gods and willing to take upon himself the mission with which nature had entrusted him. They sounded quite different from the humility (together with friendliness and kindness) that an early medieval medical text demanded of the doctor, "for humility always learns, always gains knowledge, towers over nobody,[7] offends nobody."[8] Neither Hippocrates' reply nor the Abderites' invitation mentioned compassion for poor sick Democritus as a reason for Hippocrates' going to Abdera. Yet this very un-Christian Hippocrates[9] knew that by refusing to cure Democritus, he would offend the gods who had given medicine as a favor to mankind. His obligation to heal went beyond Democritus's particular case.

Galen claimed that Hippocrates, like himself and a few others of the ancients, practiced medicine for the sake of philanthropy.[10] Galen's interpretation of Hippocrates' outlook and activities, including his treatment of poor people on Thasos and other islands, thus has to be seen as philanthropic, and the same holds true of the broader outlook under which the Abderites appealed to Hippocrates. He was to come to Abdera for the sake of their city, for the sake of culture (*paideia*) and of future generations.[11] Hippocrates saw himself as fulfilling nature's mission in curing Democritus. In the late anonymous preface to *Aphorisms*, Hippocrates, as "nature incarnate," fulfilled the divine mission of saving mankind from destruction. There was here a parallel with Jesus, "the word . . . made flesh" (John 1:14), who carried out God's mission of mercy.[12] Intentionally or not, this was a christianized Hippocrates, whose admirable work had its source in God's compassion for man. Galen's philanthropy likewise was not limited to helping needy patients. He was zealous in establishing truth; he had "slaved in the service of the art and [had] served friends, relatives, and fellow-citizens in many respects,"[13] and he had written some of his main works with an eye to posterity.[14]

As long as the physician was not compared to a healing god or

7. *Nullum excedit* (?). Text and translation are uncertain.

8. Hirschfeld (313), *Epistula ad Nepotianum;* p. 361, ll. 12–13. See also MacKinney's ([435], p. 11) translation.

9. Although this Hippocrates does not accept a fee, his motivation stands in stark contrast to that of the Christian anargyroi; see above, chap. 12.C, especially the text to nn. 107–10.

10. Galen (248), *De placitis Hippocratis et Platonis* 9.5.6; 2:565, ll. 26–30.

11. Hippocrates (307), Pseudepigrapha 10; p. 5, ll. 16–31.

12. See above, chap. 4, n. 47.

13. Galen (243), *De sanitate tuenda* 5.1; p. 136, ll. 21–22.

14. On Galen's philanthropy, see Temkin (667), pp. 47–50.

glorified as a savior, his philanthropy in the service of mankind was hardly objectionable to Christians. The *Vita* and his reply to the king of Persia portrayed Hippocrates' philanthropy as limited to the Greeks,[15] but Greek patriotism was of little interest to Galen, to the Romans,[16] or to the Byzantines who called themselves Romans and whose Christianity favored a universalistic outlook.

The Hippocrates of the oath does not mention philanthropy and patriotism. The oath, in its single-minded attention to the patient's welfare and insistence on proper behavior in the patient's house, made the doctor the servant of his art. It went further, and its specific prohibition of any involvement in murder, suicide, and abortion was to meet with Christian ethical standards. Yet it was not a Christian oath, not only because it called on pagan gods but also because the doctor's reward was worldly success, and his punishment for breaking the oath was worldly failure. The Hippocrates of the oath, with his strict rules for accepting pupils, was not the same as Plato's Hippocrates, who resembled a Sophist in his willingness to teach medicine to anyone for pay. Nor was he the Hippocrates of the oath as interpreted by Scribonius Largus.[17] The latter Hippocrates was an educator who guided physicians toward humaneness, and his art was the protector of human life.

Whereas the Hippocratic oath was silent regarding the patient's economic and social condition as well as the doctor's remuneration, for Hippocrates the author of *Precepts,* these matters were to be approached with a philanthropic attitude.[18] He was not above demanding his fee, but in this and in his relationship to patients, consideration for them came first. The Hellenist inscriptions, *Precepts,* as well as the writings of Scribonius Largus, Celsus, Soranus, and Aretaeus, attest that concern for the sick and for helpless strangers was expected of doctors, and that some doctors made it their compassionate concern. Christianity was to make this expectation an obligation.

The many faces of Hippocrates correspond to the plurality of potential relationships of Hippocratic physicians to Christianity. There is no sense in asking how close *the* Hippocratic doctor came to anticipating Christian ideals. However, it is valid to ask whether there were specifically Christian demands that were not met by any pagan doctor.

Jesus had come to show mercy to sinners (Matt. 9:13), but no Hip-

15. See above, chap. 6.A, especially text to nn. 34, 35, and 37; and chap. 6.B.1.

16. To some of whom his Greek patriotism appeared in a very sinister light; see above, chap. 6.B.1, especially text to nn. 63–74.

17. See above, chap. 6, text to nn. 76–77.

18. See above, chap. 3.

pocrates, except the christianized, had come to show mercy to the sick. Hippocratic philanthropy was the practice of medicine in the service of mankind (or, more narrowly, of the Greeks) or it was concern and compassion for one's patients.[19] On the Christian side there stood Basil, who founded a leprosarium in order to take care of those expelled from human society; and the monks of Cassiodorus's Vivarium, who "devote[d] the services of holy piety to those who [took] refuge in the abodes of the saints."[20] Basil and the other founders of early hospitals, the monks of Cassiodorus, and the priests, who were—or became—physicians, were Christians whose charity took the form of providing medical care. The layman who chose medicine as a profession in order to serve the needy sick, at home or abroad, was to make his appearance later.[21] It is only necessary to think of the miraculous healings at places of pilgrimage dedicated to saints or harboring holy relics to realize that the influence of Christianity on healing in the broad sense went beyond its influence on Hippocratic medicine. Regarding the latter, it gave and it received. Medicine made contributions to Christian anthropology, it was useful in theological debates,[22] and—its greatest gift—it constituted the necessary worldly analogue for spiritual medicine.

As a human being, the Hippocratic doctor, if an earnest convert to Christianity, entered a new religious world. His traditional science remained intact, but he would be careful not to allow its naturalism to tinge his religious beliefs. As a practitioner, he learned to give God the credit for any cures he achieved. Perhaps the original complaint about the doctor's lot changed to a professional requirement under Christian influence.[23] The doctor might also be more charitable to indigent pa-

---

19. Amundsen and Ferngren (26), p. 12, have pointed out "the great gap that existed between the classical concept of *philanthropia* and the Christian idea of *agape* as the dynamic of ethics." The study of medicine because of love for the sick probably is a Christian phenomenon (see below, text to n. 21). Nevertheless, Origen's [509], *Contra Celsum* 3.74; col. 1016C–D) reference to the "philanthropic physician [who] looks for the sick that he may bring them the remedies and make them strong" (see above, chap. 11, n. 99; and cf. Amundsen and Ferngren [26], pp. 16–17) suggests that as far as medicine is concerned, the gap may not have been quite as wide.

20. See above, chap. 12, text to n. 74.

21. He is the secularized descendent of Christian missionary doctors and possibly of the anargyroi and priest-physicians of late Antiquity; cf. Amundsen (17), p. 321.

22. Cf. above, chap. 11.

23. Cf. above, chap. 11, text to n. 98. I think it more likely that this metamorphosis had already occurred in pagan times.

tients than he had been before.[24] But by and large his science remained the same, and his practice did not have to undergo a revolution. What shook the world did not shake everything in it in equal measure.

An imaginary situation and a few hypothetical questions may show that the path of Hippocrates from pagan to Christian was not as well marked as characterizations of paganism and Christianity might make us believe. Supposing that Hippocrates had found a stranger, wounded and robbed, lying by the wayside. Would Hippocrates the craftsman have passed him by because he was not his client and no fee was to be expected? Would the Hippocrates of the oath have declined to help him because the man was not *his* patient? Would the Hippocrates of the legend have cured him because he felt an obligation to mend nature's damaged work? Would the Hippocrates of *Precepts* have played the good Samaritan? And, for good measure, what would a modern doctor do, mindful of the Hippocratic oath and of ethical codes but also aware that his assistance might be requited by a malpractice suit?

Whatever replies, if any at all, are given to those questions will have to depend not so much on inferences from philosophical and religious systems and socially accepted ideals and taboos, as on the interpretation of the medical texts that are at our disposal. Thus, the admonition in *Precepts* that the physician should help needy strangers will do more to answer one of the above questions than will debatable interpretations of Stoic philanthropy.[25] The answers will gain in clarity if they are not couched in abstractions but are offered in comparisons with the practices of modern doctors. Our frequent inability to give satisfactory answers might be enlightening because it might point out where our ignorance lies.

24. Concrete evidence for the changes the doctor underwent as a result of his conversion is more likely to be found in letters and other personal documents than in the extant medical literature, which does not show any influence of Christian ideals on medical practice; cf. Amundsen and Ferngren (26), p. 17; also idem (23), p. 15.

25. Is *Precepts* to be related to the old Stoicism of Chrysippus (Edelstein [198], p. 330, n. 20), to the middle Stoicism of Panaetius, or to the late Stoicism of Seneca? (For these divisions, cf. Pohlenz (564), vol. 1. See also above, chap. 3.)

The fable of the good Samaritan presents Christian agape more concretely than does the more abstract Pauline notion. I have used it as a touchstone for our convictions regarding pagan medical attitudes rather than relying on discussions of pagan and Christian ethics. Edelstein (198), p. 322, conceded "that even in the classical period there may have been men who dedicated themselves to medicine out of an instinctive compassion for the sufferings of their fellow men." I believe that such compassion existed and that many Hippocratic doctors would have stopped and attended to the wounded man, just as modern doctors probably would do.

Medicine is a sphere of life and a part of our social institutions. But it has sufficient autonomy that its history can be said to be associated with, yet not determined by, general social, philosophical, and religious movements. To say that medicine is a sphere of life means that it has a special place within all that is human.[26] "Health is the object of medicine and the possession [of health] its accomplishment," according to a fundamental definition of Galen's.[27] Moreover, Dogmatic Hippocratic medicine studied "the nature of the body which it endeavors to heal, and the forces of all the causes by which the body, being daily exposed to them, becomes healthier or more sickly as related to itself."[28] Like secular medicine in general, Hippocratic medicine asserted the value of the human body and its functions, and it did so on a naturalistic basis.

However, just as Hippocratic naturalism left it open whether nature was to be thought of as divine or as God's creation, so Hippocratic medicine had no answer to the question of the meaning of life, or that of why health and the healthy body should be valued as a good. The Cynic pagan Democritus laughed at the foolish doings of mankind and implicitly at Hippocrates, who was helping the world to go on with its silly ways.[29] The Christian theologian Gregory of Nazianzus, having praised the devotion of doctors to their patients, then asked: "And all this to what purpose? . . . What profit accrues from a life the release from which is the highest and safest good to be striven after by a man who is truly healthy and intelligent?"[30]

The legendary Hippocrates was converted by Democritus, which left the question open as to how, as a Cynic, Hippocrates could possibly practice medicine. And what was a Hippocratic doctor to reply to Gregory? What was he to tell Christian ascetics who broke every rule of dietetic medicine, tormented their bodies, and claimed by such discipline to be led back to a pristine state of health?[31] A Hippocratic doctor could be a sincere and devout Christian, but it is hard to imagine him entering the ascetic's world.

Philosophers might evaluate health in various ways. But the Hippocratic physician did not have to read the philosophers' works to find support for his stance. The pagan cultures of Greece and Rome found

26. For medicine as a sphere of human life, see Temkin (665), pp. 13–16, and in more detail my "Studien zum 'Sinn'-Begriff in der Medizin," *Kyklos* 2 (1929): 21–105.

27. Galen (242), *De sectis ad introducendos* 1; 3:1, ll. 1–3.

28. Ibid. 3; p. 4, ll. 18–22.

29. See above, chap. 6.B.2.

30. See above, chap. 11, text to n. 81, for the full quotation.

31. See above, chap. 12, n. 29.

their values in this life. "To the Greek of the 5th century B.C. and long thereafter health appeared as the highest good." [32] Within the Christian culture oriented toward the kingdom of God, health became problematic. Healing was good; it was part of the love for one's neighbor, and Jesus had likened himself to a physician. Hospitals with medical attendants came into existence; ascetics and holy men healed, even though they might look askance at secular healers. But to be healed, unless by God and His servants, was not generally accepted as good. Rigorous ascetics refused to have doctors attend them. Disease could be a well-deserved punishment for sin, or it could be a test, and had not Paul taken pleasure in infirmities? What was at issue was not healing; Hippocratic science was accepted by the church, both for the theoretical support it offered and as an instrument for practicing charity and compassion. But on what could the Hippocratic doctor lean for whom medicine was a profession or a trade, compassionate and merciful toward his patients though he might be? His strongest support came from the human attachment to health and to life and from the trust that people retained in secular medicine. This trust had maintained medicine side by side with the cult of Asclepius.[33] It also was behind the lack of sufficient faith in God and Jesus that—as Origen, Macarius, and Diadochus conceded—made medicine necessary.[34]

Naturalistic medicine withstood complete assimilation to the Christian world not only in that it left open the possibility that its practitioners might deviate from the teachings of the church. It also offered a counterbalance to complete devotion to a life of the spirit.[35] Hippocratic medicine sided with the majority of people—for whom eating, drinking, procreating, and the other activities that Democritus had derided were part of normal life. In this sense, too, medicine was not neutral, since passively it sided with the rationally disciplined[36] claims of the flesh and against the suppression of the flesh by the spirit. Throughout the world of pagans and Christians, Hippocrates represented the autonomy of medicine as a sphere of life. With his system and many of its practices discarded, he has yet not ceased to do so.

32. Sigerist (624), p. 68.
33. See above, chap. 7.
34. See above, chap. 12.B.
35. On the Christian view of the body and its relation to society as bequeathed to the Middle Ages, see Brown (115), epilogue, pp. 428–47.
36. Rationally disciplined by dietetic medicine; cf. above, chap. 2, especially text to nn. 19–22, for Galen's views.

LIST OF ABBREVIATIONS

Apostolic Fathers
   The Apostolic Fathers. With an English translation by Kirsopp Lake. 2 vols.
   Loeb Classical Library. London: William Heinemann; New York: G. P. Put-
   nam's Sons, 1925 and 1924.

AV
   The Holy Bible: Containing the Old and New Testaments. Authorized
   (King James) Version. Philadelphia: National Bible Press, 1970.

Catholic Encyclopedia
   The Catholic Encyclopedia. 15 vols. and index. New York: Universal
   Knowledge Foundation, 1907–14.

CAG
   Commentaria in Aristotelem Graeca. 23 vols. in 29 pts. Berlin: Georg Reimer, 1882–1909.

CMG
   Corpus Medicorum Graecorum. Leipzig-Berlin, 1908–.

CML
   Corpus Medicorum Latinorum. Leipzig-Berlin, 1915–.

Colloque hippocratique de Paris
   *Hippocratica: Actes du colloque hippocratique de Paris (4–9 septembre
   1978).* Edited by M. D. Grmek. Paris: Éditions du Centre National de la
   Recherche Scientifique, 1980.

Dietz, AC

Dietz, Fridericus Reinholdus (ed.). *Apollonii Citiensis, Stephani, Palladii, Theophili, Meletii, Damascii, Ioannis, aliorum Scholia in Hippocratem et Galenum.* 2 vols. Königsberg: Bornträger, 1834.

Fathers of the Church

The Fathers of the Church: A New Translation. New York: Fathers of the Church.

Loeb

Loeb Classical Library. Cambridge: Harvard University Press; London: William Heinemann; New York: Macmillan; New York: G. P. Putnam's Sons. Dates listed are those appearing on the title page of the volume.

Migne, PG

Jacques Paul Migne. *Patrologiae cursus completus . . . series Graeca.* 161 vols. Paris: Garnier, 1857–1866.

Migne, PL

Jacques Paul Migne. *Patrologiae cursus completus . . . series Latina.* 221 vols. Paris, 1844–1855.

NEB

The New English Bible with the Apocrypha. Oxford University Press and Cambridge University Press, 1970.

NTM

NTM: Schriftenreihe für Geschichte der Naturwissenschaften, Technik und Medizin (Leipzig).

Nutton, GPP

Nutton, Vivian (ed.). *Galen's Problems and Prospects: A Collection of Papers Submitted at the 1979 Cambridge Conference.* London: Wellcome Institute for the History of Medicine, 1981.

PW

Pauly's Real-Encylopädie der classischen Altertumswissenschaft. Rev. ed. by Georg Wissowa, Stuttgart, 1894–.

Scarborough, Symposium

Scarborough, John (ed.). *Symposium on Byzantine Medicine.* Dumbarton Oaks Papers, no. 38 (1984). Washington, D.C.: Dumbarton Oaks Library and Collection, 1985.

Sudhoffs Archiv

Archiv für Geschichte der Medizin, and *Sudhoffs Archiv: Zeitschrift für Wissenschaftsgeschichte.*

T

T followed by a number refers to the testimonies in Edelstein and Edelstein (197), vol. 1.

The Vulgate
Biblia Sacra iuxta Vulgatam Clementinam. New ed. Edited by Alberto Colunga and Laurentius Turrado. Madrid: Bibloteca de Autores Cristianos, 1953.

BIBLIOGRAPHY

1. Ackroyd, P. R., and Evans, C. F. (eds.). *The Cambridge History of the Bible*. Vol. 1. Cambridge: Cambridge University Press, 1970.
2. Aetius Amidenus. *Libri medicinales*. Edited by Alexander Olivieri. *CMG*, vols. 8.1 (books 1–4) and 8.2 (books 5–8). 1935 and 1950.
3. Agnellus of Ravenna. *Lectures on Galen's De sectis*. Latin text and translation by Seminar Classics 609, State University of New York at Buffalo. Arethusa Monographs, no. 8. Buffalo: Department of Classics, State University of New York, 1981.
4. Agrimi, Jole, and Crisciani, Chiara. "Medicina del corpo e medicina dell' anima: Note sul saperi del medico fino all'inizio del sec. XIII." *Episteme* 10 (1976): 5–102.
5. Alexander of Aphrodisias. *In Aristotelis Metaphysica commentaria*. Edited by Michael Hayduck. *CAG*, vol. 1. 1891.
6. ———. *In Aristotelis Topicorum libros octo commentaria*. Edited by Maximilian Wallies. *CAG*, 2.2. 1891.
7. Alexander of Tralles. *Alexander von Tralles*. Edited with a German translation by Theodor Puschmann. 2 vols. Vienna: Wilhelm Braunmüller, 1878.
8. Alexanderson, Bengt. *Die hippokratische Schrift Prognostikon: Überlieferung und Text*. Studia graeca et latina Gothoburgensia, no. 17. Göteborg: Elanders, 1963.
9. Ambrose. *Exameron, De paradiso, De Cain et Abel, De Noe, De Abraham, De Isaac, De bono mortis*. In *Sancti Ambrosii Opera*. Corpus scriptorum

ecclesiasticorum Latinorum, vol. 32.1, edited by Karl Schenkl. Vienna, 1897.

10. ———. *Letters.* Translated by Sister Mary Melchior Beyenka. Fathers of the Church, vol. 26. 1954.

11. ———. *Saint Ambrose: Hexameron, Paradise, and Cain and Abel.* Translated by John J. Savage. Fathers of the Church, vol. 42. 1961.

12. *Ammianus Marcellinus.* With an English translation by John C. Rolfe. 3 vols. Vol. 2. Loeb. 1937.

13. Ammonius. *In Porphyrii Isagogen sive V voces.* Edited by Adolf Busse. CAG, vol. 4.3. 1891.

14. Amundsen, Darrel W. "Casuistry and Professional Obligations: The Regulation of Physicians by the Court of Conscience in the Late Middle Ages, Parts I and II." *Transactions and Studies of the College of Physicians of Philadelphia* 3 (1981): 22–39 and 93–112.

15. ———. "The Liability of the Physician in Classical Greek Legal Theory and Practice." *Journal of the History of Medicine and Allied Sciences* 32 (1977): 172–203.

16. ———. "Medicine and Faith in Early Christianity." *Bulletin of the History of Medicine* 56 (1982): 326–50.

17. ———. "Medicine and Religion in Western Traditions." In *The Encyclopedia of Religion,* edited by Mircea Eliade, 9:319–24. New York: Macmillan, 1987.

18. ———. "The Physician's Obligation to Prolong Life: A Medical Duty without Classical Roots." *Hastings Center Report* (August 1978): 23–30.

19. ———. "Physician, Patient and Malpractice: An Historical Perspective." In *The Law-Medicine Relation: A Philosophical Exploration,* edited by S. F. Spicker, J. M. Healey, and H. T. Engelhardt, pp. 255–58. Dordrecht: D. Reidel, 1981.

20. ———. "Romanticizing the Ancient Medical Profession: The Characterization of the Physician in the Graeco-Roman Novel." *Bulletin of the History of Medicine* 48 (1974): 320–37.

21. ———. "Visigothic Medical Legislation." *Bulletin of the History of Medicine* 45 (1971): 553–69.

22. Amundsen, Darrel W., and Ferngren, Gary B. "The Early Christian Tradition." In *Caring and Curing: Health and Medicine in the Western Religious Tradition,* edited by Ronald L. Numbers and Darrel W. Amundsen, pp. 40–63. New York: Macmillan, 1986.

23. ———. "Evolution of the Patient-Physician Relationship: Antiquity through the Renaissance." In *The Clinical Encounter: The Moral Fabric of the Patient-Physician Relationship,* edited by Earl E. Shelp, pp. 3–46. Philosophy and Medicine, vol. 14. Dordrecht: D. Reidel, 1983.

24. ———. "Medicine and Religion: Early Christianity through the Middle Ages." In *Health/Medicine and the Faith Traditions,* edited by Martin E. Marty and Kenneth L. Vaux, pp. 93–131. Philadelphia: Fortress Press, 1982.

25. ———. "Medicine and Religion: Pre-Christian Antiquity." In *Health/Med-*

icine and the Faith Traditions, edited by Martin E. Marty and Kenneth L. Vaux, pp. 53–92. Philadelphia: Fortress Press, 1982.

26. ———. "Philanthropy in Medicine: Some Historical Perspectives." In *Beneficence and Health Care,* edited by Earl E. Shelp, pp. 1–31. Dordrecht: D. Reidel, 1982.

27. ———. "Virtue and Medicine from Early Christianity through the Sixteenth Century." In *Virtue and Medicine: Explorations in the Character of Medicine,* edited by Earl E. Shelp, pp. 23–61. Philosophy and Medicine, vol. 17. Dordrecht: D. Reidel, 1985.

28. Angus, S. *The Religious Quests of the Graeco-Roman World.* New York: Charles Scribner's Sons, 1929.

29. *The Apocrypha According to the Authorized Version.* With an introduction by Robert H. Pfeiffer. London: Eyre and Spottiswoode; New York: Harper and Brothers, n.d.

30. *Apocryphal Gospels, Acts, and Revelations.* Translated by Alexander Walker. Edinburgh: T. and T. Clark, 1873.

31. Apollonius of Citium. *Kommentar zu Hippokrates über das Einrenken der Gelenke [In Hippocratis De articulis commentarius]* Edited by Jutta Kollesch and Fridolf Kudlien. *CMG,* vol. 1.1. Berlin: Akademie-Verlag, 1965.

32. *Apophthegmata patrum.* Migne, *PG,* 65:71–440.

33. *The Apostolic Constitutions,* edited by James Donaldson. Ante-Nicene Christian Library, vol. 17. Edinburgh: T. and T. Clark, 1870.

34. *The Apostolic Fathers.* With an English translation by Kirsopp Lake. 2 vols. Loeb. 1925 and 1924.

35. *Appian's Roman History.* With an English translation by Horace White. 4 vols. Vol. 2. Loeb. 1912.

36. Apuleius. *Apulei Platonici Madaurensis De philosophia libri.* Edited by Paul Thomas. Apulei opera quae supersunt, vol. 3. Leipzig: B. G. Teubner, 1921.

37. ———. *The Golden Ass: Being the Metamorphoses of Lucius Apuleius.* With an English translation by W. Adlington (1566); revised by S. Gasclee. Loeb. 1928.

38. Arbesmann, Rudolph. "The Concept of 'Christus Medicus' in St. Augustine." *Traditio* 10 (1954): 1–28.

39. *Aretaeus.* Edited by Carl Hude. 2nd ed. *CMG,* vol. 2. Berlin: Academia Scientiarum, 1958.

40. ———. *The Extant Works of Aretaeus the Cappadocian.* Edited and translated by Francis Adams. London: Sydenham Society, 1856.

41. Aristides, Aelius. *Aristides.* Edited by Wilhelm Dindorf. Vol. 2. Leipzig: Weidmann, 1829.

42. ———. *Aristides.* 4 vols. Vol. 1. With an English translation by C. A. Behr. Loeb. 1973.

43. ———. *The Complete Works.* Vol. 2, *Orations 17–53.* Translated by Charles A. Behr. Leiden: E. J. Brill, 1981.

44. ———. *Quae supersunt omnia.* Edited by Bruno Keil. Vol. 2 (orations 17–53). 2nd ed. (photostat of 1898 ed.). Berlin: Weidmann, 1958.

45. *Aristophanes.* With an English translation by Benjamin Bickley Rogers. 3 vols. Vol. 3. Loeb. 1927.

46. Aristotle. *The "Art" of Rhetoric.* With an English translation by John Henry Freese. Loeb. 1926.

47. ———. *Meteorologica.* With an English translation by H. D. P. Lee. Loeb. 1952.

48. ———. *Parva Naturalia.* Revised text by Sir David Ross. Oxford: Clarendon Press, 1955.

49. ———. *Problems.* With an English translation by W. S. Hett. 2 vols. Loeb. 1961 and 1957.

50. Arnim, Hans von (ed.). *Stoicorum veterum fragmenta.* 4 vols. Reprint. Leipzig: B. G. Teubner, 1921–24.

51. Arnobius. *Disputationum contra gentes libri septem.* Migne, PL, 5:713–1290.

52. Asclepius. *In Aristotelis Metaphysicorum libros A–Z commentaria.* Edited by Michael Hayduck. CAG, vol. 6.2. 1888.

53. Asmus, Rudolf. *Das Leben des Philosophen Isidoros von Damaskios aus Damaskos.* Philosophische Bibliothek, vol. 125. Leipzig: Meiner, 1911.

54. ———. "Der Neuplatoniker Asklepiodotos d. Gr." *Sudhoffs Archiv* 7 (1914): 26–42.

55. Athanasius. *The Life of Saint Antony.* Translated by Robert T. Meyer. Ancient Christian Writers, no. 10. Westminster, Md.: Newman Press, 1950.

56. Athenaeus. *The Deipnosophists.* With an English translation by Charles Burton Gulick. 7 vols. Vols. 4 and 7. Loeb. 1930 and 1941.

57. Athenagoras. *Embassy for the Christians, The Resurrection of the Dead.* Translated by Joseph Hugh Crehan. Ancient Christian Writers, no. 23. Westminster, Md.: Newman Press; London: Longmans, Green, 1956.

58. Augustine. *The City of God by Saint Augustine.* Translated by Marcus Dods. 1872. Reprint (2 vols.). New York: Hafner, 1948.

59. ———. *The City of God against the Pagans.* With an English translation by William M. Green. 7 vols. Vols. 2 and 7. Loeb. 1963 and 1972.

60. ———. *Confessions.* With an English translation by William Watts. 2 vols. Loeb. 1922–25.

61. ———. *Contra Faustum.* Edited by Joseph Zycha. Corpus Scriptorum Ecclesiasticorum Latinorum, vol. 25, pp. 249–797. Vienna: F. Tempsky, 1981.

62. ———. *St. Augustine on the Psalms.* Translated by Scholastica Hebgin and Felicitas Corrigan. Vol. 1 (Psalms 1–29). Ancient Christian Writers, no. 29. Westminster, Md.: Newman Press; London: Longmans Green, 1960.

63. ———. *Quaestiones in Heptateuchum libri VII.* Corpus Christianorum, Series latina, no. 33. Turnholt: Brepols, 1958.

64. Ausonius. With an English translation by Hugh G. Evelyn White. 2 vols. Vol. 1. Loeb. 1919.

65. Baader, Gerhard. "Der ärztliche Stand in der Antike." In *Jahrbuch der Universität Düsseldorf 1977–78,* pp. 301–15. Düsseldorf: Triltsch.

66. ———. "Die Entwicklung der medizinischen Fachsprache in der Antike

und im frühen Mittelalter." In *Medizin im mittelalterlichen Abendland,* edited by Gerhard Baader and Gundolf Keil, pp. 417–42. Wege der Forschung, vol. 363. Darmstadt: Wissenschaftliche Buchgesellschaft, 1982.

67. ———. "Gesellschaft, Wirtschaft und ärztlicher Stand im frühen und hohen Mittelalter." *Medizinhistorisches Journal* 14 (1979): 176–85.

68. ———. "Handschrift und Frühdruck als Überlieferungsinstrumente der Wissenschaften." *Berichte zur Wissenschaftsgeschichte* 3 (1980): 7–22.

69. ———. "Die Schule von Salerno." *Medizinhistorisches Journal* 13 (1978): 124–45.

70. Baader, Gerhard, and Keil, Gundolf. "Mittelalterliche Diagnostik: Ein Bericht." In *Medizinische Diagnostik in Geschichte und Gegenwart: Festschrift für Heinz Goerke zum sechzigsten Geburtstag,* edited by Christa Habrich, Frank Marguth, and Jörn Henning Wolf, pp. 121–44. Munich: Fritsch, 1978.

71. Baffioni, Giovanni. "Inediti di Archelao da un codice Bolognese." In *Bolletino del Comitato per la preparazione della edizione nazionale dei classici greci e latini,* n.s., fasc. 3, pp. 57–73. Rome: Academia Nazionale dei Lincei, 1954.

72. Baldwin, Barry. "Beyond the House Call: Doctors in Early Byzantine History and Politics." In Scarborough, *Symposium,* pp. 15–19.

73. ———. "The Career of Oribasius." *Acta Classica* 18 (1975): 85–97.

74. Balestri, P. J. "Cyrus and John, Saints." In *Catholic Encyclopedia,* 4:597.

75. Barnabas. *The Epistle of Barnabas.* In *Apostolic Fathers,* 1:337–409.

76. Barnes, Timothy D. *Constantine and Eusebius.* Cambridge: Harvard University Press, 1981.

77. Baron, Salo Wittmayer. *A Social and Religious History of the Jews.* 2nd ed. Vol. 2. New York: Columbia University Press, 1952.

78. Bartels, Klaus, and Huber, Ludwig. *Veni, vidi, vici: Geflügelte Worte aus dem Griechischen und Lateinischen.* 2nd ed. Zurich: Artemis, 1967.

79. Baruk, H. "La médecine hébraïque face à la médecine hippocratique." In *La collection hippocratique et son rôle dans l'histoire de la médecine: Colloque de Strasbourg (23–27 octobre 1972).* Leiden: E. J. Brill, 1975.

80. Basil. *Constitutiones asceticae ad eos qui simul aut solitarie vivunt.* Migne, *PG,* 31:1321–1428.

81. ———. *The Letters.* With an English translation by Roy J. Deferrari. 4 vols. Loeb. 1926–34.

82. ———. *Quod Deus non est auctor malorum.* Migne, *PG,* 31:329–54.

83. ———. *Regulae brevius tractatae.* Migne, *PG,* 31:1051–1320.

84. ———. *Regulae fusius tractatae.* Migne, *PG* 31:889–1052.

85. ———. *Sur l'origine de l'homme (Hom. X et XI de l'Hexaéméron).* With French translation by Alexis Smets and Michel van Esbroeck. Sources Chrétiennes, no. 160. Paris: Éditions du Cerf, 1970.

86. Beccaria, Augusto. *I codici di medicina del periodo presalernitano (secoli IX, X, XI).* Rome: Storia e Letteratura, 1956.

87. Behr, C. A. *Aelius Aristides and The Sacred Tales.* Chicago: Argonaut, 1967.

88. Below, Karl-Heinz. *Der Arzt im römischen Recht.* Münchener Beiträge zur Papyrusforschung und antiken Rechtsgeschichte, fasc. 37. Munich: C. H. Beck, 1953.

89. Benedict. S. *Benedicti regula monasteriorum.* Edited by Benno Linderbauer. Florilegium Patristicum, vol. 17. Bonn: Hanstein, 1928.

90. Benedum, Christa. "Asklepiosmythos und archaeologischer Befund." *Medizinhistorisches Journal* 22 (1987): 48–61.

91. Betz, Hans Dieter (ed.). *The Greek Medical Papyri in Translation.* Chicago: University of Chicago Press, 1986.

92. [The Bible.] *Biblia Sacra iuxta Vulgatam Clementinam.* New ed. Edited by Alberto Colunga and Laurentius Turrado. Madrid: Biblioteca de Auctores Cristianos, 1953.

93. ———. *The Holy Bible: Containing the Old and the New Testament.* Authorized (King James) Version. Philadelphia: National Bible Press, 1970.

94. ———. *The New English Bible with the Apocrypha.* Oxford: Oxford University Press; Cambridge: Cambridge University Press, 1970.

95. *Biblia Hebraica.* Edited by Rud. Kittel. 2 vols. 2nd ed. reprinted. Stuttgart: Württ. Bibelanstalt, 1925.

96. Bidez, Joseph, and Cumont, Franz. *Les mages hellénisés.* 2 vols. Paris: Les Belles Lettres, 1938.

97. Bieler, Ludwig. Θεῖος ἀνήρ: *Das Bild des "göttlichen Menschen" in Spätantike und Frühchristentum.* Vol. 1. Vienna: Oskar Höfels, 1935.

98. Biesterfeldt, Hans Heinrich. "Ǧalīnūs Quwā n-nafs." *Der Islam* 63 (1986): 119–36.

99. ———. "Some Opinions on the Physician's Remuneration in Medieval Islam." *Bulletin of the History of Medicine* 58 (1984): 16–27.

100. Biesterfeldt, Hans Heinrich, and Gutas, Dimitri. "The Malady of Love." *Journal of the American Oriental Society* 104 (1984): 21–55.

101. Bloch, Herbert. "The Pagan Revival in the West at the End of the Fourth Century." In *The Conflict Between Paganism and Christianity in the Fourth Century,* edited by Arnaldo Momigliano, pp. 193–218. Oxford: Clarendon Press, 1963.

102. Bloch, Iwan. "Byzantinische Medizin." In *Handbuch der Geschichte der Medizin,* edited by Max Neuburger and Julius Pagel, 1:492–568. Jena: Fischer, 1902.

103. Boardman, John, Griffin, Jasper, and Murray, Oswyn (eds.). *The Oxford History of the Classical World.* Oxford: Oxford University Press, 1986.

104. Boas, George. *Vox Populi: Essays in the History of an Idea.* Baltimore: Johns Hopkins Press, 1969.

105. Boethius. *The Theological Tractates and The Consolation of Philosophy.* With an English translation by S. J. Tester. Loeb. 1973.

106. Bolkestein, Hendrik. *Wohltätigkeit und Armenpflege im vorchristlichen Altertum.* Utrecht: A. Oosthoek, 1939.

107. Bonner, Campbell. *Studies in Magical Amulets: Chiefly Graeco-Egyptian.* Ann Arbor: University of Michigan Press, 1950.

108. Bourgey, Louis. "La relation du médecin au malade dans les écrits de l'école de Cos." *La collection hippocratique et son rôle dans l'histoire de la médecine: Colloque de Strasbourg (23–29 octobre 1972), pp. 209–27.* Leiden: E. J. Brill, 1975.

109. Bowersock, G. W. *Greek Sophists in the Roman Empire.* Oxford: Clarendon Press, 1969.

110. ———. *Julian the Apostate.* Cambridge: Harvard University Press, 1978.

111. Bowker, John. *Problems of Suffering in Religions of the World.* 1970. Reprint. Cambridge: Cambridge University Press, 1975.

112. Brain, P. "Galen on the Ideal of the Physician." *South African Medical Journal* 52 (1977): 936–38.

113. Brock, Arthur J. *Greek Medicine: Being Extracts Illustrative of Medical Writers from Hippocrates to Galen.* London: J. M. Bent; New York: E. P. Dutton, 1929.

114. Brown, Peter. *Augustine of Hippo: A Biography.* London: Faber and Faber, 1967.

115. ———. *The Body and Society: Men, Women and Sexual Renunciation in Early Christianity.* New York: Columbia University Press, 1988.

116. ———. *The Cult of the Saints: Its Rise and Function in Latin Christianity.* Chicago: University of Chicago Press, 1981.

117. ———. *The Making of Late Antiquity.* Cambridge: Harvard University Press, 1978.

118. ———. "The Rise and Function of the Holy Man in Late Antiquity." *Journal of Roman Studies* 61 (1971): 80–101 (reprinted in [119], pp. 103–52).

119. ———. *Society and the Holy in Late Antiquity.* Berkeley and Los Angeles: University of California Press, 1982.

120. ———. *The World of Late Antiquity: From Marcus Aurelius to Muhammad.* London: Thames and Hudson, 1971.

121. Browning, Robert. "The 'Low Level' Saint's Life in the Early Byzantine World." In *The Byzantine Saint: University of Birmingham Fourteenth Spring Symposium of Byzantine Studies,* edited by Sergei Hackel, pp. 117–27. Studies Supplementary to *Sobornost* 5. London: Fellowship of St. Alban and St. Sergius, 1981.

122. Broydé. "Demonology." In *The Jewish Encyclopedia,* vol. 4, pp. 514–21. New York: Funk and Wagnalls, 1903.

123. Brunn, L. von. "Hippokrates und die meteorologische Medizin." *Gesnerus* 3 (1946): 151–73 and 4 (1947): 1–18.

124. Buchmann, Georg. *Geflügelte Worte und Zitatenschatz.* Im Bertelsmann-Lesering, 1958.

125. Burford, Alison. *Craftsmen in Greek and Roman Society.* Ithaca: Cornell University Press, 1972.

126. Burton, Robert [Democritus Junior]. *The Anatomy of Melancholy.* London: Peter Parker, 1676.

127. ———. *The Anatomy of Melancholy.* Edited with an introduction by Holbrook Jackson. New York: Random House, Vintage Books, 1977.

128. Burton, R. W. B. *Pindar's Pythian Odes: Essays in Interpretation.* Oxford: Oxford University Press, 1962.

129. Bylebyl, Jerome J. "Galen on the Non-Natural Causes of Variation in the Pulse." *Bulletin of the History of Medicine* 45 (1971): 482–85.

130. Caelius Aurelianus. *On Acute Diseases and On Chronic Diseases.* Edited and translated by I. E. Drabkin. Chicago: University of Chicago Press, 1950.

131. Cameron, Averil. *Agathias.* Oxford: Clarendon Press, 1970.

132. Cantinat, Jean. *Les épitres de Saint Jacques et de Saint Jude.* Sources bibliques. Paris: Librairie Le Coffre, 1973.

133. Cassiodorus. *Institutiones.* Edited by R. A. B. Mynors. Oxford: Clarendon Press, 1937.

134. Cassius Felix. *De medicina ex Graecis logicae sectae auctoribus liber translatus sub Artabure et Calepio Consulibus (anno 447).* Edited by Valentin Rose. Leipzig: B. G. Teubner, 1879.

135. *Catalogus codicum astrologorum Graecorum,* vols. 8.3 and 8.4. *Codicum Parisinorum,* 3rd and 4th pts., edited by Pierre Boudreaux. Brussels: Lamartine, 1912–21.

136. *The Catholic Encyclopedia.* 15 vols. and index. New York: Universal Knowledge Foundation, 1907–14.

137. Celsus, A. Cornelius. *De medicina.* With an English translation by W. G. Spencer. 3 vols. Loeb. 1935–38.

138. Chadwick, Henry. *The Early Church.* Pelican History of the Church, vol. 1. Baltimore: Penguin Books, 1967.

139. ———. "Pachomios and the Idea of Sanctity." In *The Byzantine Saint: University of Birmingham Fourteenth Spring Symposium of Byzantine Studies,* edited by Sergei Hackel, pp. 11–24. Studies Supplementary to *Sobornost* 5. London: Fellowship of St. Alban and St. Sergius, 1981.

140. Chitty, Derwas J. *The Desert a City: An Introduction to the Study of Egyptian and Palestinian Monasticism under the Christian Empire.* Crestwood, N.Y.: St. Vladimir's Seminary Press, 1977.

141. Ciavolella, Massimo. *La "malattia d'amore" dell'Antichità al Medievo.* Strumenti di Ricerca, nos. 12–13. Rome: Bulzoni, 1976.

142. Cicero, Marcus Tullius. *De natura deorum.* With the commentary of G. F. Schoemann; translated by Austin Stickney. Boston: Ginn and Heath, 1885.

143. ———. *De officiis.* With an English translation by Walter Miller. Loeb. 1956.

144. ———. *De oratore.* With an English translation by E. W. Sutton and H. Rackham. Loeb. 1942.

145. ———. *De senectute, De amicitia, De divinatione.* With an English translation by William Armistead Falconer. Loeb. 1927.

146. ———. *Letters to Atticus.* With an English translation by E. O. Winstedt. 3 vols. Loeb. 1925.

147. ———. *Tusculan Disputations.* With an English translation by J. E. King. Loeb. 1966.

148. Clement. *The First Epistle of Clement to the Corinthians.* In *Apostolic Fathers,* 1:3–121.

149. ——. *The Second Epistle of Clement to the Corinthians.* In *Apostolic Fathers,* 1:125–63.

150. Clement of Alexandria. *Le pédagogue.* With a French translation; Greek text edited by Henri-Irénée Marrou et al. 3 vols. Sources Chrétiennes, nos. 70, 108, and 158. Paris: Éditions du Cerf, 1960–70.

151. ——. *Stromata.* Migne, *PG,* vols. 8 and 9.

152. ——. *The Writings of Clement of Alexandria.* Translated by William Wilson. 2 vols. Ante-Nicene Christian Library, vols. 4 and 12. Edinburgh: T. and T. Clark, 1871–72.

153. Codex Theodosianus. *Theodosiani libri XVI cum constitutionibus Sirmondianis et leges novellae ad Theodosianum pertinentes.* Edited by Theodor Mommsen and Paul M. Meyer. Berlin: Weidmann, 1905.

154. Cohn-Haft, Louis. *The Public Physicians of Ancient Greece.* Smith College Studies in History, vol. 42. Northampton, Mass.: Department of History of Smith College, 1956.

155. Constantelos, Demetrios J. *Byzantine Philanthropy and Social Welfare.* New Brunswick, N.J.: Rutgers University Press, 1968.

156. *Corpus iuris civilis.* Vol. 1, *Institutiones,* edited by Paul Krüger, and *Digesta,* edited by Theodor Mommsen, 8th ed. Vol. 2, *Codex Iustinianus,* edited by Paul Krüger, 6th ed. (stereotyped). Berlin: Weidmann, 1899 and 1895.

157. Courcelle, Pierre. "Anti-Christian Arguments and Christian Platonism: From Arnobius to St. Ambrose." In *The Conflict between Paganism and Christianity in the Fourth Century,* edited by Arnaldo Momigliano, pp. 151–92. Oxford: Clarendon Press, 1963.

158. ——. "Gefängnis (der Seele)." In *Reallexikon für Antike und Christentum,* Lieferung 66, cols. 294–318. Stuttgart: Anton Hiersemann, 1973.

159. ——. "Tradition platonicienne et traditions chrétiennes du corpsprison (Phédon 62b; Cratyle 400c)." *Revue des études latines* 43 (1965): 406–43.

160. Daniélou, Jean, and Marrou, Henri. *The First Six Hundred Years.* Translated by Vincent Cronin. Christian Centuries, vol. 1. New York: McGraw-Hill, 1964.

161. Daremberg, Ch. "Aurelius de acutis passionibus." *Janus* 2 (1847): 468–77. Reprint. Leipzig: Lorentz, 1931.

162. Dawes, Elizabeth, and Baynes, Norman H. (trans.). *Three Byzantine Saints: Contemporary Biographies Translated from the Greek.* Oxford: Basil Blackwell, 1948.

163. Degen, Rainer. "Galen im Syrischen: Eine Übersicht über die syrische Ueberlieferung der Werke Galens." In Nutton, *GPP,* pp. 131–66.

164. Deichgräber, Karl. *Die Epidemien und das Corpus Hippocraticum.* Enlarged ed. Berlin: Walter de Gruyter, 1971.

165. ——. *Die griechische Empirikerschule.* Berlin: Weidmann, 1965.

166. ——. *Hippokrates' De humoribus in der Geschichte der griechischen*

Medizin. Abhandlungen der Geistes- und sozialwissenschaftlichen Klasse, 1972, Nr. 14. Mainz: Akademie der Wissenschaften und der Literatur, 1972.

167. ———. *Medicus gratiosus: Untersuchungen zu einem griechischen Arztbild. Mit dem Anhang, Testamentum Hippocratis und Rhazes' De indulgentia medici.* Abhandlungen der Geistes- und sozialwissenschaftlichen Klasse, Jahrgang 1970, Nr. 3. Mainz: Akademie der Wissenschaften und der Literatur, 1970.

168. De Renzi, Salvatore. *Collectio Salernitana.* 5 vols. Naples: Filiatre Sebezio, 1852–59.

169. Deubner, Ludwig. *Kosmas und Damian: Texte und Einleitung.* Leipzig: B. G. Teubner, 1907.

170. Diadochus of Photica. *Oeuvres spirituelles.* Edited with French translation by Edouard des Places. Sources Chrétiennes, no. 5 bis. Paris: Éditions du Cerf, 1955.

171. Dibelius, Martin. *James: A Commentary on the Epistle of James.* Revised by Heinrich Greeven; translated by Michael A. Williams. Hermeneia: A Critical and Historical Commentary on the Bible. Philadelphia: Fortress Press, 1976.

172. *The Didache, or Teaching of the Twelve Apostles.* In *Apostolic Fathers,* 1:308–33.

173. Didymus Alexandrinus. *Fragmenta in Job.* Migne, *PG,* 39:1119–54.

174. Diels, Hermann. *Die Fragmente der Vorsokratiker.* 4th ed. 2 vols. Berlin: Weidmann, 1922.

175. Dietz, Fridericus Reinholdus (ed.). *Apollonii Citiensis, Stephani, Palladii, Theophili, Meletii, Damascii, Ioannis, aliorum Scholia in Hippocratem et Galenum.* 2 vols. Königsberg: Bornträger, 1834.

176. Di Lella, Alexander A. *The Hebrew Text of Sirach: A Text-Critical and Historical Study.* The Hague: Mouton, 1966.

177. Diller, Hans. *Kleine Schriften zur antiken Literatur.* Edited by Hans-Joachim Newiger and Hans Seyffert. Munich: C. H. Beck, 1971.

178. ———. *Kleine Schriften zur antiken Medizin.* Edited by Gerhard Baader and Hermann Grensemann. Ars medica, 2. Abteilung, Band 3. Berlin: Walter de Gruyter, 1973.

179. ———. *Wanderarzt und Aitiologe: Studien zur hippokratischen Schrift* Περὶ ἀέρων ὑδάτων τόπων. Philologus, supplementary vol. 26, fasc. 3. Leipzig: Dieterich, 1934.

180. *Dio Chrysostom.* With an English translation by J. W. Cohoon and H. Lamar Crosby. 5 vols. Vol. 3. Loeb. 1940.

181. *Diodorus of Sicily.* With an English translation by C. H. Oldfather. 12 vols. Vols. 1 and 6. Loeb. 1933 and 1954.

182. Diogenes Laertius. *Lives of Eminent Philosophers.* With an English translation by R. D. Hicks. 2 vols. Loeb. 1925.

183. [Diognetus.] *The Epistle to Diognetus.* In *Apostolic Fathers,* 2:348–79.

184. Dioscorides. *Pedanii Dioscuridis Anazarbei De materia medica libri quinque.* Edited by Max Wellmann. 3 vols. Berlin: Weidmann, 1907–14.

185. ———. *Des Pedanios Dioskurides aus Anazarbos Arzneimittellehre in*

fünf Büchern. German translation by J. Berendes. Stuttgart: Ferdinand Enke, 1902.

186. Dodds, E. R. *The Ancient Concept of Progress and Other Essays on Greek Literature and Belief.* Oxford: Clarendon Press, 1973.

187. ———. *The Greeks and the Irrational.* Sather Classical Lectures, vol. 25. Berkeley and Los Angeles: University of California Press, 1951.

188. ———. *Pagan and Christian in an Age of Anxiety.* Cambridge: Cambridge University Press, 1965.

189. Dols, Michael W. "The Origins of the Islamic Hospital: Myth and Reality." *Bulletin of the History of Medicine* 61 (1987): 367–90.

190. Drachmann, A. B. *Atheism in Pagan Antiquity.* London: Gyldendal, 1922.

191. Drijvers, Hans J. W. "Hellenistic and Oriental Origins." In *The Byzantine Saint: University of Birmingham Fourteenth Spring Symposium of Byzantine Studies,* edited by Sergei Hackel, pp. 25–33. Studies Supplementary to *Sobornost* 5. London: Fellowship of St. Alban and St. Sergius, 1981.

192. Duffy, John. "Byzantine Medicine in the Sixth and Seventh Centuries: Aspects of Teaching and Practice." In Scarborough, *Symposium,* pp. 21–27.

193. *Ecclesiasticus, or The Wisdom of Jesus Son of Sirach.* With commentary by John G. Snaith. Cambridge: Cambridge University Press, 1974.

194. ———. *The Hebrew Text of the Book of Ecclesiasticus.* Edited by Israel Lévi. Semitic Study Series, no. 3. Leiden: E. J. Brill, 1904.

195. *L'école de Salerne: Traduction en vers français.* Paris: Baillière, 1880.

196. Eddy, Mary Baker. *Science and Health with Key to the Scriptures.* Reprint. Boston: Trustees under the Will of Mary Baker G. Eddy, 1934.

197. Edelstein, Emma J., and Edelstein, Ludwig. *Asclepius: A Collection and Interpretation of the Testimonies.* 2 vols. Baltimore: Johns Hopkins Press, 1945.

198. Edelstein, Ludwig. *Ancient Medicine: Selected Papers of Ludwig Edelstein.* Edited by Owsei Temkin and C. Lilian Temkin; translations from the German by C. Lilian Temkin. Baltimore: Johns Hopkins Press, 1967.

199. ———. "Antike Diätetik." *Die Antike* 7 (1931): 255–70.

200. ———. "Hippokrates von Kos." *PW,* suppl. 6 (1935), cols. 1290–1345.

201. ———. *Der hippokratische Eid: Mit einem forschungsgeschichtlichen Nachwort von Hans Diller.* Lebendige Antike. N.p.: Artemis, 1969.

202. ———. *The Meaning of Stoicism.* Martin Classical Lectures, vol. 21. Cambridge: Harvard University Press (for Oberlin College), 1966.

203. ———. "Motives and Incentives for Science in Antiquity." In *Scientific Change,* edited by A. C. Crombie, pp. 15–41. New York: Basic Books, 1963.

204. ———. Περὶ ἀέρων *und die Sammlung der hippokratischen Schriften.* Problemata, fasc. 4. Berlin: Weidmann, 1931.

205. ———, and Kidd, J. G. (eds.). *Posidonius: 1. The Fragments.* Cambridge: Cambridge University Press, 1972.

206. Epictetus. *The Discourses as Reported by Arrian, The Manual, and Frag-*

ments. With an English translation by W. A. Oldfather. 2 vols. Loeb. 1926–28.

207. *The Epistles of James, Peter, and Jude.* Introduction, translation, and notes by Bo Reicke. Anchor Bible. Garden City, N.Y.: Doubleday, 1964.

208. Erotianus. *Vocum Hippocraticarum collectio.* Edited by Ernst Nachmanson. Collectio scriptorum veterum Upsaliensis. Goteburg-Upsala: Eranos, 1918.

209. Eunapius. *Lives of the Philosophers and Sophists.* In *Philostorgius and Eunapius: The Lives of the Sophists,* with an English translation by Wilmer Cave Wright. Loeb. 1952.

210. Euripides. *The Daughters of Troy.* In *Euripides,* with an English translation by Arthur S. Way. Vol. 1. Loeb. 1925.

211. Eusebius. *The Ecclesiastical History.* With an English translation. 2 vols. Vol. 1 translated by Kirsopp Lake. Vol. 2 translated by J. E. L. Oulton and H. J. Lawlor. Loeb. Vol. 1, 1965; vol. 2, 1964.

212. ———. *The Treatise of Eusebius, the Son of Pamphilus, against the Life of Apollonius of Tyana Written by Philostratus.* With an English translation by F. C. Conybeare. In Philostratus (543), 2:483–605.

213. Eyben, E. "Die Einteilung des menschlichen Lebens im römischen Altertum." *Rheinisches Museum für Philologie,* n.s., 116 (1973): 150–90.

214. Fabricius, Cajus. *Galens Exzerpte aus älteren Pharmakologen.* Ars medica, 2. Abteilung, Band 2. Berlin: Walter de Gruyter, 1972.

215. Ferguson, John. *Moral Values in the Ancient World.* London: Methuen, 1958.

216. ———. *The Religions of the Roman Empire.* Ithaca: Cornell University Press, 1970.

217. Ferngren, Gary B. "The Imago Dei and the Sanctity of Life: The Origins of an Idea." In *Euthanasia and the Newborn: Conflicts Regarding Saving Lives,* edited by Richard C. McMillan, H. Tristram Engelhardt, Jr., and Stuart F. Spicker, pp. 23–45. Dordrecht: D. Reidel, 1987.

218. ———. "Roman Lay Attitudes towards Medical Experimentation." *Bulletin of the History of Medicine* 59 (1985): 495–505.

219. Ferngren, Gary B., and Amundsen, Darrel W. "Virtue and Health— Medicine in pre-Christian Antiquity." In *Virtue and Medicine: Explorations in the Character of Medicine,* edited by Earl E. Shelp, pp. 3–22. Dordrecht: Reidel, 1985.

220. Festugière, André-Jean. "L'expérience religieuse du médecin Thessalos." Reprinted in *Hermétisme et mystique paienne,* pp. 141–80. Paris: Aubier-Montaigne, 1963.

221. ———. *Personal Religion among the Greeks.* Sather Classical Lectures. Berkeley and Los Angeles: University of California Press, 1960.

222. ———. *La révélation d'Hermès Trismégiste.* 4 vols. Paris: J. Gabalda. Vol. 1, 3rd ed., 1950; vol. 2, 3rd ed., 1949; vol. 3, 1953; vol. 4, 2nd ed., 1949.

223. Fichtner, Gerhard. "Christus als Arzt: Ursprünge und Wirkungen eines Motivs." *Frühmittelalterliche Studien* (Münster) 16 (1982): 1–18.

224. ———. "Das verpflanzte Mohrenbein—zur Interpretation der Kosmas and Damian–Legende." In *Medizin im mittelalterlichen Abendland,* edited by Gerhard Baader and Gundolf Keil, pp. 324–43. Wege der Forschung, vol. 365. Darmstadt: Wissenschaftliche Buchgesellschaft, 1982.

225. Finley, M. I. *The Ancient Economy.* Berkeley and Los Angeles: University of California Press, 1973.

226. Fischer, Klaus-Dietrich. "Zur Entwicklung des ärztlichen Standes im römischen Kaiserreich." *Medizinhistorisches Journal* 14 (1979): 165–75.

227. Flashar, Hellmut. "Beiträge zur spätantiken Hippokratesdeutung." *Hermes* 90 (1962): 402–18.

228. ———. *Melancholie und Melancholiker in den medizinischen Theorien der Antike.* Berlin: Walter de Gruyter, 1966.

229. Fleischer, Ulrich. *Untersuchungen zu den pseudohippokratischen Schriften* Παραγγελίαι, Περὶ ἰητροῦ *und* Περὶ εὐσχημοσύνης. Neue Deutsche Forschungen: Abteilung klassische Philologie, vol. 10. Berlin: Junker und Dünnhaupt, 1939.

230. Fox, Robin Lane. *Pagans and Christians.* New York: Alfred A. Knopf, 1987.

231. Fox, Ruth A. *The Tangled Chain: The Structure of Disorder in The Anatomy of Melancholy.* Berkeley, Los Angeles, and London: University of California Press, 1976.

232. Frank, Jerome D. *Persuasion and Healing.* Rev. ed. Baltimore: Johns Hopkins University Press, 1973.

233. Fredrich, Carl Johann. *Hippokratische Untersuchungen.* Berlin: Weidmann, 1899.

234. Freind, John. *The History of Physick; from the Time of Galen to the Beginning of the Sixteenth Century.* 2 vols. London: J. Walther, 1725–26.

235. French, Roger, and Greenaway, Frank (eds.). *Science in the Early Roman Empire.* Totowa, N.J.: Barnes and Noble, 1986.

236. Frend, W. H. C. *The Rise of Christianity.* Philadelphia: Fortress Press, 1984.

237. ———. "The Rise of Christianity." *American Scholar* 54 (1985): 397–402.

238. Frings, Hermann-Josef. "Aus Fremden Leiden eigene Sorgen." *Sudhoffs Archiv* 43 (1959): 1–12.

239. ———. *Medizin und Arzt bei den griechischen Kirchenvätern bis Chrysostomos.* Diss., University of Bonn, 1959.

240. Fulgentius. *Opera.* Edited by Rudolf Helm. Stuttgart: B. G. Teubner, 1970.

241. Galen. *Claudii Galeni Opera omnia.* Edited by Carl Gottlob Kühn. 22 vols. Leipzig: Cnobloch, 1821–33.

242. ———. *Claudii Galeni Pergameni Scripta minora.* Edited by J. Marquardt, I. Müller, and G. Helmreich. 3 vols. Leipzig: B. G. Teubner, 1884–93. Reprint. Amsterdam: Adolf M. Hakkert, 1967.

243. ———. *De sanitate tuenda, De alimentorum facultatibus, De bonis ma-*

lisque sucis, De victu attenuante, De pisana. Edited by K. Koch, G. Helmreich, K. Kalbfleisch, O. Hartlich. *CMG,* vol. 5.4.2. Leipzig: B. G. Teubner, 1923.

244. ———. *De usu partium libri XVII.* Edited by Georg Helmreich. 2 vols. Leipzig: B. G. Teubner, 1907–9.

245. ———. *In Hippocratis De natura hominis, In Hippocratis de victu acutorum, De diaeta Hippocratis in morbis acutis.* Edited by J. Mewaldt, G. Helmreich, and J. Westenberger. *CMG,* 5.9.1. Leipzig: B. G. Teubner, 1914.

246. ———. *In Hippocratis Epidemiarum librum VI commentaria I–VIII.* Edited by Ernst Wenkebach and Franz Pfaff. 2nd (photostatic) ed. *CMG,* vol. 5.10.2.2. Berlin: Academia Litterarum, 1956.

247. ———. *In Hippocratis Prorrheticum I Comm. III.* Edited by H. Diels. *De comate secundum Hippocratem.* Edited by J. Mewaldt. *In Hippocratis Prognosticum.* Edited by J. Heeg. *CMG,* vol. 5.9.2. Leipzig: B. G. Teubner, 1915.

248. ———. *On the Doctrines of Hippocrates and Plato [De placitis Hippocratis et Platonis].* Edited and translated by Phillip De Lacy. *CMG* 5.4.1 and 5.4.2. 2 pts. Pt. 1 (books 1–5), 3rd ed. Pt. 2 (books 6–9), 2nd ed. Berlin: Akademie-Verlag, 1984.

249. ———. *On the Natural Faculties.* With an English translation by Arthur John Brock. Loeb. 1928.

250. ———. *On Prognosis [De praecognitione].* Edited and translated by Vivian Nutton. *CMG,* vol. 5.8.1. Berlin: Akademie-Verlag, 1979.

251. ———. *On the Usefulness of the Parts of the Body.* Translated with introduction and commentary by Margaret Tallmadge May. 2 vols. Ithaca, N.Y.: Cornell University Press, 1968.

252. ———. *Subfiguratio emperica.* In Deichgräber (165), pp. 42–90.

253. García Ballester, Luis. *Alma y enfermedad en la obra de Galeno.* Cuadernos Hispanicos de historia de la medicina y de la ciencia, no. 12. Valencia-Granada, 1972.

254. ———. "La 'psique' en el somaticismo médico de la antiguedad: La actitud de Galeno." *Episteme* 3 (1969): 195–209.

255. Garrison, Fielding H. *An Introduction to the History of Medicine.* 4th ed. Philadelphia: W. B. Saunders, 1929.

256. Geffken, Johannes. *The Last Days of Greco-Roman Paganism.* Translated by Sabine MacCormack. Amsterdam: North Holland, 1978.

257. Gellius, Aulus. *The Attic Nights of Aulus Gellius.* With an English translation by John C. Rolfe. 3 vols. Loeb. 1927–28.

258. Gesenius, Wilhelm. *Hebräisches und Aramäisches Handwörterbuch über das Alte Testament.* Edited by Frants Buhl. 17th ed. 1915. Reprint. Berlin-Göttingen: Springer, 1949.

259. Gibbon, Edward. *The Decline and Fall of the Roman Empire.* 2 vols. New York: Modern Library, 1932.

260. Gil, Luis. "Ärztlicher Beistand und attische Komödie." *Sudhoffs Archiv* 57 (1973): 255–74.

261. Gilbert, Otto. *Die meteorologischen Theorien des griechischen Altertums*. Leipzig: B. G. Teubner, 1907.

262. Gill, Christopher. "Ancient Psychotherapy." *Journal of the History of Ideas* 46 (1985): 307–25.

263. Gomperz, Theodor. *Griechische Denker*. 3 vols. Leipzig: Veit and Comp., 1896–1909.

264. Goodspeed, Edgar J. (ed.). *Die ältesten Apologeten: Texte mit kurzen Einleitungen*. Göttingen: Vandenhoeck und Ruprecht, 1914.

265. *The Gospel According to John (i–xii)*. Introduction, translation, and notes by Raymond E. Brown. Anchor Bible. Garden City, N.Y.: Doubleday, 1966.

266. Gourevitch, Danielle. "Déontologie médicale: quelques problèmes." *Mélanges d'archéologie et d'histoire*, fasc. 81. Publiés par l'École Française de Rome. Paris, 1969.

267. ———. *Le triangle hippocratique dans le monde gréco-romain: Le malade, sa maladie et son médecin*. Rome: École Française de Rome, 1984.

268. Grant, Robert M. *Miracle and Natural Law in Graeco-Roman and Early Christian Thought*. Amsterdam: North-Holland, 1952.

269. *The Greek Anthology*. With an English translation by W. R. Paton. 5 vols. Loeb. 1925–27.

270. Gregory of Nazianzus. *Funeral Orations by Saint Gregory Nazianzen and Saint Ambrose*. Translation by Leo P. McCauley, John J. Sullivan, Martin R. P. McGuire, and Roy J. Deferrari. Fathers of the Church, vol. 22, 1953.

271. ———. *Oratio II—Apologetica*. Migne, *PG*, 35:407–514.

272. ———. *Oratio VII—Funebra in laudem Caesarii fratris*. Migne, *PG*, 35:755–88.

273. ———. *Oratio XLIII—Funebris oratio in laudem Basilii Magni*. Migne, *PG*, 36:493–606.

274. Gregory of Nyssa. *La création de l'homme*. French translation by Jean Laplace; notes by Jean Daniélou. Sources Chrétiennes, no. 6. Paris: Éditions du Cerf, 1944.

275. ———. *In Scripturae verba: Faciamus hominem ad imaginem et similitudinem nostram, oratio 1*. Migne, *PG*, 44:257–78.

276. Grensemann, Hermann. *Die hippokratische Schrift "Über die heilige Krankheit."* Ars medica, 2. Abteilung, Band 1. Berlin: Walter de Gruyter, 1968.

277. ———. *Knidische Medizin*. Teil I: *Die Testimonien zur ältesten knidischen Lehre und Analysen knidischer Schriften im Corpus Hippocraticum*. Ars Medica, 2. Abteilung, Band 4.1. Berlin: Walter de Gruyter, 1975.

278. Grmek, Mirko D. *Diseases in the Ancient Greek World*. Translated by Mirelle Muellner and Leonard Muellner. Baltimore: Johns Hopkins University Press, 1989.

279. Guthrie, W. K. C. *A History of Greek Philosophy*. 5 vols. Cambridge: Cambridge University Press, 1962–78.

280. Hähnel, Ruth. "Der künstliche Abortus im Altertum." *Sudhoffs Archiv* 29 (1937): 224–55.
281. Hamilton, Edith (trans.). *Three Greek Plays.* New York: W. W. Norton, 1937.
282. Hamilton, J. S. "Scribonius Largus on the Medical Profession." *Bulletin of the History of Medicine* 60 (1986): 209–16.
283. Hands, A. R. *Charities and Social Aid in Greece and Rome.* Ithaca: Cornell University Press, 1968.
284. Harig, Georg. "Die Diätetik der römischen Enzyklopädisten." *NTM* 13 (1976): 1–15.
285. ———. "Die Galenschrift 'De simplicium medicamentorum temperamentis ac facultatibus' und die 'Collectiones medicae' des Oribasius." *NTM* 3 (1966): 3–26.
286. Harig, Georg, and Kollesch, Jutta. "Galen und Hippokrates." In *La collection hippocratique et son rôle dans l'histoire de la médecine: Colloque de Strasbourg (23–27 octobre 1972),* pp. 257–74. Leiden: E. J. Brill, 1975.
287. ———. "Der hippokratische Eid." *Philologus* 122 (1978): 157–76.
288. Harnack, Adolf. *The Expansion of Christianity in the First Three Centuries.* English translation by James Moffatt. Vol. 1. Theological Translation Library, vol. 19. New York: G. P. Putnam's Sons; London: Williams and Norgate, 1904.
289. ———. *Die griechische Uebersetzung des Apologeticus Tertullian's, Medicinisches aus der ältesten Kirchengeschichte.* Texte und Untersuchungen zur Geschichte der altchristlichen Literatur, vol. 8. Leipzig: J. C. Hinrich, 1892.
290. Harvey, Susan Ashbrook. "Physicians and Ascetics in John of Ephesus: An Expedient Alliance." In Scarborough, *Symposium,* pp. 87–93.
291. Heidel, William Arthur. *Hippocratic Medicine: Its Spirit and Method.* New York: Columbia University Press, 1941.
292. Heinimann, Felix. "Eine vorplatonische Theorie der *techne.*" *Museum Helveticum* 18 (1961): 105–30.
293. ———. *Nomos und Physis.* Schweizerische Beiträge zur Altertumswissenschaft, fasc. 1. Basel: Friedrich Reinhardt, 1945.
294. Heliodorus. *Aethiopica.* Edited by Aristides Colonna. Scriptores graeci et latini consilio R. Academiae Lynceorum editi. Rome, 1938.
295. ———. *Die Abenteuer der schönen Chariklea.* German translation by Rudolf Reymer. Zurich: Artemis, 1950.
296. Hempel, Johannes. *Heilung als Symbol und Wirklichkeit im biblischen Schrifttum.* 2nd ed. Göttingen: Vandenhoeck und Ruprecht, 1965.
297. *Hermetica.* Edited and with an English translation by Walter Scott. Vol. 1. Oxford: Clarendon Press, 1924.
298. *Herodotus.* With an English translation by A. B. Godley. 4 vols. Loeb. 1921–28.
299. ———. *Historiarum libri IX.* 2 vols. Leipzig: B. G. Teubner, 1825–26.

300. Herzog, Rudolf. *Die Wunderheilungen von Epidauros. Philologus,* suppl. 22, fasc. 3. Leipzig: Dieterich, 1931.

301. *Hesiod.* Translation by Richmond Lattimore. Ann Arbor: University of Michigan Press, 1959.

302. Hippocrates. *Hippocrates.* With an English translation. 4 vols. Volumes 1, 2, and 4 translated by W. H. S. Jones. Vol. 3 translated by E. T. Withington. Loeb. 1957–59.

303. ———. *Hippocratis quae geruntur omnia.* Edited by Hugo Kühlewein. 2 vols. Leipzig: B. G. Teubner, 1894–1902.

304. ———. *Die hippokratische Schrift von der Siebenzahl in ihrer vierfachen Überlieferung.* Edited by W. H. Roscher. Paderborn: Ferdinand Schöningh, 1913.

305. ———. *Hippocratis et aliorum medicorum veterum reliquiae.* Edited by Franciscus Zaccharias Ermerins. Vol. 1. Utrecht: Kemink, 1859.

306. ———. *Indices librorum, Iusiurandum, Lex, De arte, De medico, De decente habitu, Praeceptiones, De prisca medicina, De aere locis aquis, De alimento, De liquidorum usu, De flatibus.* Edited by I. L. Heiberg. *CMG,* vol. 1.1. Leipzig: B. G. Teubner, 1927.

307. ———. *Hippocratis quae feruntur epistulae ad codicum fidem recensitae.* Edited by Walther Putzger. Wissenschaftliche Beilage zum Jahresbericht des kgl. Gymnasiums zu Wurzen, Ostern 1914. Wurzen, 1914.

308. ———. *The Medical Works of Hippocrates.* Translated by John Chadwick and W. N. Mann. Springfield, Ill. Charles C Thomas, 1950.

309. ———. *Oeuvres complètes d'Hippocrate.* French translation with the Greek text on opposite pages, by É. Littré. 10 vols. Paris: J.-B. Baillière, 1839–61.

310. ———. *Schriften: Die Anfänge der abendländischen Medizin.* Translated into German by Hans Diller. Reinbeck bei Hamburg: Rowohlt, 1962.

311. ———. *Über die Umwelt* [*De aere aquis locis*]. Edited with a German translation by Hans Diller. *CMG,* vol. 1.1.2. Berlin: Akademie-Verlag, 1970.

312. Hippolytus. *Philosophumena ou réfutation de toutes les hérésies.* French translation by A. Siouville. 2 vols. Les Textes du Christianisme, no. 6. Paris: Rieder, 1928.

313. Hirschfeld, Ernst. "Deontologische Texte des frühen Mittelalters." *Sudhoffs Archiv* 20 (1928): 353–71.

314. Honecker, Martin. "Christus medicus." In *Der kranke Mensch in Mittelalter und Renaissance,* edited by Peter Wunderli, pp. 27–43. Studia humaniora, vol. 5. Düsseldorf: Droste, 1986.

315. Hopfner. "Mageia." *PW,* 27. Halbband (1928), cols. 301–93.

316. Horace. *Opera omnia.* Edited by Wilhelm Dillenburger. 4th ed. Bonn: Adolph Marcus, 1860.

317. Horden, Peregrine. "Saints and Doctors in the Early Byzantine Empire: The Case of Theodore of Sykeon." *Studies in Church History* 19 (1982): 1–13.

318. Hunger, Herbert. *Die hochsprachliche profane Literatur der Byzantiner.* 2 vols. Byzantinisches Handbuch im Rahmen des Handbuchs der Altertumswissenschaft, 12. Abteilung, Vol. 5, pt. 5, vols. 1–2. Munich: C. H. Beck, 1978.

319. Hunger, Herbert, Stegmüller, Otto, Erbse, Hartmut, Imhof, Max, Büchner, Karl, Beck, Hans-Georg, and Rüdiger, Horst. *Geschichte der Textüberlieferung der antiken und mittelalterlichen Literatur.* Vol. 1. Zurich: Atlantis, 1961.

320. Ibn abī Uṣaibi ʿah. ʿUyūn al-ʾanbāʾ fī ṭabaqāt al-ʾaṭibbāʾ. [Cairo], 1882.

321. Ignatius. *Epistles.* In *Apostolic Fathers,* 1:172–277.

322. Ioannes Chrysostomus. *Homilia in paralyticum per tectum demissum.* Migne, *PG,* 51: 47–64.

323. Ioannes Philoponus. *De opificio mundi.* Edited by G. Reichardt. Leipzig: B. G. Teubner, 1897.

324. ———. *In Aristotelis libros De generatione et corruptione commentaria.* Edited by Jerome Vitelli. CAG, vol. 14, pt. 2. 1897.

325. ———. *In Aristotelis Physicorum libros tres priores commentaria.* Edited by Hieronymus Vitelli. CAG, vol. 16. 1887.

326. Iohannes Alexandrinus. *Commentaria in librum De sectis Galeni.* Edited by C. D. Pritchet. Leiden: E. J. Brill, 1982.

327. ———. *Commentaria in sextum librum Hippocratis Epidemiarum.* Edited by C. D. Pritchet. Leiden: E. J. Brill, 1975.

328. Irenaeus. *Contra haereses libri quinque.* Migne. *PG,* 7:433–1224.

329. ———. *Contre les hérésies.* Livre 4. Edited by Adelin Rousseau. 2 vols. Sources Chrétiennes, no. 100. Paris: Éditions du Cerf, 1965.

330. ———. *The Writings of Irenaeus.* Translated by Alexander Roberts and W. H. Rambaut. 2 vols. Ante-Nicene Christian Library, vols. 5 and 9. Edinburgh: T. and T. Clark, 1874.

331. Isidore of Pelusium. *Epistolarum libri quinque.* Migne, *PG,* 78:177–1674.

332. Isidore of Seville, *Etymologiarum sive originum libri XX.* Edited by W. M. Lindsay. 2 vols. Oxford: Oxford University Press, 1911.

333. ———. *Isidore of Seville: The Medical Writings.* An English translation with an introduction and commentary by William D. Sharpe. Transactions of the American Philosophical Society, n.s., vol. 54, pt. 2, 1964. Philadelphia: American Philosophical Society, 1964.

334. Iskandar, Albert Zaki. "An Attempted Reconstruction of the Late Alexandrian Medical Curriculum." *Medical History* 20 (1976): 235–58.

335. Jaeger, Werner. *Early Christianity and Greek Paideia.* Cambridge: Harvard University Press, 1961.

336. ———. *Paideia: The Ideals of Greek Culture.* Translated by Gilbert Highet. Vol. 3. New York: Oxford University Press, 1944.

337. ———. *The Theology of the Early Greek Philosophers.* 1947. Reprint. Oxford: Clarendon Press, 1948.

338. Jakobovits, Immanuel. *Jewish Medical Ethics: A Comparative and His-*

torical Study of the Jewish Religious Attitude to Medicine and Its Practice. New York: Bloch, 1959.

339. Jerome. *Epistulae.* Edited by Isidor Hilberg. Corpus scriptorum ecclesiasticorum Latinorum, vol. 54. Vienna: Tempsky und Freytag, 1916.

340. ———. *Epistulae.* Migne, *PL,* vol. 22.

341. ———. *Select Letters of St. Jerome.* With an English translation by F. A. Wright. Loeb. 1933.

342. ———. *Vita S. Hilarionis.* Migne, *PL,* 23:29–54.

343. Joly, Robert. "Esclaves et médecins dans la Grèce antique." *Sudhoffs Archiv* 53 (1969): 1–14.

344. ———. "Hippocrates and the School of Cos: Between Myth and Skepticism." In *Nature Animated,* edited by Michael Ruse, pp. 29–47. Dordrecht: D. Reidel, 1983.

345. ———. "Hippocrates of Cos." In *Dictionary of Scientific Biography,* vol. 6, pp. 418–31. New York: Charles Scribner's Sons, 1972.

346. ———. *Le niveau de la science hippocratique: Contribution à la psychologie de l'histoire des sciences.* Paris: Les Belles Lettres, 1966.

347. ———. "Platon, Phèdre et Hippocrate: Vingt ans après." In *Formes de pensée dans la collection hippocratique: Actes du IVᵉ colloque international hippocratique (Lausanne, 21–26 septembre 1981),* edited by François Lasserre and Philippe Mudry, pp. 407–21. Geneva: Droz, 1983.

348. ———. "Un peu d' épistémologie historique pour hippocratisants." *Colloque hippocratique de Paris,* pp. 371–91.

349. Jones, A. H. M. *The Later Roman Empire 284–602: A Social, Economic and Administrative Survey.* 2 vols. Norman: University of Oklahoma Press, 1964.

350. Jones, W. H. S. *The Doctor's Oath: An Essay in the History of Medicine.* Cambridge: Cambridge University Press, 1924.

351. Jonsen, Albert R. "Do No Harm." *Annals of Internal Medicine* 88 (1978): 827–32.

352. *Josephus.* With an English Translation. Vol. 2, *The Jewish War, Books I–III,* translated by H. St. J. Thackeray. Vol. 9, *Jewish Antiquities, Books XVIII–XX,* translated by Louis A. Feldman. Loeb. 1927 and 1965.

353. Julian. *The Works of the Emperor Julian.* With an English translation by Wilmer Cave Wright. 3 vols. Loeb. Vols. 1 and 2, 1913; vol. 3, 1923.

354. Justin Martyr. *Apologiae duae.* Edited and with a Latin translation by Gerard Rauschen. Florilegium Patristicum. Bonn: Hanstein, 1911.

355. ———. *The Writings of Justin Martyr and Athenagoras.* Translation by Marcus Dods, George Reith, and B. P. Pratten. Ante-Nicene Christian Library, vol. 2. Edinburgh: T. and T. Clark, 1874.

356. Justin (pseud.). *Responsiones ad orthodoxos.* Migne, *PG,* 6:1249–1400.

357. *Juvenal and Persius.* With an English translation by G. G. Ramsay. Loeb. 1961.

358. Kee, Howard Clark. *Medicine, Miracle, and Magic in New Testament Times.* Cambridge: Cambridge University Press, 1986.

359. ──────. *Miracle in the Early Christian World.* New Haven: Yale University Press, 1983.

360. Keenan, Sister Mary Emily. "St. Gregory of Nazianzus and Early Byzantine Medicine." *Bulletin of the History of Medicine* 9 (1941): 8–30.

361. ──────. "St. Gregory of Nyssa and the Medical Profession." *Bulletin of the History of Medicine* 15 (1944): 150–61.

362. Kind, Ernst. "Marcellus Empiricus oder Burdigalensis." *PW*, 14 (1930), cols. 1498–1503.

363. Kingsbury, John M. *Poisonous Plants of the United States and Canada.* Englewood Cliffs, N.J.: Prentice Hall, 1964.

364. Kirk, G. S., and Raven, J. E. *The Presocratic Philosophers: A Critical History with a Selection of Texts.* 1957. Reprint. Cambridge: Cambridge University Press, 1962.

365. Kitto, H. D. F. *The Greeks.* Baltimore: Penguin Books, 1965.

366. Knowles, David. *Christian Monasticism.* World University Library. New York: McGraw-Hill, 1969.

367. Kocher, Paul H. *Science and Religion in Elizabethan England.* San Marino, Calif.: Huntington Library, 1953.

368. Koelbing, Huldrych M. *Arzt und Patient in der antiken Welt.* Zurich: Artemis, 1977.

369. Kollesch, Jutta. "Arztwahl und ärztliche Ethik in der römischen Kaiserzeit." *Das Altertum* (Berlin: Akademie-Verlag) 18 (1972): 27–30.

370. ──────. "Galen und die zweite Sophistik." In Nutton, *GPP*, pp. 1–11.

371. Kollesch, Jutta, and Kudlien, Fridolf. "Bemerkungen zum Περὶ ἄρ-Θρων—Kommentar des Apollonius von Kition." *Hermes* 89 (1961): 322–32.

372. Kornexl, Elmar. *Begriff und Einschätzung der Gesundheit des Körpers in der griechischen Literatur von ihren Anfängen bis zum Hellenismus.* Commentationes Aenipontanae, vol. 21. Innsbruck: Universitätsverlag Wagner, 1970.

373. Kotelmann, L. *Gesundheitspflege im Mittelalter.* Hamburg: Leopold Voss, 1890.

374. Kottek, Samuel. "The Essenes and Medicine." *Clio Medica* 18 (1983): 81–99.

375. ──────. "Physicians and Healing Personnel in the Works of Flavius Josephus." *Gesnerus* 42 (1985): 41–55.

376. Kristeller, Paul Oskar. "The School of Salerno." *Bulletin of the History of Medicine* 17 (1945): 138–94.

377. Kroll, Jerome, and Bachrach, Bernard. "Sin and the Etiology of Disease in pre-Crusade Europe." *Journal of the History of Medicine and Allied Sciences* 41 (1986): 395–414.

378. Kudlien, Fridolf. "Anatomie." *PW*, suppl. 11 (1968), cols. 38–48.

379. ──────. "*Anniversarii vicini*: Zur freien Arbeit im römischen Dorf." *Hermes* 112 (1984): 66–84.

380. ──────. "Antike Anatomie und menschlicher Leichnam." *Hermes* 97 (1969): 78–94.

381. ———. "Der antike Arzt vor der Frage des Todes." In *Der Grenzbereich zwischen Leben und Tod: Vorträge gehalten auf der Tagung der Jungius Gesellschaft . . . am 9/10 Oktober 1975*, pp. 68–81. Göttingen, 1976.

382. ———. "Der Arzt des Körpers und der Arzt der Seele." *Clio Medica* 3 (1968): 1–20.

383. ———. *Der Beginn des medizinischen Denkens bei den Griechen von Homer bis Hippokrates.* Zurich: Artemis, 1967.

384. ———. "Dialektik und Medizin in der Antike." *Medizinhistorisches Journal* 9 (1974): 187–200.

385. ———. "Dogmatische Ärzte." *PW*, suppl. 10 (1965), cols. 179–80.

386. ———. "Galen's Religious Belief." In Nutton, *GPP*, pp. 117–30.

387. ———. "Gesundheit." *Reallexikon für Antike und Christentum* 10:902–45. Stuttgart: Anton Hiersemann, 1978.

388. ———. "Das Göttliche und die Natur im hippokratischen Prognostikon." *Hermes* 105 (1977): 268–74.

389. ———. "Jüdische Ärzte im römischen Reich." *Medizinhistorisches Journal* 20 (1985): 36–57.

390. ———. "Medical Ethics and Popular Ethics in Greece and Rome." *Clio Medica* 5 (1970): 91–121.

391. ———. "Medicine as a 'Liberal Art' and the Question of the Physician's Income." *Journal of the History of Medicine and Allied Sciences* 31 (1976): 448–59.

392. ———. "Medizinische Aspekte der antiken Unsterblichkeitsvorstellung." *Rheinisches Museum für Philologie*, n.s., 121 (1978): 218–25.

393. ———. "Mutmassungen über die Schrift Περὶ ἰητροῦ." *Hermes* 94 (1966): 54–59.

394. ———. "Paetus." *PW*, suppl. 10 (1965), cols. 473–74.

395. ———. "Pneumatische Ärzte." *PW*, suppl. 11 (1968), cols. 1097–1108.

396. ———. "Poseidonios und die Ärzteschule der Pneumatiker." *Hermes* 90 (1962): 419–29.

397. ———. *Die Stellung des Arztes in der römischen Gesellschaft.* Forschungen zur antiken Sklaverei, vol. 18. Stuttgart: Franz Steiner, 1986.

398. ———. "The Third Century A.D.—A Blank Spot in the History of Medicine." In *Medicine, Science, and Culture: Historical Essays in Honor of Owsei Temkin*, edited by Lloyd G. Stevenson and Robert P. Multhauf, pp. 25–34. Baltimore: Johns Hopkins Press, 1968.

399. ———. "Überlegungen zu einer Sozialgeschichte des frühgriechischen Arztes und seines Berufs." *Hermes* 114 (1986): 129–46.

400. ———. "Die Unschätzbarkeit ärztlicher Leistung und das Honorarproblem." *Medizinhistorisches Journal* 14 (1979): 3–16.

401. ———. *Untersuchungen zu Aretaios von Kappadokien.* Mainz: Akademie der Wissenschaften und der Literatur. Abhandlungen der Geistes- und Sozialwissenschaftlichen Klasse 1963, no. 11. Wiesbaden: Franz Steiner, 1963.

402. ———. "Zum Thema 'Homer und die Medizin.'" *Rheinisches Museum für Philologie*, n.s., 108 (1965): 293–299.

403. ———. "Zur Interpretation eines hippokratischen Aphorismus." *Sudhoffs Archiv* 46 (1962): 289–94.

404. ———. "Zwei Interpretationen zum hippokratischen Eid." *Gesnerus* 35 (1978): 253–63.

405. Ladner, Gerhart B. "The Philosophical Anthropology of Saint Gregory of Nyssa." *Dumbarton Oaks Papers* 12 (1958): 59–94.

406. La Fontaine, Jean de. *Fables de La Fontaine*. Illustrated by J.-J. Grenville. With notes and a biography by Auger. Paris: Garnier Frères, n.d.

407. Laín Entralgo, Pedro. "Hippocratica Varia." In *Homenaje a Antonio Tovar*, pp. 231–41. Madrid: Editorial Gredos, 1972.

408. ———. *La medicina hipocrática*. Madrid: Revista de Occidente, 1970.

409. ———. "Quaestiones hippocraticae disputatae tres." In *La collection hippocratique et son rôle dans l'histoire de la médecine: Colloque de Strasbourg (23–27 octobre 1972)*, pp. 305–19. Leiden: E. J. Brill, 1975.

410. ———. *The Therapy of the Word in Classical Antiquity*. Edited and translated by L. J. Rather and John M. Sharp. New Haven: Yale University Press, 1970.

411. Latte, Kurt. "Griechische und römische Religiosität." In *Kleine Schriften zu Religion, Recht, Literatur und Sprache der Griechen und Römer*, by Kurt Latte, edited by O. Gigon, W. Buchwald, and W. Kunkel, pp. 48–59. Munich: C. H. Beck, 1968.

412. Laux, Rudolf. "Ars medicinae: Ein frühmittelalterliches Kompendium der Medizin." *Kyklos* 3 (1930): 417–34.

413. Laws, Sophie. *A Commentary on the Epistle of James*. Harper's New Testament Commentaries. San Francisco: Harper and Row, 1980.

414. Leibowitz, J. O. "Medical Ethics and Etiquette in Jewish History." *Medica Judaica* 1, no. 3 (March-April 1971). Unpaginated reprint.

415. Leisegang, H. "Platon." *PW*, 40. Halbband (1950), cols. 2342–3537.

416. Leitner, Helmut. *Bibliography to the Ancient Medical Authors*. Bern: Hans Huber, 1973.

417. Lemerle, Paul. *Le premier humanisme byzantin: Notes et remarques sur enseignement et culture à Byzance des origines au Xe siècle*. Bibliothèque byzantine: Études, no. 6. Paris: Presses Universitaires de France, 1971.

418. Lewis, Naphtali. "Exemption of Physicians from Liturgy." *Bulletin of the American Society of Papyrologists* 2 (1965): 87–92.

419. ———. *Life in Egypt under Roman Rule*. Oxford: Clarendon Press, 1983.

420. Libanius. Κατὰ ἰατροῦ φαρμακέως. In *Libanii opera*, edited by Richard Foerster, vol. 8, pp. 182–94. Leipzig: B. G. Teubner, 1915.

421. Lichtenthaeler, Charles. *Der Eid des Hippokrates: Ursprung und Bedeutung*. Cologne: Deutscher Ärzte-Verlag, 1984.

422. Lieber, Elinor. "Galen in Hebrew: The Transmission of Galen's Works in the Medieval Islamic World." In Nutton, *GPP*, pp. 167–86.

423. Lietzmann, Hans (ed.). *Das Leben des heiligen Symeon Stylites*. With a German translation of the Syriac biography and the letters by Heinrich

Hilgenfeld. Texte und Untersuchungen zur Geschichte der altchristlichen Literatur, 3rd ser. vol. 2. Leipzig: J. C. Hinrich, 1908.

424. Lindberg, David C. "Science and the Early Church." In *God and Nature: Historical Essays on the Encounter between Christianity and Science,* edited by David C. Lindberg and Ronald L. Numbers, pp. 19–48. Berkeley, Los Angeles, and London: University of California Press, 1986.

425. Lloyd, G. E. R. "The Hippocratic Question." *Classical Quarterly,* n.s., 25–26 (1975): 177–92.

426. ———. *Magic, Reason, and Experience: Studies in the Origin and Development of Greek Science.* Cambridge: Cambridge University Press, 1979.

427. ———. *Science, Folklore, and Ideology: Studies in the Life Sciences in Ancient Greece.* Cambridge: Cambridge University Press, 1983.

428. Lloyd-Jones, Hugh. *The Justice of Zeus.* Sather Classical Lectures, vol. 41. Berkeley, Los Angeles, and London: University of California Press, 1971.

429. Lonie, Iain M. "De natura pueri, ch. 13." In *Corpus Hippocraticum: Colloque de Mons, Septembre 1975,* pp. 123–35. Mons: Université de Mons, 1977.

430. ———. *The Hippocratic Treatises "On Generation," "On the Nature of the Child," "Diseases IV": A Commentary.* Ars Medica, 2. Abteilung, Band 7. Berlin: Walter de Gruyter, 1981.

431. ———. "The Paradoxical Text 'On the Heart'," pt. 2. *Medical History* 17 (1973): 136–53.

432. *Lucian.* With an English translation. 8 vols. Vols. 1–5 translated by A. M. Harmon. Vol. 6 translated by A. Kilburn. Vols. 7–8 translated by M. D. Macleod. Loeb. Vols. 1–4, 1921–27; vols. 5–8, 1936–61.

433. Macarius. *Die 50 geistlichen Homilien des Makarios.* Edited by Hermann Dörries, Erich Klostermann, and Matthias Kroeger. Patristische Texte und Studien, vol. 4. Berlin: Walter de Gruyter, 1964.

434. MacKinney, Loren C. *Early Medieval Medicine.* Hideyo Noguchi Lectures, vol. 3. Baltimore: Johns Hopkins Press, 1937.

435. ———. "Medical Ethics and Etiquette in the Early Middle Ages: The Persistence of Hippocratic Ideals." *Bulletin of the History of Medicine* 26 (1952): 1–31.

436. MacMullen, Ramsay. *Christianizing the Roman Empire (A.D. 100–400).* New Haven: Yale University Press, 1984.

437. ———. *Paganism in the Roman Empire.* New Haven: Yale University Press, 1981.

438. Magoulias, H. J. "The Lives of the Saints as Sources of Data for the History of Byzantine Medicine in the Sixth and Seventh Centuries." *Byzantinische Zeitschrift* 57 (1964): 127–50.

439. Maloney, Gilles, and Frohn, Winnie (eds.). *Concordance des oeuvres hippocratiques.* 5 vols. N.p.: Les Editions du Sphinx, 1984.

440. Manetti, Daniela. "Tematica filosofica e scientifica nel papiro Fiorentino

115." In *Studi su papiri greci di logica e medicina,* by W. Cavini, M. C. Donnini Maccio, M. S. Funghi, and D. Manetti, pp. 173–206. Florence: Olschki, 1985.

441. Mansfeld, Jaap. "Theoretical and Empirical Attitudes in Early Greek Scientific Medicine." *Colloque hippocratique de Paris,* pp. 371–91.

442. Manuel, Frank E. "The Use and Abuse of Psychology in History." *Daedalus* 117, no. 3 (Summer 1988): 199–225. (Reprinted from Winter 1971 issue.)

443. Marcellus. *De medicamentis liber.* 2nd ed. Edited by Eduard Liechtenhan. With a German translation by Jutta Kollesch and Diethard Nickel. 2 vols. *CML,* vol. 5. Berlin: Akademie-Verlag, 1968.

444. Marcus Aurelius Antoninus. *The Communings with Himself.* Revised text with an English translation by C. R. Haines. Loeb. 1979.

445. Marrou, Henri Irénée. "Synesius of Cyrene and Alexandrian Neoplatonism." In *The Conflict between Paganism and Christianity in the Fourth Century,* edited by Arnaldo Momigliano, pp. 126–50. Oxford: Clarendon Press, 1963.

446. Martial. *Epigrams.* With an English translation by Walter C. A. Ker. 2 vols. Loeb. 1920.

447. *Matthew.* In *The Interpreter's Bible,* vol. 7, Nashville: Abingdon, 1979.

448. Mayr-Harting, Henry. "Jesus, Scourge of Money-Grubbers." *Times Literary Supplement,* December 26, 1986, p. 1447.

449. Meeks, Wayne A. *The First Urban Christians: The Social World of the Apostle Paul.* New Haven: Yale University Press, 1983.

450. Meier, Gabriel. "Cosmas and Damian, Saints." In *Catholic Encyclopedia,* 4:403–4.

451. Meier, John P. "Jesus among the Historians." *New York Times Book Review,* December 21, 1986, pp. 1 and 16–19.

452. *La mélancolie dans la relation de l'âme et du corps.* Littérature, Médecine, Société, no. 1. University of Nantes, 1979.

453. Melito. *Fragmentum ex Apologia Melitonis ad Antonium Caesarem.* Migne, *PG,* 5:1225–32. (This is a Latin version from Cureton's *Specilegium Syriacum,* London, 1855.)

454. Mesulam, Marek-Marsel, and Perry, Jon. "The Diagnosis of Love-Sickness: Experimental Psychophysiology without the Polygraph." *Psychophysiology* 9 (1972): 546–51.

455. Methodius. *De resurrectione.* Edited by D. G. Nathanael Bonwetsch. In *Die griechischen christlichen Schriftsteller der ersten drei Jahrhunderte,* vol. 27. Leipzig: Hinrich, 1917.

456. ———. *Convivium.* Migne, *PG,* 18:27–220.

457. Meyer, Theodor. *Geschichte des römischen Ärztestandes.* Habilitationsschrift Jena. Kiel: Graphische Kunstanstalt L. Handorff, 1907.

458. ———. *Theodorus Priscianus und die römische Medizin.* Jena: Fischer, 1909.

459. Meyer-Steineg, Theodor. "Hippokrates-Erzählungen." *Sudhoffs Archiv* 6 (1912): 1–11.

460. Michler, Markwart. "Die praktische Bedeutung des normativen Physis-Begriffes in der hippokratischen Schrift De Fracturis—De Articulis." *Hermes* 90 (1962): 385–401.

461. Millar, Fergus; with Berciu, D., Frye, Richard N., Kossak, Georg, and Rice, Tamara Talbot. *The Roman Empire and Its Neighbours.* London: Weidenfeld and Nicolson, 1967.

462. Miller, Harold W. "The Concept of the Divine in De morbo sacro." *Transactions of the American Philological Association* 84 (1953): 1–15.

463. Miller, Timothy S. *The Birth of the Hospital in the Byzantine Empire.* Henry E. Sigerist Supplements to the *Bulletin of the History of Medicine,* n.s., no. 10. Baltimore: Johns Hopkins University Press, 1985.

464. ———. "Byzantine Hospitals." In Scarborough, *Symposium,* pp. 53–61.

465. Minucius Felix. *Octavius.* With an English translation by W. C. A. Kerr. Loeb. 1931.

466. Momigliano, Arnaldo. *Cassiodorus and Italian Culture of His Time.* Italian Lecture, British Academy, 1955. London: Oxford University Press. (Proceedings of the British Academy, 41: 207–45.)

467. ———. "How Roman Emperors Became Gods." *American Scholar* 55 (Spring 1986): 181–93.

468. ———. "Pagan and Christian Historiography in the Fourth Century A.D." In *The Conflict between Paganism and Christianity in the Fourth Century,* edited by Arnaldo Momigliano, pp. 79–99. Oxford: Clarendon Press, 1963.

469. Moraux, Paul. *Der Aristotelismus bei den Griechen von Andronikos bis Alexander von Aphrodisias.* 2 vols. Peripatoi, vols. 5 and 6. Berlin: Walter de Gruyter, 1973–84.

470. ———. "Galien comme philosophe: La philosophie de la nature." In Nutton, *GPP,* pp. 87–116.

471. Morrison, Karl F. (ed.). *The Church in the Roman Empire.* University of Chicago Readings in Western Civilization, vol. 3. Chicago: University of Chicago Press, 1986.

472. ———. "Incentives for Studying the Liberal Arts." In *The Seven Liberal Arts in the Middle Ages,* edited by David L. Wagner, pp. 32–57. Bloomington: Indiana University Press, 1983.

473. Müller, Gerhard. "Arzt, Kranker und Krankheit bei Ambrosius von Mailand (334–397)." *Sudhoffs Archiv* 51 (1967): 193–216.

474. Müri, Walter. *Der Arzt im Altertum: Griechische und lateinische Quellenstücke von Hippokrates bis Galen mit der Übertragung ins Deutsche.* 3rd ed. Munich: Ernst Heimeran, 1962.

475. Nachmanson, Ernst. "Hippocratea: Aus Aufzeichnungen und Vorarbeiten." In *Symbolae philologicae O. A. Danielson octogenario dicatae,* pp. 185–202. Upsala: A. B. Lundequist, 1932.

476. ———. "Zum Nachleben der Aphorismen." *Quellen und Studien zur Geschichte der Naturwissenschaften und der Medizin* 3, no. 4 (1933): 92–107 (pp. 300–315 of the whole vol.).

477. Nemesius Emesenus. *De natura hominis: graece et latine.* Edited by Chris-

tian Friedrich Matthaei. Halle: Joan. Jac. Gebauer, 1802. Reprint. Hildesheim: Georg Olms, 1967.

478. Nestle, Wilhelm. "Die Haupteinwände des antiken Denkens gegen das Christentum." In *Griechische Studien,* by Wilhelm Nestle, pp. 597–660. Stuttgart, 1948. Reprint. Aalen: Scientia Verlag Aalen, 1968.

479. ———. "Hippocratica." *Hermes* 73 (1938): 1–38.

480. Neuburger, Max. *Geschichte der Medizin.* 2 vols. Stuttgart: Ferdinand Enke, 1906–11.

481. Nilsson, Martin Persson. *Greek Piety.* Translated by Herbert Jennings Rose. New York: Norton Library, 1969.

482. ———. *Greek Popular Religion.* New York: Columbia University Press, 1940.

483. Nock, Arthur Darby. *Conversion: The Old and the New in Religion from Alexander the Great to Augustine of Hippo.* Oxford: Clarendon Press, 1933.

484. ———. *Essays on Religion and the Ancient World.* Selected and edited by Zeph Stewart. Vol. 1. Cambridge: Harvard University Press, 1972.

485. Nörenberg, Heinz-Werner. *Das Göttliche und die Natur in der Schrift Über die heilige Krankheit.* Bonn: Habelt, 1968.

486. Noorda, Sijbolt. "Illness and Sin, Forgiving and Healing: The Connection of Medical Treatment and Religious Beliefs in Ben Sira 38, 1–15." In *Studies in Hellenistic Religions,* edited by M. S. Vermaseren, pp. 215–24. Leiden: E. J. Brill, 1979.

487. Nutton, Vivian. "Ammianus and Alexandria." *Clio Medica* 7 (1972): 165–76.

488. ———. "Archiatri and the Medical Profession in Antiquity." *Papers of the British School at Rome* 45 (1977): 191–226.

489. ———. "From Galen to Alexander: Aspects of Medicine and Medical Practice in Late Antiquity." In Scarborough, *Symposium,* pp. 1–14.

490. ———. "Galen in the Eyes of His Contemporaries." *Bulletin of the History of Medicine* 58 (1984): 315–24.

491. ———. (ed.). *Galen: Problems and Prospects. A Collection of Papers Submitted at the 1979 Cambridge Conference.* London: Wellcome Institute for the History of Medicine, 1981.

492. ———. "Galen's Philosophical Testament: 'On My Own Opinions.' " In *Aristoteles: Werk und Wirkung,* vol. 2, edited by Jürgen Wiesner, pp. 27–51. Berlin: Walter de Gruyter, 1987.

493. ———. "Murders and Miracles: Lay Attitudes towards Medicine in Classical Antiquity." In *Patients and Practitioners: Lay Perceptions of Medicine in Pre-Industrial Society,* edited by Roy Porter, pp. 23–53. Cambridge: Cambridge University Press, 1985.

494. ———. "The Perils of Patriotism: Pliny and Roman Medicine." In *Science in the Early Roman Empire: Pliny the Elder, His Sources and Influence,* edited by Roger French and Frank Greenaway, pp. 30–58. Totowa, N.J.: Barnes and Noble, 1986.

495. ———. Review of *The Birth of the Hospital in the Byzantine Empire*, by Timothy S. Miller. *Medical History* 30 (1986): 218–21.

496. ———. "Two Notes on Immunities: Digest 27, 1, 6, 10 and 11." *Journal of Roman Studies* 61 (1971): 52–63.

497. Oberhelman, Steven M. "The Diagnostic Dream in Ancient Medical Theory and Practice." *Bulletin of the History of Medicine* 61 (1987): 47–60.

498. Oliver, James H. "Two Athenian Poets." *Hesperia,* suppl. 8, pp. 243–58. American School of Classical Studies at Athens, 1949.

499. Oliver, James H., and Maas, Paul Lazarus. "An Ancient Poem on the Duties of a Physician." *Bulletin of the History of Medicine* 7 (1939): 315–23.

500. Oliver, John Rathbone. "The Sacrificing Women in the Temple of Asklepios: The Fourth Mime of Herondas, an Early Coan Literary Document." *Bulletin of the History of Medicine* 2 (1934): 504–11.

501. Olympiodorus. *In Aristotelis Meteora commentaria.* Edited by Wilhelm Stüve. CAG, vol. 12.2. 1900.

502. ———. *Prolegomena et in Categorias commentarium.* Edited by Adolf Busse. CAG, vol. 12.1. 1902.

503. Onions, Richard Broxton. *The Origins of European Thought about the Body, the Mind, the Soul, the World, Time, and Fate.* Cambridge: Cambridge University Press, 1951.

504. Opelt, Ilona. *Hieronymus' Streitschriften.* Heidelberg: Carl Winter, 1973.

505. Oribasius. *Collectionum medicarum reliquiae.* Edited by Johannes Raeder. 4 vols. CMG, vols. 6.1.1, 6.1.2, 6.2.1, and 6.2.2. Leipzig: B. G. Teubner, 1928–33.

506. ———. *Oeuvres d'Oribase.* Edited with a French translation by Bussemaker and Daremberg. 6 vols. Paris: Imprimerie Nationale, 1851–76.

507. ———. *Synopsis ad Eustathium, Libri ad Eunapium.* Edited by Johannes Raeder. CMG, vol. 6.3. Leipzig: B. G. Teubner, 1926.

508. Origen. *Commentarium in Evangelium secundum Matthaeum.* Migne, PG, 13:1253–1362.

509. ———. *Contra Celsum.* Migne, PG, 11:637–1632.

510. ———. *Contra Celsum.* Translated by Henry Chadwick. Cambridge: Cambridge University Press, 1953.

511. ———. *Contra haereses.* Migne, PG, vol. 16.3, pp. 3009–3454.

512. ———. *Ex Origenis commentariis in Exodum: In illud: Induravit Dominus cor Pharaonis.* Migne, PG, 12:263–82.

513. ———. *Explanatio super psalmum tricesimum septimum, qui dicitur: Domine, ne in furore, etc.* Migne, PG, 12:1369–90.

514. ———. *In Jeremiam homiliae* 14. Migne, PG, 13:403–28.

515. ———. *In Numeros homiliae* 18. Migne, PG, 12:712–19.

516. ———. *Origène contra Celse.* Vol. 1 (books 1 and 2). With a French translation by Marcel Borret. Sources Chrétiennes, no. 132. Paris: Éditions du Cerf. 1967.

517. Orr, William F., and Walther, James Arthur. *1 Corinthians: A New Translation with a Study of the Life of Paul, Notes, and Commentary.* Anchor Bible. Garden City, N.Y.: Doubleday, 1976.

518. Pachomius. *S. Pachomii abbatis Tabennensis Regulae monasticae.* Edited by Paul Bruno Albers. Florilegium Patristicum, n.s., no. 16. Bonn: Peter Hanstein, 1923.

519. Pack, Roger. "Note on a Progymnasma of Libanius." *American Journal of Philology* 69 (1948): 299–304.

520. Pagels, Elaine. "The Defeat of the Gnostics." *New Yorker,* December 6, 1979, pp. 43–52.

521. ———. *The Gnostic Gospels.* New York: Random House, Vintage Books, 1989.

522. ———. "The Threat of the Gnostics." *New Yorker,* November 8, 1979, pp. 37–45.

523. Palladius. *Dialogus de vita S. Joannis Chrysostomi.* Edited by P. R. Coleman-Norton. Cambridge: Cambridge University Press, 1928.

524. ———. *The Lausiac History.* Translated and annotated by Robert T. Meyer. Ancient Christian Writers, no. 34. Westminster, Md.: Newman Press; London: Longmans, Green and Co., 1965.

525. Palladius (Iatrosophist). *Commentarii in Hippocratis librum sextum De morbis popularibus.* In Dietz, AC, 2:1–204.

526. ———. *Kommentar zu Hippokrates "De fracturis" und seine Parallelversion unter dem Namen des Stephanus von Alexandria.* Edited with German translations by Dieter Irmer. Hamburger Philologische Studien, no. 45. Hamburg: Helmut Buske, 1977.

527. Palm, Adolf. *Studien zur hippokratischen Schrift Περὶ διαίτης.* Diss., University of Tübingen, 1933.

528. Papadopoulos-Kerameus, A. *Varia graeca sacra: Sbornik grečeskich neizdannych bogoslovskich tekstov IV–XV vekov.* Subsidia byzantina lucis ope iterata, vol. 6. Leipzig: Zentralantiquariat, 1975.

529. Paracelsus. *Theophrast von Hohenheim gen. Paracelsus. Sämtliche Werke. 1. Abteilung: Medizinische, naturwissenschaftliche und philosophische Schriften.* Edited by Karl Sudhoff, vol. 1. Munich: R. Oldenbourg, 1929.

530. Parker, Robert. *Miasma: Pollution and Purification in Early Greek Religion.* Oxford: Clarendon, 1983.

531. Patlagean, Evelyne. *Pauvreté économique et pauvreté sociale à Byzance, 4e–7e siècles.* Paris: Mouton, 1977.

532. Paul of Aegina. *Paulus Aegineta.* Edited by I. L. Heiberg. 2 vols. CMG, vols. 9.1 and 9.2. Leipzig: B. G. Teubner, 1921–24.

533. ———. *The Seven Books of Paulus Aegineta.* Translated with a commentary by Francis Adams. 3 vols. London: Sydenham Society, 1844–47.

534. Pazzini, Adalberto. *I santi nella storia della medicina.* Rome: Casa editrice Mediterranea, 1937.

535. Pease, Arthur Stanley. "Medical Allusions in the Works of St. Jerome." *Harvard Studies in Classical Philology* 25 (1914): 73–86.

536. Pelikan, Jaroslav. *The Christian Tradition.* Vol. 2, *The Emergence of the Catholic Tradition (100–600).* Chicago: University of Chicago Press, 1971.

537. Pfohl, Gerhard (ed.). *Inschriften der Griechen: Epigraphische Quellen zur Geschichte der antiken Medizin.* Darmstadt: Wissenschaftliche Buchgesellschaft, 1977.

538. Philippson, Robert. "Verfasser und Abfassungszeit der sogenannten Hippokratesbriefe." *Rheinisches Museum für Philologie,* n.s., 77 (1928): 293–328.

539. Phillips, Joanne H. "The Emergence of the Greek Medical Profession in the Roman Republic." *Transactions and Studies of the College of Physicians of Philadelphia,* ser. 5, vol. 2, no. 4 (December 1980): 267–75.

540. ———. "Lucretius on the Inefficacy of the Medical Art: 6. 1179 and 6. 1226–38." *Classical Philology* 77 (1982): 233–35.

541. *Philo.* With an English translation. 10 vols. Vols. 1 and 2, translated by F. H. Colson and G. H. Whitaker. Vol. 9, translated by F. H. Colson. Loeb. 1929 and 1941.

542. Philostorgius. *Kirchengeschichte.* Edited by Joseph Bidez, 2nd ed., edited by Friedhelm Winkelmann. In *Die griechischen christlichen Schriftsteller der ersten Jahrhunderte.* Berlin: Akademie-Verlag, 1972.

543. Philostratus. *The Life of Apollonius of Tyana, The Epistle of Apollonius, and the Treatise of Eusebius.* With an English translation by F. C. Conybeare. 2 vols. Loeb. 1917–21.

544. ———. *Lives of the Sophists.* In *Philostratus and Eunapius, The Lives of the Sophists.* With an English translation by Wilmer Cave Wright. Loeb. 1952.

545. Photius. *Bibliotheca.* Edited by Immanuel Bekker. Berlin: Reimer, 1824.

546. Pigeaud, Jackie. *La maladie de l' âme: Étude sur la relation de l' âme et du corps dans la tradition médico-philosophique antique.* Paris: Les Belles Lettres, 1981.

547. ———. "Quelques aspects du rapport de l'âme et du corps dans le corpus hippocratique." In *Colloque hippocratique de Paris,* pp. 417–32.

548. Pinault, Jody Rubin. "How Hippocrates Cured the Plague." *Journal of the History of Medicine and Allied Sciences* 41 (1986): 52–75.

549. Pindar. *The Odes of Pindar: Including the Principal Fragments.* With an English translation by John Sandys. Loeb. 1961.

550. Pines, Shlomo. "The Oath of Asaph the Physician and Yoḥanan ben Zabda: Its Relation to the Hippocratic Oath and the Doctrina duarum viarum of the Didache." *Proceedings of the Israel Academy of Sciences and Humanities* 5, no. 9 (1976): 223–64.

551. Plato. *Cratylus, Parmenides, Greater Hippias, Lesser Hippias.* With an English translation by H. N. Fowler. Loeb. 1926.

552. ———. *Euthyphro, Apology, Crito, Phaedo, Phaedrus.* With an English translation by Harold North Fowler. Loeb. 1960.

553. ———. *Gorgias.* A revised text with introduction and commentary by E. R. Dodds. Oxford: Clarendon Press, 1959.

554. ———. *Laches, Protagoras, Meno, Euthydemus*. With an English translation by W. R. M. Lamb. Loeb. 1924.

555. ———. *Plato's Theory of Knowledge: The Theaetetus and the Sophist of Plato*. Translated with a running commentary by Francis Macdonald Cornford. Library of Liberal Arts, no. 100. New York: Liberal Arts Press, 1957.

556. Pliny. *Natural History*. With an English translation. 10 vols. Vol. 2, translated by H. Rackham. Vol. 8, translated by W. H. S. Jones. Loeb. 1942 and 1963.

557. Pliny the Younger. *Letters*. With an English translation by William Melmoth, revised by W. M. L. Hutchinson. 2 vols. Loeb. 1927.

558. Pliny (pseud.). *Plinii Secundi Iunioris qui feruntur De medicina libri tres*. Edited by Alf Onnerfors. *CML*, vol. 3. Berlin: Academia Scientiarum, 1964.

559. ———. *Plinii Secundi quae fertur una cum Gargilii Martialis Medicina*. Edited by Valentin Rose. Leipzig: B. G. Teubner, 1875.

560. *Plotinus*. With an English translation by A. H. Armstrong. 6 vols. Vols. 1–3. Loeb. 1966–67.

561. Plutarch. *Lives*. With an English translation. 11 vols. Vols. 2 and 9, translated by Bernadotte Perrin. Loeb. 1914 and 1920.

562. ———. *Moralia*. With an English translation. 17 vols. Vol. 2, translated by Frank Cole Babbitt. Vol. 6, translated by W. C. Helmbold. Vol. 14, translated by Benedict Einarson and Phillip De Lacy. Loeb. 1928, 1939, and 1967.

563. Pohlenz, Max. *Hippokrates und die Begründung der wissenschaftlichen Medizin*. Berlin: Walter de Gruyter, 1938.

564. ———. *Die Stoa: Geschichte einer geistigen Bewegung*. 2 vols. 3rd ed. Göttingen: Vandenhoeck und Ruprecht, 1964.

565. Polybius. *The Histories*. With an English translation by W. R. Paton. 6 vols. Vol. 4. Loeb. 1925.

566. Polycarp. *Epistle to the Philippians*. In *Apostolic Fathers*, 1:280–301.

567. ———. *The Martyrdom of Polycarp*. In *Apostolic Fathers*, 2:309–45.

568. Praechter, Karl. *Die Philosophie des Altertums*. 12th ed. Friedrich Ueberwegs Grundriss der Geschichte der Philosophie, pt. 1. Berlin: E. W. Mittler, 1926.

569. Preisedanz, Karl (ed. and trans.). *Papyri graecae magicae: Die griechischen Zauberpapyri*. Vol. 1. Leipzig: B. G. Teubner, 1928.

570. Preuss, Julius. *Biblisch-talmudische Medizin*. Berlin: S. Karger, 1911.

571. Proclus. *Commentaire sur le Timée*. French translation by A. J. Festugière. 5 vols. Bibliothèque des textes philosophiques. Paris: J. Vrin, 1966–68.

572. ———. *In Platonis Timaeum commentaria*. Edited by Ernest Diehl. 3 vols. Leipzig: B. G. Teubner, 1903–6.

573. *Procopius*. With an English translation. 7 vols. Vols. 1–6 translated by A. B. Dewing. Vol. 7 translated by A. B. Dewing and Glanville Downey. Loeb. Vol. 1, 1914; vols. 2–5, 1916–28; vols. 6–7, 1935–40.

574. *Prudentius*. With an English translation by H. G. Thomson. 2 vols. Loeb. 1949–53.

575. Puhlmann, Walter. "Die lateinische medizinische Literatur des frühen Mittelalters." *Kyklos* 3 (1930): 390–416.

576. Quasten, Johannes. *Patrology*. 3 vols. Westminster, Md.: Newman Press, 1950–60. (The volumes have been reprinted in different years.)

577. Quintilian. *The Institutio oratoria of Quintilian*. With an English translation by H. E. Butler. 4 vols. Vol. 1. Loeb. 1920.

578. Quintus Serenus. *Liber medicinalis*. Edited by Friedrich Vollmer. *CML*, vol. 2, fasc. 3. Leipzig: B. G. Teubner, 1916.

579. Rather, Lelland J. "The Six Things Non-Natural: A Note on the Origins and Fate of a Doctrine and a Phrase." *Clio Medica* 3 (1968): 337–47.

580. Rawlings, Hunter R., III. *A Semantic Study of Prophasis to 400 B.C.* Hermes Einzelschriften, fasc. 33. Wiesbaden: Franz Steiner, 1975.

581. Reitzenstein, R. *Die hellenistischen Mysterienreligionen nach ihren Grundgedanken und Wirkungen*. 3rd ed. Leipzig: B. G. Teubner, 1927.

582. ———. *Poimandres: Studien zur griechisch-ägyptischen und frühchristlichen Literatur*. Leipzig: B. G. Teubner, 1904.

583. Rengstorf, Karl Heinrich. *Die Anfänge der Auseinandersetzung zwischen Christusglaube und Asklepiosfrömmigkeit*. Schriften der Gesellschaft zur Förderung der Westfälischen Landesuniversität zu Münster, no. 30. Münster: Aschendorff, 1953.

584. Riddle, John M. *Dioscorides on Pharmacy and Medicine*. Austin: University of Texas Press, 1985.

585. ———. "Folk Tradition and Folk Medicine: Recognition of Drugs in Classical Antiquity." In *Folklore and Folk Medicines*, edited by John Scarborough, pp. 33–61. Madison, Wisc.: American Institute of the History of Pharmacy, 1987.

586. Riese, W. "La pensée morale de Galien." *Revue philosophique de la France et de l'étranger* 153 (1963): 331–46.

587. Robinson, Robert A. "The Historical Background of Internal Fixation of Fractures in North America." *Bulletin of the History of Medicine* 52 (1978): 354–82.

588. Roesch, Paul. "Médecins publics dans l'Égypte impériale." In *Médecins et Médecine dans l'Antiquité*. Edited by G. Sabbah, pp. 119–29. Mémoirs III du Centre Jean Palerne. Saint-Étienne: Université de Saint-Étienne, 1982.

589. Rohde, Erwin. *Psyche: Seelenkult und Unsterblichkeitsglaube der Griechen*. 9th and 10th ed. 2 vols. Tübingen: J. C. B. Mohr, 1925.

590. Rose, Valentin. *Anecdota Graeca et Graecolatina*. 2 fasc. Berlin: 1864–70. Reprint (in 1 vol.). Amsterdam: Adolf M. Hakkert, 1963.

591. Rosenthal, Franz. "An Eleventh-Century List of the Works of Hippocrates." *Journal of the History of Medicine and Allied Sciences* 28 (1973): 156–65.

592. ———. *Das Fortleben der Antike im Islam*. Zurich and Stuttgart: Artemis, 1965.

593. Rostovtzeff, M. *The Social and Economic History of the Hellenistic World.* Vol. 2. Oxford: Clarendon Press, 1941.

594. Rufus of Ephesus. *Krankenjournale.* Edited with a German translation and commentary by Manfred Ullmann. Wiesbaden: Harrassowitz, 1978.

595. ———. *Oeuvres de Rufus d' Éphèse.* Edited with a French translation by Ch. Daremberg and Ch. Émile Ruelle. Paris: Imprimerie nationale, 1879.

596. ———. *Quaestiones medicinales* [*Die Fragen des Arztes an den Kranken*]. Edited with a German translation by Hans Gärtner. *CMG,* suppl. 4. Berlin: Akademie-Verlag, 1962.

597. Ryssel, Victor (trans.). "Eine syrische Lebensgeschichte des Gregorius Thaumaturgus." *Theologische Zeitschrift aus der Schweiz* 11 (1894): 228–54.

598. Saffrey, H.-D. "Le chrétien Jean Philopon et la survivance de l'école d'Alexandrie au VIᵉ siècle." *Revue des études grecques* 67 (1954): 396–410.

599. Sakalis, Dimitrios Th. "Beiträge zu den Pseudo-Hippokratischen Briefen." In *Formes de pensée dans la collection hippocratique: Actes du IVᵉ colloque international hippocratique (Lausanne, 21–26 septembre 1981),* edited by Françoise Lasserre and Philippe Mudry, pp. 499–514. Geneva: Droz, 1983.

600. Saler, Benson. "Supernatural as a Western Category." *Ethos* 5 (1977): 31–53.

601. Sallustius. *Concerning the Gods and the Universe.* Edited and translated by Arthur Darby Nock. Cambridge: Cambridge University Press, 1926.

602. Scarborough, John. "Adaptation of Folk Medicines in the Formal Materia Medica of Classical Antiquity." In *Folklore and Folk Medicines,* edited by John Scarborough, pp. 21–32. Madison, Wisc.: American Institute of the History of Pharmacy, 1987.

603. ———. Review of *The Birth of the Hospital in the Byzantine Empire,* by Timothy S. Miller. *Isis* 77 (1986): 372–73.

604. ———. *Roman Medicine.* Ithaca: Cornell University Press, 1969.

605. ———. (ed.). *Symposium on Byzantine Medicine.* Dumbarton Oaks Papers, no. 38 (1984). Washington, D.C.: Dumbarton Oaks Library and Collection, 1985.

606. Schadewaldt, Hans. "Die Apologie der Heilkunst bei den Kirchenvaetern." *Veroeffentlichungen der internationalen Gesellschaft für Geschichte der Pharmazie e. V.* 26 (1965): 115–30.

607. ———. "Das ärztliche Gewissen." *Die medizinische Welt* 37 (1986): 1521–23.

608. ———. "Arzt und Patient in antiker und fruehchristlicher Sicht." *Medizinische Klinik* 59 (1964): 146–52.

609. ———. "Asklepios und Christus." *Die medizinische Welt,* n.s., 18 (1967): 1755–61.

610. Schipperges, Heinrich. "Zur Tradition des 'Christus Medicus' im frühen Christentum und in der älteren Heilkunde." *Arzt und Christ* (Salzburg) 11 (1965): 12–20.

611. Schöne, Hermann. "Bruchstücke einer neuen Hippokratesvita." *Rheinisches Museum für Philologie*, n.s., 58 (1903): 56–66.
612. Schubring, Konrad. "Übersehene Zitate." *Hermes* 88 (1960): 451–58.
613. Schürer, Emil. *The History of the Jewish People in the Age of Jesus Christ (175 B.C.–A.D. 135)*. New English version revised and edited by Geza Vermes and Fergus Millar. 3 vols. Edinburgh: T. and T. Clark, 1973–87.
614. Scribonius Largus. *Compositiones*. Edited by Sergio Sconocchia. Leipzig: B. G. Teubner, 1983.
615. Seneca. *Ad Lucilium epistulae morales*. With an English translation by Richard M. Gummere. 3 vols. Loeb. 1920–25.
616. ———. *Moral Essays*. With an English translation by John W. Basore. 3 vols. Loeb. Vols. 1 and 2, 1928–32; vol. 3, 1935.
617. *Septuaginta*. Edited by Alfred Rahlfs. 2 vols. 9th ed. Stuttgart: Württembergische Bibelanstalt, 1935.
618. Sextus Empiricus. *Outlines of Pyrrhonism*. With an English translation by R. G. Bury. Vol. 1. Loeb. 1933.
619. Seybold, Klaus, and Mueller, Ulrich B. *Sickness and Healing*. Translated by Douglas W. Stott. Biblical Encounter Series. Nashville, Tenn.: Abingdon, 1981.
620. Sherwin-White, A. N. Review of *Jesus and the Constraints of History*, by A. E. Harvey (London, 1980). *Times Literary Supplement*, April 9, 1982, p. 408.
621. Sherwin-White, Susan M. *Ancient Cos: An Historical Study from the Dorian Settlement to the Imperial Period*. Hypomnemata, fasc. 51. Goettingen: Vandenhoeck und Ruprecht, 1978.
622. Sidonius. *Poems and Letters*. With an English translation by W. B. Anderson. 2 vols. Loeb. 1931.
623. Sigerist, Henry E. *Antike Heilkunde*. Tusculum Schriften, no. 7. Munich: Ernst Heimeran, 1927.
624. ———. *Civilization and Disease*. Ithaca: Cornell University Press, 1943.
625. ———. *The Great Doctors: A Biographical History of Medicine*. Translated by Eden and Cedar Paul. Garden City, N.Y.: Doubleday Anchor Books, 1958.
626. Simon, Jean Robert. *Robert Burton (1577–1640) et L'Anatomie de la Mélancolie*. Diss. Paris: Didier, 1964.
627. Smith, Hilton Atmore, and Jones, Thomas Carlyle. *Veterinary Pathology*. Philadelphia: Lea and Febiger, 1957.
628. Smith, Macklin. *Prudentius' Psychomachia: A Reexamination*. Princeton: Princeton University Press, 1976.
629. Smith, Wesley D. *The Hippocratic Tradition*. Ithaca: Cornell University Press, 1979.
630. ———. "Physiology in the Homeric Poems." *Transactions and Proceedings of the American Philological Association* 97 (1966): 547–56.
631. ———. "So-Called Possession in Pre-Christian Greece." *Transactions and Proceedings of the American Philological Association* 96 (1965): 403–26.

632. Smith, William. *Smaller Classical Dictionary.* Revised by E. H. Blakeney and John Warrington. New York: E. P. Dutton (Dutton Everyman Paperback), 1958.

633. *Sophocles.* With an English translation by F. Storr. 2 vols. Loeb. 1951.

634. Sophronius. *Laus SS. Martyrum Cyri et Ioannis et miraculorum quae ab eis gesta sunt ex parte narratio.* Migne, PG, 87.3:3379–3676.

635. ———.(?) *Vita et conversatio et martyrium et partialis narratio miraculorum sanctorum illustrium anargyrorum Cyri et Ioannis.* Migne, PG, 87.3:3677–90.

636. Soranus. *Gynaeciorum libri IV, De signis fracturarum, De fasciis, Vita Hippocratis secundum Soranum.* Edited by Johannes Ilberg, CMG, vol. 4. Leipzig: B. G. Teubner, 1927.

637. ———. *Soranus' Gynecology.* Translated by Owsei Temkin with the assistance of Nicholson Eastman, Ludwig Edelstein, and Alan Guttmacher. Baltimore: Johns Hopkins Press, 1956.

638. Sozomen. *The Ecclesiastical History of Sozomen, also The Ecclesiastical History of Philostorgius.* Translated by Edward Walford. London: Henry B. Bohn, 1855.

639. ———. *Kirchengeschichte.* Edited by Joseph Bidez and Günther Christian Hansen. *Die griechischen Christlichen Schriftsteller der ersten Jahrhunderte.* Berlin: Akademie-Verlag, 1960.

640. Speyer, Wolfgang. "Genealogie." *Reallexikon für Antike und Christentum* 9:1145–1268. Stuttgart: Anton Hiersemann, 1976.

641. ———. *Die literarische Fälschung im heidnischen und christlichen Altertum.* Handbuch der Altertumswissenschaft, 1. Abteilung, 2. Teil. Munich: C. H. Beck, 1971.

642. Spuler, Bertold. *The Muslim World.* Translated by F. R. C. Bagley. 2 pts. Leiden: E. J. Brill, 1960.

643. Starobinski, Jean. *Histoire du traitement de la mélancholie des origines à 1900.* Basel: Geigi, 1960.

644. Steckerl, Fritz. *The Fragments of Praxagoras of Cos and His School.* Philosophia Antiqua, no. 8. Leiden: E. J. Brill, 1958.

645. Steinschneider, Moritz. *Die hebraeischen Uebersetzungen des Mittelalters und die Juden als Dolmetscher.* Berlin: 1893.

646. *Stephanus of Athens: Commentary on Hippocrates' Aphorisms Sections I–II.* Edited and translated by Leendert G. Westerink. CMG, vol. 11.1.3.1. Berlin: Akademie-Verlag, 1985.

647. *Stephanus the Philosopher: A Commentary on the Prognosticon of Hippocrates.* Edited and translated by John M. Duffy. CMG, vol. 11.1.2. Berlin: Akademie-Verlag, 1983.

648. ———. *Stephani philosophi et medici commentarii in priorem Galeni librum therapeuticum ad Glauconem.* In Dietz, AC, 1:233–344.

649. Stone, Michael. *Scriptures, Sects, and Visions: A Profile of Judaism from Ezra to the Jewish Revolts.* Oxford: Basil Blackwell, 1980.

650. Strabo. *The Geography.* With an English translation by Horace Leonard Jones. 6 vols. Vol. 6. Loeb. 1929.

651. Strohmaier, Gotthard. "Galen in Arabic: Prospects and Projects." In Nutton, *GPP*, pp. 187–96.

652. ———. Tentative German translation from the Arabic version of Galen's commentary on Hippocrates' *De aeris, aquis, locis,* chap. 22. Manuscript.

653. [Suda, or Souda.] *Suidae Lexicon.* Edited by Ada Adler. 5 vols. Leipzig: B. G. Teubner, 1928–38.

654. ———. *Suidae Lexicon.* Edited by Immanuel Bekker. Berlin: Georg Reimer, 1854.

655. Sudhoff, Karl. "Aus der Geschichte des Krankenhauswesens im frühen Mittelalter in Morgenland und Abendland." *Sudhoffs Archiv* 21 (1929): 164–203.

656. ———. "Eine mittelalterliche Hippokratesvita." *Sudhoffs Archiv* 8 (1915): 404–13.

657. ———. "Eine Verteidigung der Heilkunde aus den Zeiten der Mönchsmedizin." *Sudhoffs Archiv* 7 (1913): 223–37.

658. ———. "Handanlegung des Heilgottes auf attischen Weihetafeln." *Sudhoffs Archiv* 18 (1926): 235–50 and tables 9–12.

659. *Suetonius.* With an English translation by J. C. Rolfe. 2 vols. Loeb. 1965.

660. Sulpicius Severus. *Vie de Saint Martin.* Edited with introduction and French translation by Jacques Fontaine. 3 vols. Sources Chrétiennes, nos. 133, 134, 135. Paris: Les Éditions du Cerf, 1967–69.

661. Symmachus, Q. Aurelius. *Relationes.* Edited by Wilhelm Meyer. Leipzig: B. G. Teubner, 1872.

662. Tacitus. *The Histories.* With an English translation by Clifford H. Moore. *The Annals.* With an English translation by John Jackson. 4 vols. Vol. 4. Loeb. 1937.

663. ———. *Opera.* Edited by Franz Ritter. Leipzig: W. Engelmann, 1864.

664. Tatian. *Oratio ad Graecos and Fragments.* Edited and translated by Molly Whittaker. Oxford: Clarendon Press, 1982.

665. Temkin, Owsei. *The Double Face of Janus and Other Essays in the History of Medicine.* Baltimore: Johns Hopkins University Press, 1977.

666. ———. *The Falling Sickness: A History of Epilepsy from the Greeks to the Beginnings of Modern Neurology.* 2nd ed. Baltimore: Johns Hopkins University Press, 1971.

667. ———. *Galenism: Rise and Decline of a Medical Philosophy.* Ithaca: Cornell University Press, 1973.

668. ———. "Geschichte des Hippokratismus im ausgehenden Altertum." *Kyklos* 4 (1932): 1–80.

669. ———. "Guillaume Ader and His Contribution to Biblical Medicine." *Bulletin of the History of Medicine* 5 (1937): 247–58.

670. ———. "Hippocrates as the Physician of Democritus." *Gesnerus* 42 (1985): 455–64.

671. ———. "The Idea of Respect for Life in the History of Medicine." In *Respect for Life in Medicine, Philosophy, and the Law,* by Owsei Temkin,

William K. Frankena, and Sanford H. Kadish, pp. 1–23. Baltimore: Johns Hopkins University Press, 1977.

672. ———. "Medical Ethics and Honoraria in Late Antiquity." In *Healing and History: Essays for George Rosen,* edited by Charles Rosenberg, pp. 6–26. Kent: Dawson; New York: Science History Publications, 1979.

673. Tertullian. *Apology.* With an English translation by T. R. Glover. Loeb. 1931.

674. ———. *De anima.* Edited with introduction and commentary by J. H. Waszink. Amsterdam: J. M. Meulenhoff, 1947.

675. Theodoretus. *Epistolae.* Migne, *PG,* 83:1171–1494.

676. ———. *Graecarum affectionum curatio.* Migne, *PG,* 83:783–1152.

677. ———. *Thérapeutique des maladies helléniques.* Edited with a French translation by Pierre Canivet. 2 vols. Sources Chrétiennes, no. 57. Paris: Éditions du Cerf, 1958.

678. Theodorus Priscianus. *Euporiston libri III: Cum Physicorum fragmento et Additamentis Pseudo-Theodoreis.* Edited by Valentin Rose. Leipzig: B. G. Teubner, 1894.

679. Theophanes. *Chronographia.* Edited by C. Boor. 2 vols. Leipzig, 1883–85.

680. Theophilus. *De excrementis.* In *Physici et medici minores,* edited by Julius Ludwig Ideler. 2 vols. 1:397–408. 1842. Reprint. Amsterdam: Adolf M. Hakkert, 1963.

681. Theophilus of Antioch. *Trois livres à Autolycus.* Edited by G. Bardy, French translation by Jean Sender, introduction and notes by Gustav Bardy. Sources Chrétiennes, no. 20. Paris: Éditions du Cerf, 1948.

682. Theophrastus. *Opera quae supersunt omnia.* Edited by Fr. Wimmer. Paris: Ambrosius Firmin Didot, 1861.

683. Thivel, Antoine. "Le 'divin' dans la collection hippocratique." *La Collection hippocratique et son rôle dans l'histoire de la médecine: Colloque de Strasbourg (23–27 octobre 1972),* pp. 57–76. Leiden: E. J. Brill, 1975.

684. Thucydides. *Thucydides.* With an English translation by Charles Forster Smith. 4 vols. Vol. 1. Loeb. 1928.

685. ———. *De bello Peloponnesiaco libri octo.* Edited by Godfried Boehme. 2 vols. Leipzig: B. G. Teubner, 1889–90.

686. Thurston, Herbert. "Simeon Stylites the Elder," and "Simeon Stylites the Younger." In *Catholic Encyclopedia,* 13:795–96.

687. *Tibullus.* Translated by J. P. Postgate. In *Catullus, Tibullus and Pervigilium Veneris.* Loeb. 1928.

688. Todd, Robert B. "Philosophy and Medicine in John Philoponus' Commentary on Aristotle's *De anima.*" In Scarborough, *Symposium,* pp. 103–10.

689. Toellner, Richard. "Heilkunde/Medizin II. Historisch." *TRE: Theologische Realenzyklopädie,* vol. 14.5, pp. 743–52.

690. Tomlinson, R. A. *Epidauros.* Austin: University of Texas Press, 1983.

691. Toner, P. J. "Extreme Unction." In *Catholic Encyclopedia,* 5:716–30.

692. Toomer, G. J. "Galen on the Astronomers and Astrologers." *Archive for History of Exact Sciences* 32 (1985): 193–206.

693. Triebel-Schubert, Charlotte. "Bemerkungen zum Hippokratischen Eid." *Medizinhistorisches Journal* 20 (1985): 253–60.

694. *Tusculum: Lexikon griechischer und lateinischer Autoren des Altertums und des Mittelalters*. Revised by Wolfgang Buchwald, Armin Hohlweg, and Otto Prinz. Munich: Heimeran, 1963.

695. Tzetzes. *Ioannis Tzetzae Historiae*. Edited by Petrus Aloisius Leone. Naples: Libreria Scientifica, 1968.

696. Ullmann, Manfred. "Galen's Kommentar zu der Schrift 'De aere aquis locis.'" In *Corpus Hippocraticum: Colloque de Mons, Septembre 1975*, pp. 353–65. Mons: Université de Mons, 1977.

697. ———. "Zwei spätantike Kommentare zu der hippokratischen Schrift 'De morbis muliebribus.'" *Medizinhistorisches Journal* 12 (1977): 245–62.

698. Van der Horst, P. W. *Aelius Aristides and the New Testament*. Studia ad Corpus Hellenisticum Novi Testamenti, vol. 6. Leiden: E. J. Brill, 1980.

699. Van der Loos, H. *The Miracles of Jesus*. Leiden: E. J. Brill, 1965.

700. Varro. *On the Latin Language*. With an English translation by Roland G. Kent. 2 vols. Loeb. 1938.

701. Vermes, Geza. *Jesus and the World of Judaism*. London: SCM Press, 1983.

702. ———. *Jesus the Jew: A Historian's Reading of the Gospels*. New York: Macmillan, 1973.

703. Vikan, Gary. "Art, Medicine, and Magic in Early Byzantium." In Scarborough, *Symposium*, pp. 65–86.

704. Visky, Károly. "Die 'artes liberales' in den römischen Rechtsquellen unter Berücksichtigung der Ulpianstelle D 50, 13, 1 pr." In *Gesellschaft und Recht im griechisch-römischen Altertum*, edited by Michail Andreev, Johannes Irmscher, Elemér Pólay, and Witold Warkallo, pt. 1, pp. 268–95. Berlin: Akademie-Verlag, 1968.

705. Vlastos, Gregory. *Plato's Universe*. Seattle: University of Washington Press, 1975.

706. Vogt, Joseph. *Sklaverei und Humanität: Studien zur antiken Sklaverei und ihrer Erforschung*. Historia, Einzelschriften, fasc. 8. Wiesbaden: Franz Steiner, 1965.

707. Volk, Robert. *Gesundheitswesen und Wohltätigkeit im Spiegel der byzantinischen Klostertypika*. Munich: Institut für Byzantinistik und neugriechische Philologie der Universität, 1983.

708. Wallis, R. T. *Neo-Platonism*. Classical Life and Letters. New York: Scribner's, 1972.

709. Walzer, R. *Galen on Jews and Christians*. Oxford: Oxford University Press; London: Geoffrey Cumberlege, 1949.

710. Wanner, Hermann. *Studien zu Περὶ ἀρχαίης ἰατρικῆς*. Diss., University of Zurich, 1939.

711. *Webster's New Collegiate Dictionary*. Springfield, Mass.: G. and C. Merriam, 1981.

712. Weinreich, Otto. *Antike Heilungswunder: Untersuchungen zum Wunderglauben der Griechen und Römer*. Religionsgeschichtliche Versuche und Vorarbeiten, vol. 8, fasc. 1. Giessen: Alfred Töpelmann, 1909.

713. Wellmann, Max. *Die Fragmente der sikelischen Ärzte Akron, Philistion und des Diokles von Karystos*. Berlin: Weidmann, 1901.

714. ———. *Die pneumatische Schule bis auf Archigenes in ihrer Entwickelung dargestellt*. Philologische Untersuchungen, fasc. 14. Berlin: Weidmann, 1895.

715. Wenkebach, Ernst. "Galens Protreptikosfragment." In *Quellen und Studien zur Geschichte der Naturwissenschaften und der Medizin* 4, no. 3 (1935): 169–75.

716. ———. "Der hippokratische Arzt als das Ideal Galens." *Quellen und Studien zur Geschichte der Naturwissenschaften und der Medizin* 3, no. 4 (1933): 169–75.

717. Westerink, L. G. "Academic Practice about 500: Alexandria." Manuscript.

718. Whittaker, Thomas. *The Neo-Platonists: A Study in the History of Hellenism*. 4th ed. 1928. Reprint. Hildesheim: Georg Olms, 1961.

719. Wickersheimer, Ernest. "Légendes hippocratiques du moyen-âge." *Sudhoffs Archiv* 45 (1961): 164–75.

720. Wieland, Christoph Martin. *Geschichte der Abderiten*. Edited by Wolfgang Jahn. Munich: Wilhelm Goldmann, n.d.

721. Wilamowitz-Moellendorff, Ulrich von. *Der Glaube der Hellenen*. 2 vols. Berlin: Weidmann, 1931–32.

722. ———. *Griechisches Lesebuch*. Berlin: Weidmann. Vol. 1.2, *Text*, 6th ed. Vol. 2.2, *Erläuterungen*, 4th ed. Vol. 1.2, 1926; vol. 2.2, 1923.

723. ———. *Griechische Verskunst*. Berlin: Weidmann, 1921. (Pp. 595–607 deal with the poetry of Mesomedes.).

724. Wittern, R. "Die Unterlassung ärztlicher Hilfeleistung in der griechischen Medizin der klassischen Zeit." *Münchner medizinische Wochenschrift* 121 (1979): 731–34.

725. Woodhead, A. G. "The State Health Service in Ancient Greece." *Cambridge Historical Journal* 10 (1952): 235–53.

726. *The Writings of Justin Martyr and Athenagoras*. Translated by Marcus Dods, George Reith, and B. P. Pratten. Ante-Nicene Christian Library, vol. 2. Edinburgh: T. and T. Clark, 1874.

727. *The Writings of Tatian and Theophilus; and The Clementine Recognitions*. Translated by B. P. Pratten, Marcus Dods, and Thomas Smith. Ante-Nicene Christian Library, vol. 3. Edinburgh: T. and T. Clark, 1875.

728. Xenophon. *Memorabilia and Oeconomicus*. With an English translation by E. C. Marchant. Loeb. 1923.

729. Z. F. Review of "Ein neuplatonischer Galenkommentar auf Papyrus," by E. Nachmanson. *Byzantinische Zeitschrift* 26 (1926): 432–33.

730. Zuger, Abigail, and Miles, Steven H. "Physicians, AIDS, and Occupational Risk: Historic Traditions and Ethical Obligations." *JAMA* 258 (1987): 1924–28.

INDEX

OWSEI TEMKIN, who was born in Russia (in 1902) and educated in Germany, came to the United States in 1932. He is a member of the National Academy of Sciences and recipient of the Prize for Distinguished Scholarship in the Humanities from the American Council of Learned Societies. Dr. Temkin, who holds his medical degree from the University of Leipzig, is William H. Welch Professor Emeritus of the History of Medicine at Johns Hopkins, where he was also director of the Institute of the History of Medicine. Among his previous books are *The Falling Sickness: A History of Epilepsy from the Greeks to the Beginning of Modern Neurology* and *The Double Face of Janus and Other Essays in the History of Medicine.*

Designed by Martha Farlow

Composed by Graphic Composition, Inc., in Sabon

Printed by The Maple Press Company, Inc., on 50-lb. Glatfelter Eggshell Cream
and bound in IGC Arrestox A and Rainbow Linique with Rainbow endsheets